# Current Progress in Urology

# Current Progress in Urology

Editor: Ezra Martin

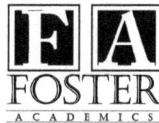

FA

FOSTER
ACADEMICS

www.fosteracademics.com

www.fosteracademics.com

**FA** **FOSTER**
ACADEMICS

Cataloging-in-Publication Data

Current progress in urology / edited by Ezra Martin.
    p. cm.
Includes bibliographical references and index.
ISBN 978-1-63242-967-4
1. Urology. 2. Genitourinary organs--Diseases. 3. Urinary organs--Diseases. I. Martin, Ezra.
RC871 .C87 2020

616.6--dc23

Foster Academics,
118-35 Queens Blvd., Suite 400,
Forest Hills, NY 11375, USA

ISBN 978-1-63242-967-4 (Hardback)

# Contents

**Permissions**

**List of Contributors**

**Index**

# Preface

Urology is a medical specialty which is involved in the diagnosis and treatment of the diseases and disorders of the urinary tract and the male reproductive organs. Urology encompasses the management of both medical and surgical conditions. Medical conditions that can be treated non-surgically include benign prostatic hyperplasia and urinary-tract infections. Surgical interventions are needed for the treatment of prostate cancer, kidney stones, bladder cancer, traumatic injury, congenital abnormalities and stress incontinence. Some of the subspecialties of this domain are endourology, urogynecology, pediatric urology, transplant urology, androurology, sexual medicine, etc. Circumcision, male genital surgery and male genital modification are certain procedures of male genitalia. This book is a valuable compilation of topics, ranging from the basic to the most complex advancements in the field of urology. Its objective is to give a general view of the different urological conditions and their treatment strategies. In this book, using case studies and examples, constant effort has been made to make the understanding of the difficult concepts of urology as easy and informative as possible, for the readers.

This book is the end result of constructive efforts and intensive research done by experts in this field. The aim of this book is to enlighten the readers with recent information in this area of research. The information provided in this profound book would serve as a valuable reference to students and researchers in this field.

At the end, I would like to thank all the authors for devoting their precious time and providing their valuable contribution to this book. I would also like to express my gratitude to my fellow colleagues who encouraged me throughout the process.

**Editor**

# TOT Approach in stress urinary incontinence (SUI) – outcome in obese female

Carsten Frohme[1*†], Friederike Ludt[1], Zoltan Varga[2], Peter J Olbert[1], Rainer Hofmann[1] and Axel Hegele[1†]

## Abstract

**Background:** Only limited data are available on the outcome of tension-free obturator tape (TOT) procedures in overweight and obese women. We would like to verify the objective and subjective outcomes of TOT in women with a higher body mass index (BMI).

**Methods:** We evaluated the records of 116 patients who had undergone TOT, stratifying by BMI into normal weight (n = 31), overweight (n = 56), and obese (n = 29) groups. We compared pre- and postoperative evaluations, including subjective and objective outcome of TOT, complications, and quality of life assessed by validated questionnaires (ICIQ-SF and KHQ).

**Results:** The median follow-up was 21 months. There were no significant differences between different groups in terms of objective cure rate and subjective success, quality of life scores and postoperative complications.

**Conclusions:** Our data demonstrate that TOT procedure is safe and effective. BMI did not influence the outcome of TOT procedures at a median of 21 months after surgery and represents no contraindication for continence surgery. The success of the outcome of TOT procedure in females and the occurrence of complications are not negatively affected by obesity.

**Keywords:** Body mass index, Obesity, Obese female, Stress urinary incontinence, Transobturator tape (TOT)

## Background

Stress urinary incontinence (SUI) is the complaint of involuntary loss of urine on effort or physical exertion (e.g. sporting activities), or on sneezing or coughing [1]. Usually it is caused by weak or damaged muscles and connective tissues in the pelvic floor, compromising urethral support, or by weakness of the urethral sphincter itself [2,3]. Among the main risk factors are age, pregnancy, childbirth, obesity and poor collagen turnover [4]. Typically, the first-line treatment is conservative, which includes pelvic floor training, electrical stimulation and biofeedback. In addition, Duloxetine has been licensed for treatment of SUI in women and has been shown to improve quality of life [5] but it is unclear whether the benefit is lasting [6]. If the condition does not improve, surgical alternatives can be offered. These include retropubic colposuspension, slings and urethral bulking in-jections [7]. Of these types of operations, the midurethral sling is currently the most common procedure performed either alone or along with concomitant pelvic floor or abdominal surgery. Transobturator tape (TOT) is similar to the initial tension free vaginal tape (TVT), but a different technique is used to insert the tape [8] However, TVT and TOT showed no significant difference concerning to the cure rate. The procedures may be comparable in terms of patient satisfaction after more than 24 month of follow-up [9,10]. The transobturator technique has the potential to reduce the incidence of significant complications associated with the retropubic approach. This technique has been further refined by the availability of the Monarc Subfascial Hammock (American Medical Systems, Inc., Minnetonka, MN, USA). Also obesity represents a risk factor for SUI [11] today there are only limited data available concerning safety, efficacy and outcome of TOT sling procedure in obese females. The aim of our study was to evaluate the clinical outcome after TOT procedure with special interest concerning different weight levels of women. A comparison of efficacy and safety of TOT between overweight and normal weight patients was performed.

* Correspondence: frohme@med.uni-marburg.de
†Equal contributors
[1]Department of Urology and Pediatric Urology, University hospital Marburg, Philipps University, Marburg, Germany
Full list of author information is available at the end of the article

## Methods
### Patient data
All consecutive women who underwent a TOT procedure at the University hospital Marburg, Department of Urology and Pediatric Urology, between January 2004 and January 2011 were retrospectively assessed (patients history, level of SUI, age, body weight etc.). They all had undergone conservative therapy options over minimal three months including urotherapy (meaning behavioural training) and pelvic floor workout. All patients signed an informed consent for the collection and analysis of their data.

The patients were classified into 3 groups according to the WHO body mass index (BMI): Group A (normal BMI <25kg/m$^2$), Group B (overweight BMI 25-30kg/m$^2$), Group C (obese BMI > 30kg/m$^2$).

### Preoperative diagnostics
All patients were urodynamically diagnosed with SUI. If mixed symptoms were present, like urgency, frequency or nocturia, the stress urinary incontinence predominated on review of the patient's history. Patients with mixed or isolated urge incontinence were excluded. Multichannel urodynamic testing included post void residual urine (PVR) determination, multichannel cystometrogram (CMG), and uroflowmetry. Patients were excluded if PVR exceeded 100 ml or CMG had detrusor overactivity. Mixed incontinence was defined by the presence of sensory urge incontinence or detrusor overactivity as well as stress incontinence during urodynamic examination.

### Surgical technique
TOT was performed using the "Monarc Subfascial Hammock" (American Medical Systems, USA). The Monarc® system includes a specially designed helical needle, which uses a transobturator-to-vagina (outside-in technique) approach for mesh placement. The procedures were performed with the patient in high lithotomy position and under spinal or general anesthesia, according to patient's preference. All received single-shot broad-spectrum intravenous antibiotics. Patients were instructed to avoid heavy lifting, exercise, and sexual intercourse for a minimum of 4 weeks postoperatively.

### Postoperative evaluation
Intraoperative events including blood loss, time for Monarc® implantation, any complications, and additional procedures were recorded. Subjects were seen at routinely scheduled 12 and 52 weeks postoperatively. Some patients took also different dates for personal reasons. Information regarding continence status was obtained and recorded. Standardized incontinence and quality of life questionnaires as the ICI Questionnaire Short Form (ICIQ-SF) and the King's Health questionnaire (KHQ) were used. Repeat urodynamics were not utilized. Cure was defined as no leakage (dry), or minimal leakage not requiring protection (substantially dry), reported by the patient, along with no leakage seen during an in office stress test. Also improvement was defined as a reduction in the use of pads of about 50% or more. Outcome measures reported include continence status, pad use, urinary urgency, need for medication for urgency, urinary retention (PVR >100 ml), and any healing difficulties. All terminology was in accordance with current ICS terminology, except where noted differently [12].

### Statistics
Patient demographics, clinical history, preoperative, surgical, and postoperative data were summarized using descriptive statistics for continuous variables and frequency tables for categorical variables (SPSS for Windows®, Version 17.0).

## Results
### General data
A total of 116 sequential female patients with symptomatic SUI underwent a TOT procedure at the University hospital Marburg, Deptartment of Urology and Pediatric Urology between January 2004 and January 2011. Mean age was 62.5 years (range 36–83).

Concomitant surgery with anterior or/and posterior colporrhaphy were preformed during TOT procedure in 19 women (anterior = 16, posterior =1, both = 2). Additionally in 1 patient a simultaneous resection of a urethral polyp was performed.

The range of BMI in the patients was 18–47 kg/m$^2$ with a median BMI of 27.5 kg/m$^2$. The patients were followed up between 2 and 56 months with a median follow up of 21 months.

### BMI-Groups
Dividing the women concerning their body weight there were 31 women in Group A (normal BMI <25kg/m$^2$), 56 women in Group B (overweight BMI 25-30kg/m$^2$) and 29 women in Group C (obese BMI >30kg/m$^2$) with a mean age of 62 years (37–80) in Group A, 63 years (36–83) in Group B and 60 years (38–78) in Group C. The median BMI was 23,4 kg/m$^2$ (18–24.8) in Group A, 28,1 kg/m$^2$ (25,1-30) in Group B and 35,4 kg/m$^2$ (30.1-47.2) in Group C. 25% of the patients in Group A underwent a co-therapy, 20% in Group B but only 7% in Group C.

### Operation time
Overall operation time including the cases with concomitant surgery was 40 min (10–120). No significant differences were detectable between the groups: 38.5

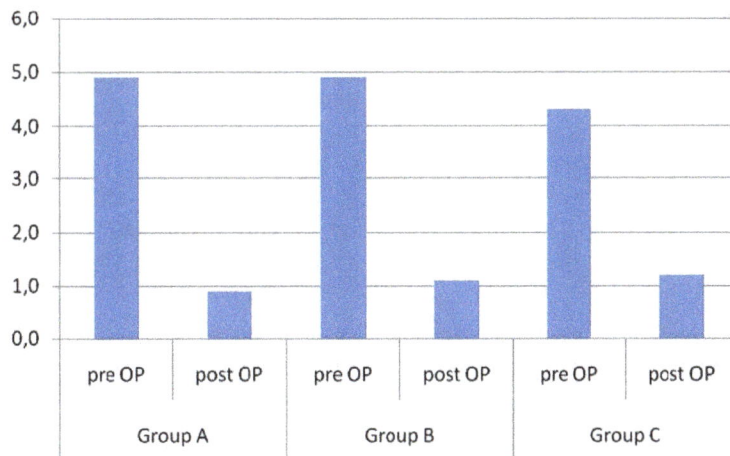

**Figure 1** Pad consumption before and after surgery broken down by groups.

min (18–85) in Group A, 43.6 min (10–120) in Group B and 36 min (15–120) in Group C.

### Success of procedure

After TOT-procedure the used median pads/day significantly reduced from baseline 4 (1–16) to 0 (0–9) ($p < 0.01$), without showing some significant differences between the BMI-groups. We found a significant improvement after surgery without significant differences between the groups (Figure 1).

Used pads/day after 6, 12, 24 and 36 months showed a significant reduction compared to baseline in every group without significant differences between the respective BMI-groups. Comparing possible impairment during time period (6, 12, 24, 36 months) no significant increase of pads/day were evident in every group and between Group A, Group B and Group C (Table 1).

Success rate was 93% with a cure rate of 83% and improvement in 10% of the women. No significant differences were evident between the groups (Group A: 96%, Group B: 94%, Group C: 91%).

Logistic analysis also revealed that BMI, history of previous pelvic surgery, concomitantly performed pelvic surgery, or occurrence of complications did not affect cure rates.

### Complications

Overall complication rate was 23.2% (27/116) including 1 major (bleeding) and 26 minor complications (see Table 2). Postoperative temporary voiding difficulty was the main postoperative complication (n = 21, 18.1%). We found appearance of de-novo-urge in 15 women (12.9%) and temporary obstructive voiding in 6 women (5.2%) with a urinary retention in 2 women (1.7%). Mean residual urine volume increased to 75 ml, only 3 patients showed an increase above 100 ml (up to 330 ml). Voiding was not impaired by reduction of the flow time. There was no significant change after performing the operation while the range about the flow was 5–57 sec. Also the maximum flow was not significantly affected.

Complication rates between the BMI-groups were nearly similar without significant differences.

### Patients satisfaction

KHQ showed significant improvement in Quality of Life in all circumstances for all different groups. No significant differences between the groups were notable. Majority of women (93%) are satisfied with the TOT-procedure including individual outcome and recommend the procedure, also without significant differences between the groups (Group A: 100%, Group B: 90%, *Group C*: 89.5%). We used the question "Would you repeat this procedure?"

**Table 1** Median used pads/day 6, 12, 24 and 36 months after TOT-procedure in group A, B and C (n = number of patients, range of used pads)

|         | 6 months | 12 months | 24 months | 36 months |
|---------|----------|-----------|-----------|-----------|
| Group A | 1 (n = 30, 0-4) | 1 (n = 28, 0-4) | 1 (n = 18, 0-4) | 0 (n = 11, 0-1) |
| Group B | 0 (n = 52, 0-9) | 0 (n = 35, 0-6) | 1 (n = 23, 0-6) | 0 (n = 10, 0-3) |
| Group C | 0 (n = 25, 0-7) | 0.5 (n = 21, 0-7) | 0.5 (n = 16, 0-2) | 0 (n = 10, 0-1) |

**Table 2** Postoperative complication rate was 23.2% including 1 major and 26 minor complications

|         | Bleeding | De-novo-urge | Dyspareunia/ vaginal pain | Residual urine | Vaginal erosion |
|---------|----------|--------------|---------------------------|----------------|-----------------|
| Group A | 1 | 4 | 1 | 3 | 1 |
| Group B | Ø | 7 | 3 | 2 | Ø |
| Group C | Ø | 4 | Ø | 1 | Ø |

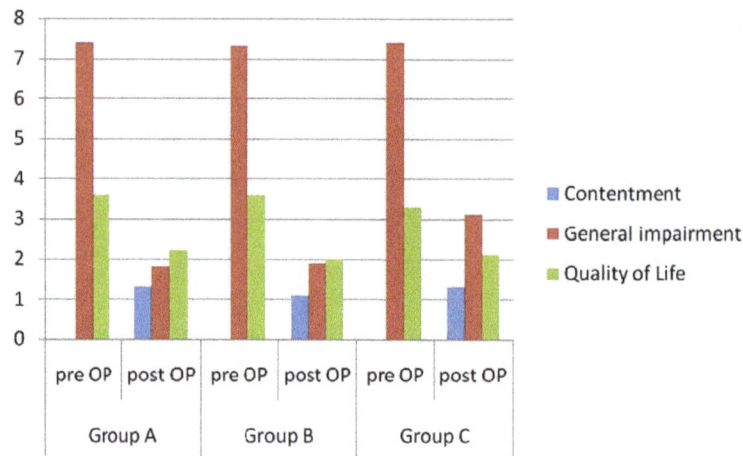

**Figure 2** KHQ showed significant improvement in QoL without differences between the three groups.

representative of contentment, so there could only be a measurement in the postoperative evaluation (Figure 2).

All relevant data, divided into different BMI-groups were summarized in Table 3.

## Discussion

This study showed that TOT was equally safe and effective for treating SUI regardless of BMI. The postoperative quality of life was similarly improved for women in each weight groups, and there were no significant differences in the complication rate.

BMI is significantly correlated with intra-abdominal pressure [13] which may increase stress on the pelvic floor, contributing to the development and recurrence of SUI. However, we did not find that women with a higher BMI were more likely to have SUI on follow-up. Results of the studies of incontinence surgery in obese patients have been contradictory. Responses to a mailed questionnaire by 970 women who underwent TVT indicated a markedly unfavorable outcome in 61 very obese women (BMI > 35 $kg/m^2$) [14]. The overall cure rate in 291 women of normal weight was 81.2%, as compared to 52.1% in the 61 very obese. In other studies these data could not be confirmed and reasons for this poor outcome are not clear. Maybe it is due to the limitations of a mailed questionnaire reflecting the general enhanced dissatisfaction of obese people [9,15]. Another study

evaluated 195 women who underwent TVT. At one year of follow-up, they found a similar surgical outcome among 68 normal-weighted, 65 overweight and 62 obese women [16]. The proportion of subjects with SUI one year after surgery was 18% in the obese, 14% in the overweight, and 19% in the normal weight groups, differences were statistically not significant. Skriapas et al. compared 31 morbidly obese patients with BMI > 40 $kg/m^2$ and 52 patients with a BMI of <30 $kg/m^2$ with a mean follow-up of 18.5 months. The objective cure rate in control group was 92.3% and 86.9% for morbidly obese group, so no significant difference was shown. They thus suggested that TVT is a good option for morbidly obese patients with severe stress incontinence [17]. Differences between the studies are caused by different lengths of follow-up, variation in the type of continence surgery, and different definitions of cure. Therefore comparability between this studies is limited (may not always be given). Also in two studies using the transobturator tape procedures no significant association between BMI and surgical outcome were found [18,19]. Even if cure was defined differently in these two studies the results are in line with our findings after a follow up of nearly 2 years. In the publication of Po-En Liu and coworkers the gain was the use of objective as well as subjective measures of cure. Compared with the normal weight group, women with a higher BMI did appear to have a lower objective cure rate. Objective cure was

**Table 3 Summarized data (divided into different BMI-groups)**

| | No | Age (years) | Median BMI ($kg/m^2$) | Op-time (min) | Compl. (n) | Success rate | Pads (n/day) Pre | Pads (n/day) Post |
|---|---|---|---|---|---|---|---|---|
| **Group A (-25 $kg/m^2$)** | 31 | 62.2 (37-80) | 23.4 (18-24.8) | 38.5 (18-85) | 10 | 96% | 4.5 (1-11) | 0.85 (0-4) |
| **Group B (25-30$kg/m^2$)** | 56 | 63 (36-83) | 28.1 (25.1-30) | 43.6 (10-120) | 12 | 94% | 4.7 (1-16) | 1.1 (0-9) |
| **Group C (>30$kg/m^2$)** | 29 | 60.3 (38-78) | 35.4 (30.1-47.2) | 36 (15-120) | 5 | 91% | 5 (3-7) | 1.4 (0-6) |
| **Σ** | 116 | **62** (36-83) | **27.5** (18-47.2) | **40** (10-120) | **27** (25.5%) | **93%** | **4** (1-16) | **0** (0-9) |

defined as no urine leakage during the stress test in the filling phase of urodynamic studies. The statistical analysis did not indicate any significant differences among the groups, although it is possible that some difference might be found if the number of cases were higher. Instead of the ICIQ-SF and KHQ they used UDI-6 and IIQ-7 scores. However, they also find a significant improvement in all compared groups so that the TOT procedure indeed improves quality of life regardless of BMI.

Liapis et al. reported an objective cure in 82.4% of 115 subjects after TOT based on the pad test finding at 4 years postoperatively [20], while there was a slightly lower objective success rate at a median of 24 months of follow-up. Albo et al. described similar objective success rates comparing TVT (77.3%) and TOT (72.3%) after 24 month follow-up in 516 women [10]. In our population success rate of 93% after 21 month of follow up was similar with cure rate of 83% and improvement of 10%.

In 2012 also a one-year outcome of mid-urethral sling procedures for stress urinary incontinence according to body mass index was published. The retrospective clinical trial was performed with 284 patients treated by the SPARC sling procedure and 49 patients also treated by the MONARC sling procedure. The women were also classified into 3 groups by BMI according to the WHO Expert Consultation. Patient's characteristics and clinical outcomes of the operation were analyzed according to BMI at 1 year after surgery but only via questionnaires and interviews. The objective and subjective cure rates for the obese group were worse after TOT procedure (96.8% vs. 66.7%) but because of the small sample size of the TOT group not statistically significant [21]. A limitation of our investigation was the duration of follow up. However, there are no publications comprising a follow up of 5 or more years also performing a differentiated approach on the outcome of obese female. So are the outcomes of transobturator tape procedure generally durable in long-term follow-up? A 5-year follow-up study comparing Burch colposuspension and transobturator tape for the surgical treatment of SUI in person without another concomitant procedure showed, that the 5-year cure rates were similar (objective cure rate, 73.9% versus 77.5%; subjective cure rate, 76.8% versus 81.7% [22]. Yonguc et al. showed in their publication that objective cure, subjective cure and patient satisfaction rates of the 126 women at 1 year after transobturator tape procedure were 89.6, 86.5 and 92% respectively. During 5-year follow-up, objective cure rate was stable with 87.3% rate, whereas subjective cure and patient satisfaction rates were decreased to 65.9 and 73%, respectively [23]. The group of Heinonen et al. evaluated 191 patients underwent TOT procedure, and thereby 139 (73%) after a mean follow-up of 6.5 years. The patient cohort was heterogeneous and consisted of patients with SUI and mixed urinary incontinence (MUI) as well as recurrent SUI. There objective and subjective cure rates were 89% and 83%, respectively. Subjective cure rate was 84% at 20-month follow-up and was maintained up to 6.5 years. At long-term follow-up, the objective cure rate was slightly greater than the subjective cure rate. In their evaluated cohort, mean body mass index BMI was 28 (range, 19–45). Patients with BMI higher 30 had significantly higher scores on condition-specific questionnaires and significantly lower scores on quality of Life questionnaires, indicating a lower general quality of life and health than in patients with BMI less or equal 30 [24]. In the subgroup analysis of our sample we could not confirm this effect for the objective cure rate.

Another limitation of our investigation was the sample size. We deliberately limited our sample to women with isolated SUI. On the other hand, our population was representative of women typically seen in the clinic complaining of isolated SUI. Our results thus help confirm the effectiveness of the TOT procedure for women in a general clinical setting.

## Conclusions

Our data demonstrate that TOT procedure is safe and effective. BMI did not influence the outcome of TOT procedures at a median of 21 months after surgery and represents no contraindication for continence surgery.

### Ethical/Institutional review board approval

There was no IRB Approval acquired for this study. An approved medical product was used. Data collections as well as pre- and postoperative investigations were performed within the usual and guideline based visits.

### Competing interest

The authors declare that they have no competing interest.

### Authors' contributions

CF: Project development, Data collection, Data analysis, Manuscript writing. FL: Data collection. ZV: Data collection, Manuscript editing. PJO: Manuscript editing. RH: Manuscript editing. AH: Project development, Data collection, Data analysis, Manuscript writing. All authors read and approved the final manuscript.

### Author details

[1]Department of Urology and Pediatric Urology, University hospital Marburg, Philipps University, Marburg, Germany. [2]Department of Urology, District hospital Sigmaringen, Sigmaringen, Germany.

### References

1. Haylen BT, de Ridder D, Freeman RM, Swift SE, Berghmans B, Lee J, Monga A, Petri E, Rizk DE, Sand PK, Schaer GN: International Urogynecological Association (IUGA)/International Continence Society (ICS) joint report on the terminology for female pelvic floor dysfunction. *Int Urogynecol J* 2010, 21:5–26.
2. Peyrat L, Haillot O, Bruyere F, Boutin JM, Bertrand P, Lanson Y: Prevalence and risk factors of urinary incontinence in young and middle-aged women. *British J Urol Int* 2002, 89:61–66.

3.  Parazzini F, Chiaffarino F, Lavezzari M, Giambanco V: **Risk factors for stress, urge or mixed urinary incontinence in Italy.** *Br J Obstet Gynaecol* 2003, 110:927–933.

4.  Edwall L, Carlstrom K, Jonasson AF: **Markers of collagen synthesis and degradation in urogenital tissue from women with and without stress urinary incontinence.** *Neurourol Urodyn* 2005, 24:319–324.

5.  Freeman R: **Initial management of stress urinary incontinence: pelvic floor muscle training and duloxetine.** *Br J Obstet Gynaecol* 2006, 113 (Suppl):10–16.

6.  Mariappan P, Ballantyne Z, N'Dow JM, Alhasso AA: **Serotonin and noradrenaline reuptake inhibitors (SNRI) for stress urinary incontinence in adults.** *Cochrane Database Syst Rev* 2005, 20:CD004742.

7.  Umoh UE, Arya LA: **Surgery in urogynecology.** *Minerva Med* 2012, 103:23–36.

8.  Delorme E, Droupy S, de Tayrac R, Delmas V: **Transobturator tape (Uratape). A new minimally invasive method in the treatment of urinary incontinence in women.** *Prog Urol* 2003, 13:656–9.

9.  Jorm AF, Korten AE, Christensen H, Jacomb PA, Rodgers B, Parslow RA: **Association of obesity with anxiety, depression and emotional well-being: a community survey.** *Aust N Z J Public Health* 2003, 27:434–40.

10. Albo ME, Litman HJ, Richter HE, Lemack GE, Sirls LT, Chai TC, Norton P, Kraus SR, Zyczynski H, Kenton K, Gormley EA, Kusek JW: **Treatment success of retropubic and transobturator mid urethral slings at 24 months.** *J Urol* 2012, 188:2281–7.

11. Lawrence JM, Lukacz ES, Liu IL, Nager CW, Luber KM: **Pelvic floor disorders, diabetes, and obesity in women: findings from the Kaiser Permanente Continence Associated Risk Epidemiology Study.** *Diabetes Care* 2007, 30:2536–41.

12. Abrams P, Cardozo L, Fall M, Griffiths D, Rosier P, Ulmsten U, *et al*: **The standardisation of terminology of lower urinary tract function: report from the standardisation sub-committee of the International Continence Society.** *Neurourol Urodyn* 2002, 21:167–178.

13. Noblett KL, Jensen JK, Ostergard DR: **The relationship of body mass index to intra-abdominal pressure as measured by multichannel cystometry.** *Int Urogynecol J Pelvic Floor Dysfunct* 1997, 8:323–6.

14. Hellberg D, Holmgren C, Lanner L, Nilsson S: **The very obese woman and the very old woman: tension-free vaginal tape for the treatment of stress urinary incontinence.** *Int Urogynecol J Pelvic Floor Dysfunct* 2007, 18:423–9.

15. Gavin AR, Simon GE, Ludman EJ: **The association between obesity, depression, and educational attainment in women: the mediating role of body image dissatisfaction.** *J Psychosom Res* 2010, 69:573–81.

16. Killingsworth LB, Wheeler TL 2nd, Burgio KL, Martirosian TE, Redden DT, Richter HE: **One-year outcomes of tension-free vaginal tape (TVT) mid-urethral slings in overweight and obese women.** *Int Urogynecol J Pelvic Floor Dysfunct* 2009, 20:1103–8.

17. Skriapas K, Poulakis V, Dillenburg W, de Vries R, Witzsch U, Melekos M, *et al*: **Tension-free vaginal tape (TVT) in morbidly obese patients with severe urodynamic stress incontinence as last option treatment.** *Eur Urol* 2006, 49:544–50.

18. Rechberger T, Futyma K, Jankiewicz K, Adamiak A, Bogusiewicz M, Skorupski P: **Body mass index does not influence the outcome of anti-incontinence surgery among women whereas menopausal status and ageing do: a randomised trial.** *Int Urogynecol J Pelvic Floor Dysfunct* 2010, 21:801–6.

19. Liu PE, Su CH, Lau HH, Chang RJ, Huang WC, Su TH: **Outcome of tension-free obturator tape procedures in obese and overweight women.** *Int Urogynecol J* 2011, 22:259–63.

20. Liapis A, Bakas P, Creatsas G: **Efficacy of inside-out transobturator vaginal tape (TVTO) at 4 years follow up.** *Eur J Obstet Gynecol Reprod Biol* 2010, 148:199–201.

21. Hwang IS, Yu JH, Chung JY, Noh CH, Sung LH: **One-year outcomes of mid-urethral sling procedures for stress urinary incontinence according to body mass index.** *Korean J Urol.* 2012, 53:171–7.

22. Asıcıoglu O, Gungorduk K, Besımoglu B, Ertas E, Yıldırım G, Celebı I, Ark C, Boran B: **A 5-year follow-up study comparing Burch colposuspension and transobturator tape for the surgical treatment of stress urinary incontinence.** *Int J Gynaecol Obstet* 2013. doi:10.1016/j.ijgo.2013.09.026

23. Yonguc T, Gunlusoy B, Degirmenci T, Kozacioglu Z, Bozkurt IH, Arslan B, Minareci S, Yılmaz Y: **Are the outcomes of transobturator tape procedure for female stress urinary incontinence durable in long-term follow-up?** *Int Urol Nephrol* 2014. doi:10.1007/s11255-013-0639-0.

24. Heinonen P, Ala-Nissilä S, Räty R, Laurikainen E, Kiilholma P: **Objective cure rates and patient satisfaction after the transobturator tape procedure during 6.5-year follow-up.** *J Minim Invasive Gynecol.* doi:10.1016/j.jmig.2012.09.007.

# 2

# Sodium hyaluronate and chondroitin sulfate replenishment therapy can improve nocturia in men with post-radiation cystitis

Mauro Gacci[1*], Omar Saleh[1], Claudia Giannessi[1], Beatrice Detti[2], Lorenzo Livi[2], Eleonora Monteleone Pasquetti[2], Tatiana Masoni[2], Enrico Finazzi Agro[3], Vincenzo Li Marzi[1], Andrea Minervini[1], Marco Carini[1], Stavros Gravas[4], Matthias Oelke[5] and Sergio Serni[1]

## Abstract

**Background:** Radiotherapy is one of the treatment options for prostate cancer (PCa) but up to 25 % of men report about severe nocturia (nocturnal voiding). The combination of hyaluronic acid (HA) and chondroitin sulfate (CS) resembles glycosaminoglycan (GAG) replenishment therapy. The aim of our study was to evaluate the impact of HA and CS on nocturia, in men with nocturia after PCa radiotherapy.

**Methods:** Twenty-three consecutive patients with symptomatic cystitis after external radiotherapy for PCa were enrolled. Patients underwent bladder instillation therapy with HA and CS weekly for the first month and, afterwards, on week 6, 8 and 12. Nocturnal voiding frequency was assessed by item 3 (Q3) of the Interstitial Cystitis Symptoms Index (ICSI) and item 2 (Q2) of the Interstitial Cystitis Problem Index (ICPI). Data were analyzed with paired-samples T-test and adjusted for age.

**Results:** Eighteen patients (78 %) reported about nocturia. Pre- and post-treatment ICSI-Q3 was $2.13 \pm 0.28$ and $1.61 \pm 0.21$ (−24.4 %, p = 0.001). With logistic regression analysis, both age and baseline ICSI-Q3 had a significant impact on nocturnal voiding frequency (r = 0.293, p = 0.011 and r = 0.970, $p < 0.001$). Pre- and post-treatment ICPI-Q2 was $1.87 \pm 0.26$ and $1.30 \pm 0.25$ (−30.5 %, p = 0.016); logistic regression analysis was without significant findings.

**Conclusion:** Bladder instillation treatment with a combination of HA and CS was effective in reducing nocturnal voiding frequency in men with post-radiation bladder pain for PCa. Randomized, controlled trials with sham treatment are needed to confirm our result.

**Keywords:** Prostate cancer, Acute radiation syndrome, Cystitis, Nocturia, Hyaluronic acid, Chondroitin sulfate

## Background

According to international prostate cancer (PCa) guidelines, external beam radiotherapy (EBRT) can be applied as primary treatment and as an alternative to radical prostatectomy in patients with low to medium risk localized PCa (Gleason score ≤7 or cT ≤ 2c or PSA ≤ 20 ng/ml) [1, 2], or can be used after surgery as adjuvant or salvage treatment, in case of biochemical relapse [3].

New PCa treatment modalities, such as intensity modulated radiation therapy (IMRT), achieve to focus the maximum administered dose more precisely on the prostate, thereby avoiding radiation damage on adjacent organs such as the bladder. Nevertheless, even with IMRT, up to 50 % of patients treated with doses >70 Gy experience lower urinary tract symptoms (LUTS), especially during the early treatment period (acute radiation toxicity). Of these patients, up to 25 % report nocturnal voiding) during or immediately after radiation therapy [4, 5]. Patients with nocturia experienced a remarkable worsening of their quality of life. Higher the nocturnal

* Correspondence: maurogacci@yahoo.it
[1]Department of Urology, University of Florence, Careggi Hospital, Largo Brambilla 3, Urologic Clinic San Luca, Florence 50100, Italy
Full list of author information is available at the end of the article

voiding frequency was, the more deteriorated the HRQoL became. The reason can be attributed to the impaired sleep caused by nocturia. Sleep disruption, in particular during the first 4 hours of slow wave sleep (SWS) period, has been implicated as a likely mechanism underlying the subjective complaints, daytime tiredness, and depressive symptoms [6, 7]. It has been hypothesized that post-radiation LUTS, including nocturnal voiding frequency (nocturia), could be caused by the damage, disruption and, consequently, discontinuation of the glycosaminoglycan (GAG) layer of the bladder mucosa [8]. Therefore, GAG replenishment therapy by instillation of hyaluronic acid (HA) with or without chondroitin sulfate (CS) has been suggested as a viable treatment option to treat post-radiation LUTS [9]. Up until now, only few clinical trials have been published which investigated GAG replenishment treatment with HA and CS combination to treat bladder pain or post-radiation LUTS [10] and no study has ever investigated nocturia/nocturnal voiding frequency in post-radiation PCa patients. Therefore, the aim of this pilot study was to evaluate the efficacy and safety of intravesical GAG replenishment treatment with HA and CS combination in men with nocturia in men after radiation therapy for prostate cancer.

## Methods
### Patient population and study design
Male patients with urinary symptoms due to post radiation cystitis and negative urine cultures after external beam radiotherapy for PCa were enrolled between May 2012 and October 2013. Men with a history of previous bladder catheterizations for acute urinary retention, urinary tract infections or bladder stones or a known malignant disease besides PCa were excluded from this study. Age and comorbidities, Gleason score and serum PSA concentration as well as radiation dose and toxicity were recorded for all patients.

Men were treated with bladder instillations containing HA and CS combination (HA 1.6 % 800 mg/50 ml and CS 2 % 1000 mg/50 ml) according only to the indication and schedule reported in the package leaflet of the manufacturer (Ialuril® Ibsa Pambio-Noranco, Switzerland). Pre- and post-treatment LUTS, including nocturnal voiding frequency, were assessed by validated questionnaires. The study protocol was reviewed and approved by the local ethic committee in Florence, Italy (A.O.U.C. Careggi ethic committee). The study did not require any deviation of the current clinical practice standards and was conducted in accordance to the principles of research, as reported in the Declaration of Helsinki or in Good Clinical Practice standards for PCa. All patients received all information about the study design and they signed informed consent. No children were included in the study.

### Radiotherapy treatment
The planning computed tomography scan was performed with 3-mm slices, with the patient in the supine position and using a leg immobilization system (Combifix-Sinmed, Civco, Kalona, IA, USA). The total dose applied was 66–70 Gy (2 Gy/fraction, five fractions weekly,). The clinical target volume (CTV) was limited to the prostatic bed and periprostatic tissue, ensuring adequate coverage of the vesico-urethral anastomosis. The planning treatment volume (PTV) included the clinical target volume, plus a 10-mm margin in all directions. For postoperative treatment, 66–70 Gy in 33–35 fractions were delivered with a tridimensional conformal technique (3DCRT).

### Hyaluronic acid and chondroitin sulfate administration and assessment of cystitis and nocturia
Three months after radiation therapy, patients with urinary symptoms due to radiation cystitis underwent intravesical administration of HA and CS weekly for the first month, and on week 6, 8 and 12 as reported in the package leaflet of the manufacturer. HA and CS was diluted in 50 ml physiologic NaCl solution, placed inside the bladder with sterile catheters (14 F) and retained for at least 1 h.

At baseline and 2 weeks after the end of treatment (week 12 + 2 = week 14), all patients were asked to complete the Interstitial Cystitis Symptom Index and Problem Index (ICSI/ICPI), initially proposed in 1997 as outcome measures in bladder pain syndrome/interstitial cystitis (BPS/IC) and currently recognized as one of the most accurate tools to identify the most relevant voiding and pain symptoms due to bladder pain [11]. In particular, the *symptom* nocturnal voiding was measured with the question 3 (Q3) of ICSI asking: *How often did you most typically get up at night to urinate?* Answers range from 0 ("not at all") to 5 ("5 or more times per night"). The *problem* associated with nocturia was measured with question 2 (Q2) of ICPI asking: *How much has getting up at night to urinate been a problem for you?* Answers range from 0 ("no problem") to 4 ("big problem").

### Statistical analyses
Correlation between symptoms and problems detected at the ICSI and ICPI total score and for the specific ICSI-Q3 and ICPI-Q2 at baseline and at the end of the study was performed with the Spearman correlation coefficient; significant data were included in an age adjusted model. Mean changes between baseline and the end of study (week 14) were assessed by a paired sample t test, for ICSI and ICPI total score and for the specific ICSI-Q3 and ICPI-Q2. A p value of 0.05 or less was considered statistically significant. All statistical analyses were done with SPSS-20®.

## Results and discussion

We included 23 consecutive patients with symptomatic cystitis and negative urine cultures after RT. Five patients (21.7 %) did not have nocturnal voiding (even if they were affected by other symptoms of cystitis), while the remaining 18 (78.3 %) presented with nocturnal voiding frequency (nocturia): 7 patients (38.9 %) 2 times per night, 10 patients (35.7 %) 3 times per night and 1 patient (3.4 %) 5 times per night. Median age of men with nocturnal voiding was $70.5 \pm 5.9$ years. Eleven were affected by high risk PCA (61 %), 6 by intermediate risk (33 %) and 1 by low risk (6 %), according to PCa risk classification [12]. Median dose that patients received was $67.9 \pm 2$ Gy and all patients reported at least grade 2 of toxicity according RTOG adverse event reporting [13].

Men with nocturnal voiding presented a statistically significant recovery of this symptom, after treatment with HA and CS (Table 1). In particular, there was a significant reduction of ICSI/ICPI total score and ICSI-Q3 and ICPI-Q2 between pre-treatment baseline and post-treatment evaluation (Fig. 1 and Table 2). Specifically regarding symptoms (ICSI Q3), 10 patients (56 %) showed improvement in the number of nocturnal voids, 8 patients (44 %) had no change and no patient reported worsening. Regarding bother (ICPI Q2), 10 patients (56 %) showed improvement, 7 patients (39 %) had no change, and only 1 patient reported worsening. At the end of bladder instillation treatment, men without nocturia at baseline continued to be without nocturia: therefore, these 5 men were excluded by further statistical analyses (Table 3).

We did not find any significant correlation between "nocturia symptom" and "nocturia bother" (ICSI-Q3 vs ICPI-Q2: baseline: $r = -0.110$, $p = 0.664$; end of study: $r = 0.549$, $p = 0.151$) before and after instillation therapy. Moreover, comorbidities, tumor characteristics, including PSA and Gleason Score, dose radiation and toxicity were not correlated with ICSI-Q3 or ICPI-Q2 (data not shown).

At baseline (after radiation therapy) ICSI-Q3 scores were correlated with ICSI total scores ($r = 0.649$, $p = 0.004$), and ICPI-Q2 scores were correlated with ICPI total scores ($r = 0.472$, $p = 0.048$). At the end of study (after instillation), ICSI-Q3 scores were correlated with ICSI total score ($r = 0.466$, $p = 0.051$), and ICPI-Q2

scores were correlated with ICPI total scores ($r = 0.808$, $p < 0.001$). Post-treatment ICSI-Q3 scores correlated with pre-treatment ICSI-Q3 scores ($r = 0.402$, $p = 0.048$), while post treatment ICPI-Q2 scores correlated with pre-treatment ICPI-Q2 scores ($r = 0.536$, $p = 0.022$).

After age adjustement, both age and baseline ICSI-Q3 correlated with post-treatment ICSI-Q3 ($r = 0.293$, $p = 0.011$ and $r = 0.970$, $p < 0.001$, respectively), while no significant data were seen in multivariate analyses for post-treatment ICPI-Q2.

Genitourinary toxicities during or after radiotherapy are a common finding for men treated for prostate cancer. In particular, up to 25 % of these patients report about nocturia as a bothersome treatment-related adverse event which can have a substantial impact on patients' quality of life [4, 14, 15]. Several factors, including comorbidities (metabolic syndrome, hearth failure, chronic renal failure), existing lower urinary tract symptoms (related to benign prostatic enlargement), or urinary tract infections can be predictive for post-radiation bladder toxicity [15]. However, the physical injury of the bladder urothelium is most likely the main pathogenetic factor of post-radiation bladder symptoms, including nocturia. The damage can be related to the volume and dose of radiation. 65 Gy has been estimated as the maximum tolerated dose for whole bladder field irradiation in order to maintain severe urinary toxicity below 5 %, while with 80 Gy the occurrence of bladder injury can be observed in up to 50 % of patients [16]. For the treatment of PCa, the bladder is only partly irradiated. However, when bladder, bladder neck and urethra receive radiation doses >70 Gy, bothersome urinary symptoms, including nocturia, are commonly observed [17].

Post-radiation injury of bladder urothelium can be caused by specific damage of the GAG layer. GAGs are a class of polysaccharides, of which HA and CS are key components. When damaging this layer, penetration of potassium into the bladder wall (interstitium) can cause activation of C-fibers which promote smooth muscle contraction, neurogenic inflammation, and hypersensitivity [18, 19]. Therefore, the aim of the treatment of radiation cystitis includes replanishment of the GAG layer of the bladder and reduction of mast cell mediated inflammatory cascades. Many other treatments have been proposed including hyperbaric oxygen therapy (HBOT) [20] since it is postulated that HBOT may result in both healing of tissues and the prevention of problems following radiotherapy; intravesical instillation with dimethyl sulfoxide [21]; or several antimuscarinic (anticholinergics) drugs such as tolterodine [22], α-adrenoceptor antagonists (α-blockers) and non-steroidal anti-inflammatory drugs. All treatments showed, however, poor clinical responses [23].

Recent papers have suggested that CS could promote regeneration of the GAG layer on the bladder

**Table 1** Number of nocturnal voids at baseline and week 14

| ICSI Q3 score | | | | |
|---|---|---|---|---|
| Baseline frequency | N | End point (week 14) | | |
| | | 1 | 2 | 3 |
| 2 | 7 | 1 | 6 | - |
| 3 | 10 | 1 | 7 | 2 |
| 4 | 0 | - | - | - |
| ≥5 | 1 | - | - | 1 |

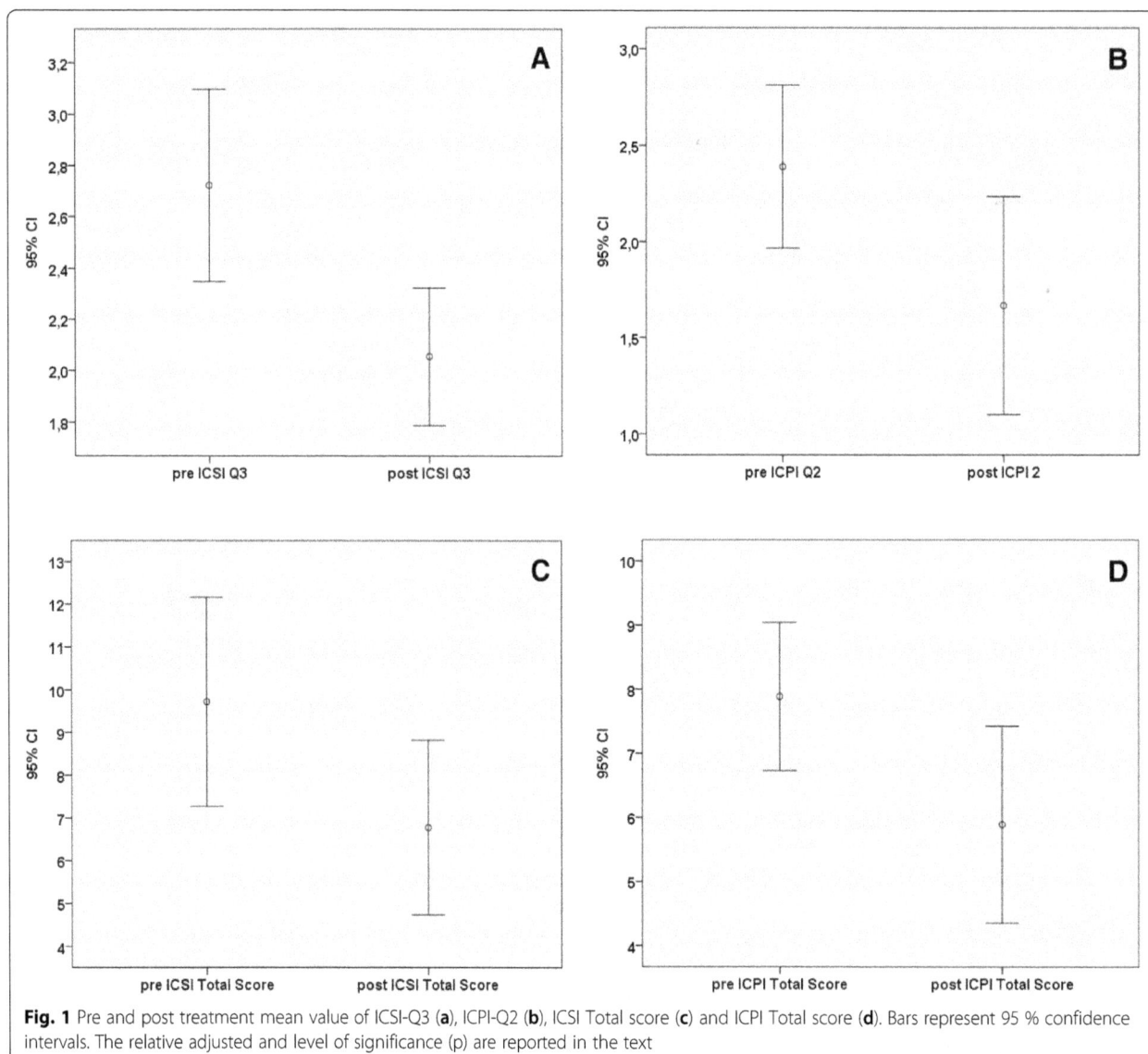

**Fig. 1** Pre and post treatment mean value of ICSI-Q3 (**a**), ICPI-Q2 (**b**), ICSI Total score (**c**) and ICPI Total score (**d**). Bars represent 95 % confidence intervals. The relative adjusted and level of significance (p) are reported in the text

urothelium and HA could have an inhibitory effect on mast cells of the bladder. In our population of men with post-radiation bladder symptoms, the severity of nocturia did not correlate with the severity of bother due to nocturia suggesting that immediately after radiation patients are more concerned by other symptoms, including

**Table 2** Pre and postoperative mean score and standard deviation of ICSI / ICPI (total score-Q3-Q2)

|  |  | Pre treatment | Post treatment | P value(pairT-test) |
|---|---|---|---|---|
| ICSI | Q3 | 2.72 ± 0.75 | 2.06 ± 0.53 | 0.001 |
|  | Total score | 9.72 ± 4.91 | 6.78 ± 4.11 | 0.004 |
| ICPI | Q2 | 2.39 ± 0.85 | 1.67 ± 1.14 | 0.015 |
|  | Total score | 7.89 ± 2.32 | 5.89 ± 3.08 | 0.006 |

.

bladder pain. Moreover, in our patients the presence of comorbidities, tumor characteristics (PSA and Gleason score), dose radiation and toxicity had a negligible influence on nocturnal voiding and nocturia-related bother.

The association between nocturnal voiding (ICSI-Q3 and ICPI-Q2) and the whole pattern of bladder pain symptoms and bother (ICSI/ICPI total scores) demonstrated that nocturnal voiding frequency (nocturia) is only one of the symptoms due to the injury of the bladder and restoration of the bladder wall after treatment allow to relief not only on nocturnal voiding, but also other post-radiation bladder symptoms. These data are confirmed by our age adjusted analysis, demonstrating that elderly men with the worst nocturnal voiding symptoms are those with poorer outcomes after instillation therapy. In these patients, the bladder damage seems to

**Table 3** Distribution of patients with improvement, no change or worsening at end of treatment, by baseline score

ICSI Q3

| Baseline frequency | N | Improvement N (%) | No change N (%) | Worsening N (%) |
|---|---|---|---|---|
| 2 | 7 | 1 (4 %) | 6 (86 %) | 0 (0 %) |
| 3 | 10 | 8 (80 %) | 2 (20 %) | 0 (0 %) |
| 4 | 0 | 0 (0 %) | 0 (0 %) | 0 (0 %) |
| ≥5 | 1 | 1 (100 %) | 0 (0 %) | 0 (0 %) |
| All | 18 | 10 (56 %) | 8 (44 %) | 0 (0 %) |

ICPI Q2

| Baseline frequency | N | Improvement N (%) | No change N (%) | Worsening N (%) |
|---|---|---|---|---|
| 0 | 1 | 0 (0 %) | 0 (0 %) | 1 (100 %) |
| 1 | 1 | 1 (100 %) | 0 (0 %) | 0 (0 %) |
| 2 | 6 | 3 (50 %) | 3 (50 %) | 0 (0 %) |
| 3 | 10 | 6 (60 %) | 4 (40 %) | 0 (0 %) |
| 4 | 0 | 0 (0 %) | 0 (0 %) | 0 (0 %) |
| All | 18 | 10 (56 %) | 7 ( 39 %) | 1 ( 5 %) |

be only partially restored by replenishment therapy, resulting in persistent nocturia. Overall, treatment with HA and CS administration was well tolerated, with no serious adverse event or early treatment discontinuations. In particular, no patients, including those without nocturnal voids, reported any worsening of their local and systemic symptoms, including the occurrence of fever or hematuria.

The main limits of our study are the small sample size, the short follow up time and the lack of a placebo arm. Our small sample size could be considered satisfactory for a "pilot study design"; however, to better understand the timing of the response to treatment with Ialuril, and to measure the difference between spontaneous recovery of urinary function vs. treatment related clinical effect, a randomized, placebo controlled trial, with several scheduled symptoms assessments and adequate follow up time is needed. The strengths are the uniformity for radiation treatment, the use of validated questionnaire and the adjustment for confounding factors.

## Conclusions

In conclusion, our pilot study demonstrated that bladder instillation with HA and CS is a safe treatment in post radiation bladder cystitis. Patients after Ialuril ® instillation reported a statistically significant reduction in symptom/bother nocturnal voiding frequency, even if the overall improvement due to the medication vs. spontaneous recovery must be confirmed by placebo controlled trials, including further assessment tools such as cystoscopy and histological evaluation.

**Abbreviation**

(PCa): Prostate cancer; (HA): Hyaluronic acid; (CS): Chondroitin sulfate; (GAG): Glycosaminoglycan; (ICSI): Interstitial Cystitis Symptoms Index; (ICPI): Interstitial Cystitis Problem Index; (EBRT): External beam radiotherapy; (IMRT): Modulated radiation therapy; (LUTS): Lower urinary tract symptoms; (CTV): Clinical target volume; (PTV): Planning treatment volume; (3DCRT): Tridimensional conformal technique; (BPS/IC): Bladder pain syndrome/interstitial cystitis; (HBOT): Hyperbaric oxygen therapy.

**Competing interests**

The authors declare that they have no competing interests.

**Authors' contributions**

MG made study conception and design. OS, CG, BD, EMP, TM and LL have made acquisition of data. MO made analysis and interpretation of data. OS has been involved in drafting of the manuscript. MO has been involved in critical revision of the manuscript for important intellectual content. MG has been involved in statistical analysis. MG gave the final approval. MG and MC have agreed to be accountable for all aspects of the work. SS, AM, VL, EFA and SG have made the supervision. All authors read and approved the final manuscript.

**Acknowledgements**

The drug was kindly provided by Ibsa Farmaceutici srl, Switzerland.

**Author details**

¹Department of Urology, University of Florence, Careggi Hospital, Largo Brambilla 3, Urologic Clinic San Luca, Florence 50100, Italy. ²Department of Radiation Therapy, University of Florence, Careggi Hospital, Largo Brambilla 3, Florence, Italy. ³Department of Urology, Tor Vergata University, Via di Tor Vergata, Rome, Italy. ⁴Department of Urology, University Hospital of Larissa, Larissa, Greece. ⁵Department of Urology, Hannover Medical School, Hannover, Germany.

**References**

1. Kuban DA, Tucker SL, Dong L, et al. Long-term results of the M. D. Anderson randomized dose-escalation trial for prostate cancer. Int J Radiat Oncol Biol Phys. 2008;70:67–74.
2. EAU guidelines http://www.uroweb.org/guidelines/online-guidelines/. Accessed 25 June 2014.
3. Bolla M, Van Poppel H, Collette L, et al. Postoperative radiotherapy after radical prostatectomy: a randomised controlled trial (EORTC trial, 22911). Lancet. 2005;366:572–8.
4. De Langhe S et al. Acute radiation-induced nocturia in prostate cancer patients is associated with pretreatment symptoms, radical prostatectomy, and genetic markers in the TGFb1 gene. Int J Radiat Oncol Biol Phys. 2013;85(2):393e399.
5. GDe Meerleer L, Vakaet S. Meersschout et al. Intensity-modulated radiotherapy as primary treatment for prostate cancer: acute toxicity in 114 patients. Phys. 2004;60:777–87.
6. Matthias O et al. Nocturia: state of the art and critical analysis of current assessment and treatment strategies. World J Urol. 2014;32:1109–17.
7. Bliwise DL, Rosen RC, Baum N. Impact of nocturia on sleep and quality of life: a brief, selected review for the international consultation on incontinence research society (ICI-RS) nocturia think tank. Neurourol Urodyn. 2014;33:S15–8.
8. Giberti C, Gallo F, Cortese P, Schenone M. Combined intravesical sodium hyaluronate/chondroitin sulfate therapy for interstitial cystitis/bladder pain syndrome: a prospective study. Ther Adv Urol. 2013;5:175–9.
9. Damiano R, Cicione A. The role of sodium hyaluronate and sodium chondroitin sulphate in the management of bladder disease. Ther Adv Urol. 2011;3:223–32.
10. Daniele P et al. Impact of intravesical hyaluronic acid and chondroitin sulfate on bladder pain syndrome/interstitial cystitis. Int Urogynecol J. 2012;23:1193–9.
11. Giannantoni A. Patient-Reported Outcomes in Bladder Pain Syndrome: Qui Auget Dolorem, Auget et Scientiam (As Pain Increases, So Increases Knowledge). Eur Urol. 2012 Feb;61(2):280-1; discussion 282-3. doi:10.1016/j.eururo.2011.10.042. Epub 2011 Nov 4.

12. D'Amico AV, Whittington R, Malkowicz SB, Cote K, Loffredo M, Schultz D, et al. Biochemical outcome after radical prostatectomy or external beam radiation therapy for patients with clinically localized prostate carcinoma in the prostate specific antigen era. Cancer. 2002;95:281–6.

13. RTOG http://www.rtog.org/ResearchAssociates/AdverseEventReporting.aspx. Accessed 11 January 2015

14. Lips IM, Dehnad H, van Gils CH, et al. High-dose intensity-modulated radiotherapy for prostate cancer using daily fiducial marker based position verification: acute and late toxicity in 331 patients. Radiat Oncol. 2008;3:15.

15. Peeters ST, Heemsbergen WD, van Putten WL, et al. Acute and late complications after radiotherapy for prostate cancer: results of a multicenter randomized trial comparing 68 Gy to 78 Gy. Int J Radiat Oncol Biol Phys. 2005;61:1019–34.

16. Emami B, Lyman J, Brown A, et al. Tolerance of normal tissue to therapeutic irradiation. Int J Radiat Oncol Biol Phys. 1991;21:109–22.

17. Fiorino C et al. Dose–volume effects for normal tissues in external radiotherapy: Pelvis. Systematic review. Radiother Oncol. 2009;93:153–67.

18. Costantini E, Lazzeri M, Porena M. GAGs and GAGs diseases: when pathophysiology supports the clinic. Urologia. 2013 Jul-Sep;80(3):173-8. doi: 10.5301/RU.2013.11500. Epub 2013 Sep 30.

19. Pier Francesco Bassi, Mauro Cervigni,Enrico Finazzi Agrò, Rocco Damiano, Roman Tomaškin. Increasing evidence of effectiveness of GAG therapy in different forms of cystitis. Eur Med J – Urol. 2013;1:33–40.

20. Fuentes-Raspall R, Inoriza JM, Rosello-Serrano A, Auñón-Sanz C, Garcia-Martin P, Oliu-Isern G. Late rectal and bladder toxicity following radiation therapy for prostate cancer: predictive factors and treatment results. Rep Pract Oncol Radiother. 2013;18:298–303.

21. Rössberger J, Fall M, Peeker R. Critical appraisal of dimethyl sulfoxide treatment for interstitial cystitis: discomfort, side-effects and treatment outcome. Scand J Urol Nephrol. 2005;39:73–7.

22. Madersbacher H, Van Ophoven A, Van Kerrebroeck PE. GAG layer replenishment therapy for chronic forms of cystitis with intravesical glycosaminoglycans — a review. Neurourol Urodyn. 2013;32:9–18.

23. Zelefsky MJ, Ginor RX, Fuks Z, et al. Efficacy of selective alpha-1 blocker therapy in the treatment of acute urinary symptoms during radiotherapy for localized prostate cancer. Int J Radiat Oncol Biol Phys. 1999;45:567–70.

**3**

# Protocol for a prospective magnetic resonance imaging study on supraspinal lower urinary tract control in healthy subjects and spinal cord injury patients undergoing intradetrusor onabotulinumtoxinA injections for treating neurogenic detrusor overactivity

Lorenz Leitner[1†], Matthias Walter[1†], Patrick Freund[1], Ulrich Mehnert[1], Lars Michels[2], Spyros Kollias[2] and Thomas M Kessler[1*]

## Abstract

**Background:** The control of the lower urinary tract is a complex, multilevel process involving both the peripheral and central nervous system. Due to lesions of the neuraxis, most spinal cord injury patients suffer from neurogenic lower urinary tract dysfunction, which may jeopardise upper urinary tract function and has a negative impact on health-related quality of life. However, the alterations to the nervous system following spinal cord injury causing neurogenic lower urinary tract dysfunction and potential effects of treatments such as intradetrusor onabotulinumtoxinA injections on lower urinary tract control are poorly understood.

**Methods/Design:** This is a prospective structural and functional magnetic resonance imaging study investigating the supraspinal lower urinary tract control in healthy subjects and spinal cord injury patients undergoing intradetrusor onabotulinumtoxinA injections for treating neurogenic detrusor overactivity.
Neuroimaging data will include structural magnetic resonance imaging (T1-weighted imaging and diffusion tensor imaging) as well as functional, i.e. blood oxygen level-dependent sensitive magnetic resonance imaging using a 3 T magnetic resonance scanner. The functional magnetic resonance imaging will be performed simultaneously to three different bladder stimulation paradigms using an automated magnetic resonance compatible and synchronised pump system.
All subjects will undergo two consecutive and identical magnetic resonance imaging measurements. Healthy subjects will not undergo any intervention between measurements but spinal cord injury patients will receive intradetrusor onabotulinumtoxinA injections for treating neurogenic detrusor overactivity.
Parameters of the clinical assessment including bladder diary, urinalysis, medical history, neuro-urological examination, urodynamic investigation as well as standardised questionnaires regarding lower urinary tract function and quality of life will serve as co-variates in the magnetic resonance imaging analysis.
(Continued on next page)

* Correspondence: tkessler@gmx.ch
†Equal contributors
[1]Neuro-Urology, Spinal Cord Injury Centre & Research, University of Zürich, Balgrist University Hospital, Forchstrasse 340, 8008 Zürich, Switzerland
Full list of author information is available at the end of the article

(Continued from previous page)

**Discussion:** This study will identify structural and functional alterations in supraspinal networks of lower urinary tract control in spinal cord injury patients with neurogenic detrusor overactivity compared to healthy controls. Post-treatment magnetic resonance imaging measurements in spinal cord injury patients will provide further insights into the mechanism of action of treatments such as intradetrusor onabotulinumtoxinA injections and the effect on supraspinal lower urinary tract control.

**Keywords:** Urinary bladder, Spinal cord injury, Neuroimaging, Magnetic resonance imaging, Neurogenic detrusor overactivity, OnabotulinumtoxinA intradetrusor injections

## Background

Spinal cord injury (SCI) is a devastating event with far-reaching consequences for the individual's health and the economic and social future. In the past, renal failure due to neurogenic lower urinary tract dysfunction (NLUTD) was a leading cause of death after SCI [1]. Furthermore, NLUTD has a highly negative impact on patients' quality of life (QoL). Acute SCI initially causes "spinal shock", characterised by an acontractile/hypocontractile detrusor and urinary retention, which in case of a suprasacral lesion (today the vast majority of SCI) is followed by development of detrusor overactivity mostly combined with detrusor sphincter dyssynergia [2]. Antimuscarinics are the pharmacological first-line treatment for detrusor overactivity although the effectiveness is limited [3]. In addition, many patients discontinue antimuscarinics due to bothersome side-effects [4]. Thus, intradetrusor onabotulinumtoxinA injections have become an established, highly effective, minimally invasive, and generally well-tolerated therapy for refractory detrusor overactivity [5] to improve patients' health and QoL [6]. Despite the popularity of intradetrusor onabotulinumtoxinA injections, the exact mechanisms of action remain to be elucidated. Nevertheless, it seems highly probable that, in addition to a direct efferent effect by blocking the presynaptic release of acetylcholine from the parasympathetic innervation resulting in temporary chemodenervation of the detrusor, onabotulinumtoxinA also modulates afferent pathways [7]. It is, however, not known whether this treatment can normalise alterations in supraspinal areas and whether supraspinal modulation correlates with clinical improvements.

The control of the lower urinary tract (LUT) is a complex, multilevel process that involves both the peripheral and central nervous system but the exact mechanisms involved in humans are still incompletely understood [8]. Neuroimaging studies over the last decade have consistently pointed to a complex supraspinal network that controls LUT function [9]. These studies tremendously increased our understanding of how human LUT function is coordinated and how it can be affected by neurological disorders. Recent neuroimaging studies demonstrated reorganisation of supraspinal activity in response to LUT stimulation tasks in patients with disorders such as Parkinson's disease [10-12] and SCI [13] as compared to healthy controls, which might represent the neural correlate of their NLUTD.

Cortical and sub-cortical (for example, brainstem) brain regions are essential for voluntary LUT control [9,14,15]. Investigation of the supraspinal regions with high-resolution imaging techniques, for example, structural magnetic resonance imaging (MRI) and functional MRI (fMRI), can significantly increase our knowledge on the effects of supraspinal lesions and alterations related to NLUTD [9,16]. Although diffusion tensor imaging (DTI) [17] is popular in other fields in neuroscience, it has only been applied in the context of supraspinal LUT control in one prospective study [18] in patients with non-neurogenic LUT symptoms.

In this study, we will first identify supraspinal areas associated with LUT control in SCI patients with neurogenic detrusor overactivity and healthy controls. Subsequently, we will investigate the effects of intradetrusor onabotulinumtoxinA injections on supraspinal areas. Task-related blood oxygen level-dependent (BOLD) fMRI will be used along structural MRI (T1-weighted and DTI). Moreover, we will examine volumetric parameters (for example, grey and white matter concentration) by voxel- (VBM) [19] and tensor-based morphometry (TBM) [20], structural integrity and connectivity of white matter tracts (DTI) as well as structural (SC) and functional connectivity (FC).

This unique and detailed multimodal imaging and clinical approach will distinguish the different structural and functional processing units involved during supraspinal LUT control and will identify dysfunctional neuronal components in SCI patients responsible for neurogenic detrusor overactivity.

For a test-retest validation, we will additionally investigate the reliability [21] of BOLD signals in task-related fMRI in healthy controls by the intra-class correlation coefficient (ICC) for absolute or consistent agreement of participants activations over two visits.

## Methods/Design

### Study design

This prospective research study will be conducted at the University of Zürich, Zürich, Switzerland in cooperation with our partner, the institute of Neuro-Radiology, University of Zürich, University Hospital Zürich, Zürich, Switzerland.

### Study location

The study has two study locations, that is, the department of Neuro-Urology, Spinal Cord Injury Centre & Research, University of Zürich, Balgrist University Hospital, Zürich, Switzerland (first and third visit, see below) and the MR-Centre, University Hospital Zürich, Zürich, Switzerland (second and third visit, see below).

### Study population and recruitment

In line with the inclusion and exclusion criteria (Table 1), we will investigate SCI patients with neurogenic detrusor overactivity and healthy controls with an unimpaired LUT function. Participants of both groups will be similar according to age and gender.

20–24 SCI patients with neurogenic detrusor overactivity refractory to antimuscarinics and scheduled for study independent intradetrusor onabotulinumtoxinA injections and 12–24 healthy controls will be recruited.

### Interventions

Subjects providing written informed consent will be invited for the following visits (Figure 1):

Screening (Visit 1): Evaluation for study eligibility will be based on medical history, urinalysis to exclude urinary tract infection (UTI) and pregnancy in female participants, 3-day bladder diary, post void residual, urodynamic parameters as well as on standardised validated questionnaires such as Qualiveen [22] and International Consultation on Incontinence modular questionnaire [(ICIQ), Bristol Urological Institute, Southmead Hospital Bristol, UK] assessing lower urinary tract symptoms (LUTS) in both woman (ICIQ-FLUTS) and men (ICIQ-MLUTS).

MRI measurements (Visit 2 and 3, Figure 1): Two MRI measurements will be performed in identically manner within a 5 to 7 weeks interval.

Both MRI measurements will be performed using a Philips Ingenia 3 Tesla MR scanner (Philips Medical Systems, Best, The Netherlands) with a 16-channel head coil to acquire the following sequences (Figure 2):

- Structural sequences will comprise T1-weighted and DTI.
- Functional sequences will comprise three different task-related fMRI paradigms (Figure 3).
  - In the first two task-related fMRI paradigms, we will examine the effect of visceral bladder sensation by automated, repetitive bladder filling with 100 mL body warm (37°C) saline starting with an

**Table 1 Inclusion and exclusion criteria for all participants**

| Groups | Inclusion criteria | Exclusion criteria |
|---|---|---|
| All participants | • MR suitability | • Pregnancy or breast feeding |
| | • Written informed consent | • Any anatomical anomaly of LUT/genitalia |
| | | • Any LUT malignancy |
| | | • Claustrophobia |
| SCI patients | • Age limit: > 18 years | • Symptomatic UTI |
| | • Neurogenic detrusor overactivity | |
| | • Refractory to antimuscarinic treatment | |
| | • Scheduled for intradetrusor onabotulinumtoxinA injections | |
| Healthy controls | • Age limits: > 18 years | • Impaired LUT function |
| | • Unimpaired LUT function | • Any LUTS (3-day bladder diary) |
| | • No LUTS (3-day bladder diary) | • Any number of episodes of urinary urgency/week |
| | • No episode of urinary urgency/week | • Urinary frequency > 8/24 h |
| | • Urinary frequency < 8/24 h | • Any craniocerebral injury or surgery |
| | | • Any permanent ferromagnetic implant |
| | | • Any previous surgery of LUT/genitalia |
| | | • UTI |
| | | • PVR > 150 mL |

LUT = lower urinary tract, LUTS = lower urinary tract symptoms, MR = magnetic resonance, PVR = post void residual, SCI = spinal cord injury, UTI = urinary tract infection.

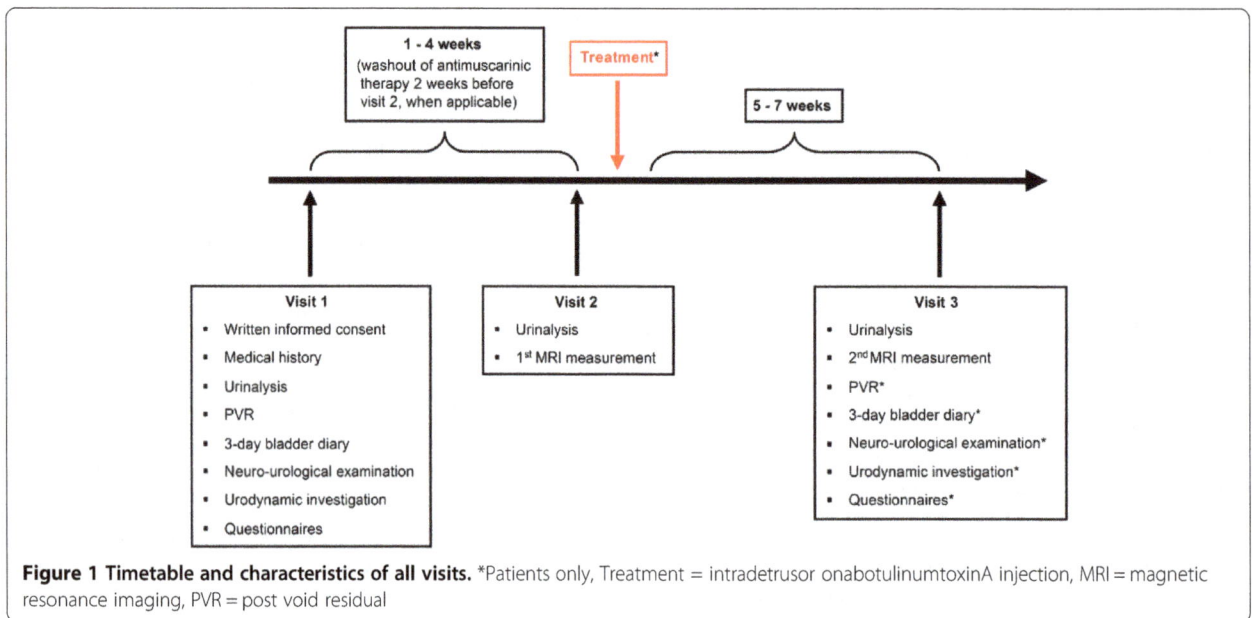

**Figure 1 Timetable and characteristics of all visits.** *Patients only, Treatment = intradetrusor onabotulinumtoxinA injection, MRI = magnetic resonance imaging, PVR = post void residual

empty bladder (first paradigm) and a bladder volume eliciting desire to void (second paradigm).

- The third task-related fMRI paradigm will contain automated, repetitive filling of 100 mL cold (4-8°C) saline starting with an empty bladder.

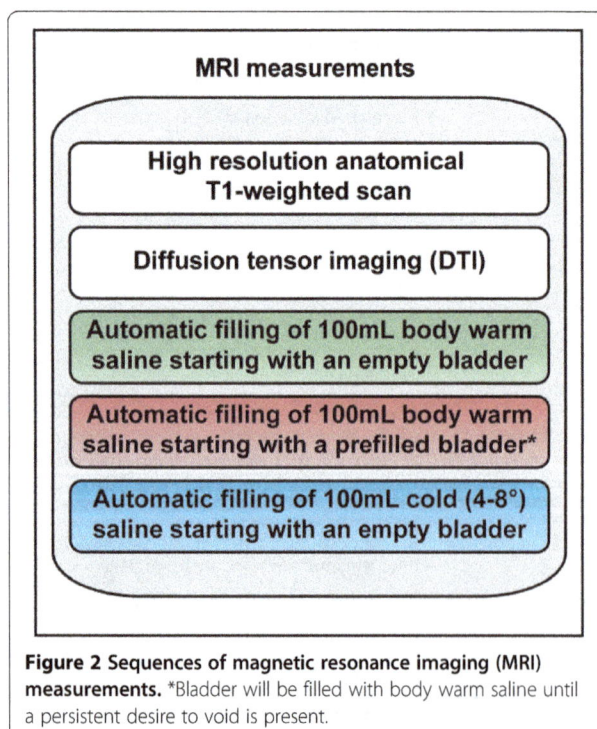

**Figure 2 Sequences of magnetic resonance imaging (MRI) measurements.** *Bladder will be filled with body warm saline until a persistent desire to void is present.

Repetitive filling will be performed using an automated MR-compatible and MR-synchronised pump system [18] to precisely fill and drain the bladder. During the MRI measurements, all participants will use an MR-compatible handheld response system [23] to rate their desire to void and level of pain on a displayed visual analogue scale.

### Study outcome measures
#### Primary

(A) Task-related BOLD signal intensity in supraspinal regions of interest (ROI) in SCI patients with neurogenic detrusor overactivity compared to healthy controls.
(B) Supraspinal morphometry of ROIs in SCI patients with neurogenic detrusor overactivity compared to healthy controls.
(C) SC and FC between ROIs of the supraspinal LUT controlling circuitries in SCI patients with neurogenic detrusor overactivity and healthy controls.
(D) Changes of task-related BOLD signal intensity, SC and FC between ROIs in SCI patients with neurogenic detrusor overactivity before and after study independent intradetrusor onabotulinumtoxinA injections.

#### Secondary

(A) Reliability of BOLD signal changes between first and second MRI measurement in healthy controls.
(B) Correlations between clinical co-variates that are bladder diary parameters, urodynamic parameters, level of desire to void during fMRI and task-related

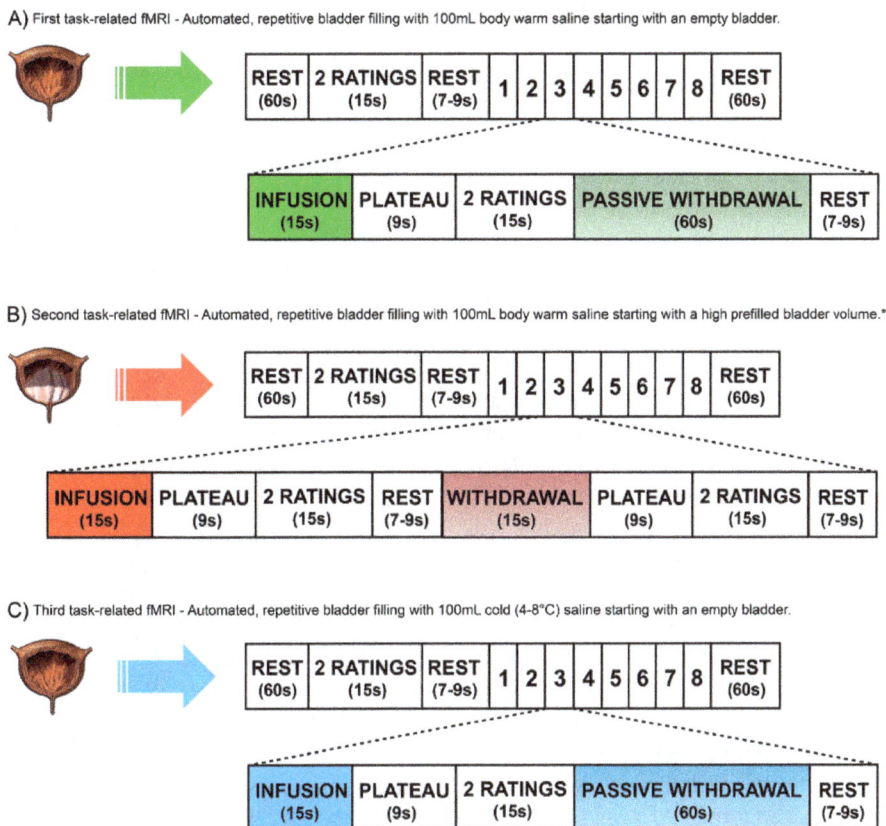

**Figure 3 Scan paradigm of three different task-related functional MRIs (fMRIs).** All task-related fMRIs identically start with a 'baseline' rest (60 s, no specific stimulus or task is performed), a 'baseline' rating (desire to void and level of pain), a short rest (jittered between 7 and 9 s in which blood oxygen level-dependent (BOLD) activation resulting from motor activity during the previous rating will return to baseline to avoid contamination of the following condition) and conclude with a 'last' rest (60 s, no specific stimulus or task is performed). All task-related fMRIs consist of eight repetitive blocks, each with either five (first and third fMRIs) or eight (second fMRI) conditions. **(A)** Conditions of the first task-related fMRIs: (1) automated infusion of 100 mL body warm saline, (2) plateau phase (bladder distention after infusion is perceived), (3) rating, (4) passive withdrawal to empty the bladder completely and (5) short rest. This task-related fMRI starts with an empty bladder. **(B)** Conditions of the second task-related fMRIs: (1) automated infusion of 100 mL warm saline, (2) plateau phase, (3) rating, (4) short rest, (5) automated withdrawal of 100 mL, (6) plateau phase (bladder distention after withdrawal is perceived), (7) rating and (8) short rest. *This task-related fMRI (B) starts with a high prefilled bladder volume, that is, the bladder will be filled with body warm saline until a persistent desire to void is present. **(C)** Conditions of the third task-related fMRIs: (1) automated infusion of 100 mL cold (4–8°C) saline, (2) plateau phase, (3) rating, (4) passive withdrawal to empty the bladder completely and (5) short rest. This task-related fMRI starts with an empty bladder.

BOLD signal intensity in supraspinal ROIs as well as structural parameters, that is, grey matter volume and number of white matter tracts between ROIs.

For the analysis of the neuroimaging data, we will use statistical parametric mapping (SPM) V.8 or newer (Wellcome Department of Imaging Neuroscience, University College London, UK) and toolboxes as appropriate.

## Data analysis

Clinical data, for example, questionnaires scores, urodynamic parameters and 3-day bladder diary outcomes will be statistically analysed and compared between groups using IBM's Statistical Package for the Social Sciences (SPSS) version 19.0 or newer (Armonk, New York, U.S.). The statistical analysis will be presented with means and standard deviations or with medians and interquartile ranges as appropriate.

## Regulatory issues

### Ethical approval

This study has been approved by the local ethics committee (Kantonale Ethikkommission Zürich, KEK-ZH-Nr. 2011–0346) and will be performed in accordance to the World Medical Association Declaration of Helsinki [24], the guidelines for Good Clinical Practice (GCP) [25], and the guidelines of the Swiss Academy of Medical Sciences [26]. Handling of all personal data will strictly comply with the federal law of data protection in Switzerland [27].

### Safety

According to the safety regulations of the MR-Centre of the University Hospital Zürich, the staff involved in this study will be instructed and trained. Prior to entering the scanner room, all participants will be asked to remove any ferromagnetic items (for example, bra, chains, earrings, rings, and piercings). All participants will be provided with standardised clinical scrubs to prevent incidental import of ferromagnetic items into the MR room. To exclude UTI or pregnancy, urinalysis will be performed on every participant before urodynamic investigations and MR measurements. In case of pregnancy, the participant will be excluded from the study and referred to a gynaecologist. In case of UTI, the participant will not undergo the experiment but will be treated appropriately. After successful treatment, a re-assignment to the study is possible.

In case of an adverse event (AE) or a severe adverse event (SAE), as defined by the International Organization for Standardization (ISO, 14155) [28] and the International Conference on Harmonisation (ICH) GCP guidelines (E6) [25], responsible authorities, that is, the principle investigator and the ethics committee will be informed. Appropriate actions will be executed. All AEs and SAEs will be followed as long as medically indicated.

### Funding

The Swiss National Science Foundation (grant number: 135774), Wings for Life, the Emily Dorothy Lagemann Stiftung and the Swiss Continence Foundation are funding this study.

## Discussion

This study will investigate structural and functional abnormalities and specific alterations in the brain networks of supraspinal LUT control in SCI patients with neurogenic detrusor overactivity compared to healthy controls using a multimodal imaging protocol. Importantly, effects on the supraspinal LUT control after treatment for neurogenic detrusor overactivity with intradetrusor onabotulinumtoxinA injections in SCI patients will be explored.

The findings will help to verify, amend, or adjust neuronal circuitry models established from findings in healthy controls, now in the context of SCI patients with neurogenic detrusor overactivity. Furthermore it will show whether neurogenic detrusor overactivity specific treatment such as intradetrusor onabotulinumtoxinA injections induce structural or functional reorganisation in supraspinal areas related to LUT control and in how far such changes correlate with improvements of clinical outcome parameters. These investigations will help us to understand how onabotulinumtoxinA modulates afferent pathways.

Advanced neuroimaging and evaluation techniques have the potential to serve as quantifiable outcome measures for therapy success and for improving our treatment strategies in this patient population.

### Trial status

The trial is in the recruiting phase at the time of manuscript submission.

### Abbreviations

AE: Adverse event; BOLD: Blood oxygen level-dependent; DTI: Diffusion tensor imaging; FA: Fractional anisotropy; FC: Functional connectivity; fMRI: Functional magnetic resonance imaging; GLM: General linear model; GCP: Good clinical practice; ICC: Intra-class correlation coefficient; ICH: International conference on harmonisation; ISO: International organization for standardization; LUT: Lower urinary tract; LUTS: Lower urinary tract symptoms; MR: Magnetic resonance; MRI: Magnetic resonance imaging; MD: Mean diffusivity; MNI: Montreal neurologic institute; NLUTD: Neurogenic lower urinary tract dysfunction; PVR: Post void residual; QoL: Quality of life; ROI: Regions of interest; SAE: Severe adverse event; SPM: Statistical parametric mapping; SC: Structural connectivity; SCI: Spinal cord injury; TBM: Tensor-based morphometry; UTI: Urinary tract infection; VBM: Voxel-based morphometry.

### Competing interests

The authors declare that they have no competing interests.

### Authors' contributions

All authors participated in creating the study design. LL, MW, and TMK drafted the manuscript. PF, UM, LM, and SK provided a critical revision of the manuscript. PF, UM, SK and TMK obtained the funding of this study. All the authors read and approved the final manuscript.

### Acknowledgements

We would like to acknowledge Wings for Life, Swiss National Science Foundation, Emily Dorothy Lagemann Stiftung, and Swiss Continence Foundation for financial support.

### Author details

[1]Neuro-Urology, Spinal Cord Injury Centre & Research, University of Zürich, Balgrist University Hospital, Forchstrasse 340, 8008 Zürich, Switzerland. [2]Institute of Neuro-Radiology, University of Zürich, University Hospital Zürich, Zürich, Switzerland.

### References

1. Hackler RH: A 25-year prospective mortality study in the spinal cord injured patient: comparison with the long-term living paraplegic. J Urol 1977, 117:486–488.
2. Pannek J, Blok B, Castro-Diaz D, del Popolo G, Groen J, Karsenty G, Kessler TM, Kramer G, Stöhrer M: Guidelines on neuro-urology, European association of urology 2014. www.uroweb.org/gls/pdf/21%20Neuro-Urology_LR.pdf.
3. Buser N, Ivic S, Kessler TM, Kessels AG, Bachmann LM: Efficacy and adverse events of antimuscarinics for treating overactive bladder: network meta-analyses. Eur Urol 2012, 62:1040–1060.
4. Kessler TM, Bachmann LM, Minder C, Lohrer D, Umbehr M, Schunemann HJ, Kessels AG: Adverse event assessment of antimuscarinics for treating overactive bladder: a network meta-analytic approach. PLoS One 2011, 6:e16718.
5. Wollner J, Kessler TM: Botulinum toxin injections into the detrusor. BJU Int 2011, 108:1528–1537.
6. Chancellor MB, Patel V, Leng WW, Shenot PJ, Lam W, Globe DR, Loeb AL, Chapple CR: OnabotulinumtoxinA improves quality of life in patients with neurogenic detrusor overactivity. Neurology 2013, 81:841–848.

7.  Apostolidis A, Dasgupta P, Fowler CJ: **Proposed mechanism for the efficacy of injected botulinum toxin in the treatment of human detrusor overactivity.** *Eur Urol* 2006, **49**:644–650.
8.  Fowler CJ, Griffiths D, de Groat WC: **The neural control of micturition.** *Nat Rev Neurosci* 2008, **9**:453–466.
9.  Fowler CJ, Griffiths DJ: **A decade of functional brain imaging applied to bladder control.** *Neurourol Urodyn* 2010, **29**:49–55.
10. Herzog J, Weiss PH, Assmus A, Wefer B, Seif C, Braun PM, Herzog H, Volkmann J, Deuschl G, Fink GR: **Subthalamic stimulation modulates cortical control of urinary bladder in Parkinson's disease.** *Brain* 2006, **129**:3366–3375.
11. Herzog J, Weiss PH, Assmus A, Wefer B, Seif C, Braun PM, Pinsker MO, Herzog H, Volkmann J, Deuschl G, Fink GR: **Improved sensory gating of urinary bladder afferents in Parkinson's disease following subthalamic stimulation.** *Brain* 2008, **131**:132–145.
12. Kitta T, Kakizaki H, Furuno T, Moriya K, Tanaka H, Shiga T, Tamaki N, Yabe I, Sasaki H, Nonomura K: **Brain activation during detrusor overactivity in patients with Parkinson's disease: a positron emission tomography study.** *J Urol* 2006, **175**:994–998.
13. Mehnert U, Michels L, Zempleni MZ, Schurch B, Kollias S: **The supraspinal neural correlate of bladder cold sensation–an fMRI study.** *Hum Brain Mapp* 2011, **32**:835–845.
14. Andrew J, Nathan PW: **Lesions on the anterior frontal lobes and disturbances of micturition and defaecation.** *Brain* 1964, **87**:233–262.
15. Holstege G: **Micturition and the soul.** *J Comp Neurol* 2005, **493**:15–20.
16. de Groat WC: **A neurologic basis for the overactive bladder.** *Urology* 1997, **50**:36–52. discussion 53–36.
17. Basser PJ, Mattiello J, LeBihan D: **MR diffusion tensor spectroscopy and imaging.** *Biophys J* 1994, **66**:259–267.
18. Walter M, Michels L, Kollias S, van Kerrebroeck PE, Kessler TM, Mehnert U: **Protocol for a prospective neuroimaging study investigating the supraspinal control of lower urinary tract function in healthy controls and patients with non-neurogenic lower urinary tract symptoms.** *BMJ Open* 2014, **4**:e004357.
19. Ashburner J, Friston KJ: **Voxel-based morphometry–the methods.** *Neuroimage* 2000, **11**:805–821.
20. Ashburner J, Friston KJ: **Diffeomorphic registration using geodesic shooting and Gauss-Newton optimisation.** *Neuroimage* 2011, **55**:954–967.
21. Caceres A, Hall DL, Zelaya FO, Williams SC, Mehta MA: **Measuring fMRI reliability with the intra-class correlation coefficient.** *Neuroimage* 2009, **45**:758–768.
22. Costa P, Perrouin-Verbe B, Colvez A, Didier J, Marquis P, Marrel A, Amarenco G, Espirac B, Leriche A: **Quality of life in spinal cord injury patients with urinary difficulties. Development and validation of qualiveen.** *Eur Urol* 2001, **39**:107–113.
23. Jarrahi B, Wanek J, Mehnert U, Kollias S: **An fMRI-compatible multi-configurable handheld response system using an intensity-modulated fiber-optic sensor.** *Conf Proc IEEE Eng Med Biol Soc* 2013, **2013**:6349–6352.
24. World Medical Association: **Declaration of Helsinki - ethical principles for medical research involving human subjects.** 1964, [http://www.wma.net/en/30publications/10policies/b3/]
25. International conference on harmonisation: **Good clinical practice guideline.** http://www.ich.org/products/guidelines/efficacy/article/efficacy-guidelines.html.
26. Swiss Academy of Medical Sciences: **Guideline - concerning scientific research involving human beings.** 2009, http://www.samw.ch/dms/en/Publications/Guidelines/e_Leitfaden_Forschung_def.pdf.
27. The Federal Authorities of the Swiss Confederation: **Bundesgesetz über den Datenschutz (DSG) vom 19. Juni 1992, Stand. 01.01.2014.** 1992, http://www.admin.ch/opc/de/classified-compilation/19920153/201401010000/235.1.pdf.
28. **International organization for standardization, ISO 14155.** http://www.iso.org/iso/catalogue_detail?csnumber=45557.

# 4

# Urinary ATP as an indicator of infection and inflammation of the urinary tract in patients with lower urinary tract symptoms

Kiren Gill[1,4*], Harry Horsley[1,4], Anthony S Kupelian[1,4], Gianluca Baio[2], Maria De Iorio[2], Sanchutha Sathiananamoorthy[1,4], Rajvinder Khasriya[1,4], Jennifer L Rohn[1,4], Scott S Wildman[3] and James Malone-Lee[1,4]

## Abstract

**Background:** Adenosine-5′-triphosphate (ATP) is a neurotransmitter and inflammatory cytokine implicated in the pathophysiology of lower urinary tract disease. ATP additionally reflects microbial biomass thus has potential as a surrogate marker of urinary tract infection (UTI). The optimum clinical sampling method for ATP urinalysis has not been established. We tested the potential of urinary ATP in the assessment of lower urinary tract symptoms, infection and inflammation, and validated sampling methods for clinical practice.

**Methods:** A prospective, blinded, cross-sectional observational study of adult patients presenting with lower urinary tract symptoms (LUTS) and asymptomatic controls, was conducted between October 2009 and October 2012. Urinary ATP was assayed by a luciferin-luciferase method, pyuria counted by microscopy of fresh unspun urine and symptoms assessed using validated questionnaires. The sample collection, storage and processing methods were also validated.

**Results:** 75 controls and 340 patients with LUTS were grouped as without pyuria (n = 100), pyuria 1-9 wbc $\mu l^{-1}$ (n = 120) and pyuria $\geq$10 wbc $\mu l^{-1}$ (n = 120). Urinary ATP was higher in association with female gender, voiding symptoms, pyuria greater than 10 wbc $\mu l^{-1}$ and negative MSU culture. ROC curve analysis showed no evidence of diagnostic test potential. The urinary ATP signal decayed with storage at 23°C but was prevented by immediate freezing at $\leq$ -20°C, without boric acid preservative and without the need to centrifuge urine prior to freezing.

**Conclusions:** Urinary ATP may have a role as a research tool but is unconvincing as a surrogate, clinical diagnostic marker.

**Keywords:** Lower urinary tract symptoms (LUTS), Adenosine-5′-triphosphate (ATP), Urinary tract infection (UTI)

## Background

"Lower Urinary Tract Symptoms" (LUTS) is a collective term describing [1] urinary storage problems such as frequency, urgency and urge incontinence; [2] voiding difficulties such as hesitancy, reduced stream, intermittency and incomplete voiding; [3] sensory symptoms that include various experiences of pain; and [4] stress urinary incontinence. There is considerable overlap between these symptoms [1] so that diagnostic categorisation is difficult. Whatever the symptom mix, the exclusion of urinary tract infection (UTI) is a mandatory first step in the assessment of all LUTS [2]. Whilst acute UTI is not diagnostically challenging, in the case of LUTS without acute frequency and dysuria, exclusion of infection poses a diagnostic challenge.

There are good reasons to scrutinise urinary adenosine-5′-triphosphate (ATP) as a possible surrogate marker of UTI since the reliability of popular diagnostic methods used to exclude UTI have been questioned [3-6]. Published guidelines across Europe, USA and the UK reveal significant discrepancies in the choice of a quantitative threshold used to define significant bacteriuria. The clean-catch, midstream urine (MSU) sample culture in the UK and Europe commonly uses the Kass (1957) [7] criterion

* Correspondence: kiren.gill@ucl.ac.uk
[1]Division of Medicine, University College London, Archway Campus, London, UK
[4]Research Department of Clinical Medicine, Division of Medicine, University College London, Wolfson House, 2 – 10 Stephenson Way, NW1 2HE London, UK
Full list of author information is available at the end of the article

of $10^5$ colony forming units (cfu) $ml^{-1}$ of a single species of a known urinary pathogen. Kass drew these data from 74 women with acute pyelonephritis and 337 normal controls, a select sample unrepresentative of wider lower urinary tract symptoms (LUTS). Despite its limitations, this criterion has become a ubiquitous reference standard and has been challenged by several groups [6,8]. The European Associate of Urology (EUA) guidelines for urological infections emphasise that no single threshold can be applied in all clinical situations. The urinary dipstick tests for nitrite and leucocyte esterase are also commonly used as a bedside screening test for infection and as a measure of a positive urine culture. However the use of urinary dipstick have been validated against the urine culture to a threshold of $10^5$ colony forming units (cfu) $ml^{-1}$ and given the recent criticism of the Kass criterion, urinary dipstick have also recently been found to be unreliable [3,4,9].

Urinary tract ATP has attracted intense interest in the last 30 years for its pharmacological and pathophysiological associations. There are great hopes that purinergic receptor manipulation might influence detrusor motor function and urothelial afferents [10], achieving therapeutic benefit. ATP is an important urothelial cell distress signal [11] and is released by inflammatory cells and bacteria [12]. Urinary tract infection featuring bacterial invasion, urothelial distress and an innate immune response involving recruitment of inflammatory cells, should be associated with increased urinary ATP levels. Indeed, high levels of ATP have been detected in the urine of patients with interstitial cystitis and acute UTI with a positive urine culture [13]. Increased ATP has also been shown to be released from cultured urothelial cells infected with uropathogenic *E.coli* (UPEC) [14], and UPEC also produce ATP when cultured *in vitro* [15]. It has been postulated that ATP may reflect microbial biomass and hence ATP increases as the amount of bacteria present increases. Currently ATP levels are used widely in the food, water and sanitation industry as a measure of bacterial contamination [16].

Given the problems with current tests [3], developing alternative diagnostic assays is a high priority. We therefore sought to scrutinise the performance of urinary ATP to test for potential as a surrogate measure of inflammation and infection when assessing patients with chronic LUTS. The experiment was divided into two parts; [1] a clinical experiment that evaluated urinary ATP in patients with LUTS and controls, comparing urinary ATP with symptoms, microscopic pyuria and urine culture results; and [2] a laboratory experimental series that explored the factors that could influence sample collection, storage and preservation. As urine contains native ATPase activity, the time-decay curve of urinary ATP from collection to processing was evaluated. Boric acid crystals, which

are commonly used as a urinary preservative, have been shown to prevent microbial swarming [17] and boric acid has a preservative influence on white cells [18]. We therefore studied the effects of the use of urinary preservative boric acid, storage temperature and the effect of centrifugation on urinary ATP concentration.

## Methods
### Ethical approval
Ethical committee approval for this study, including all study documentation, was obtained from the Whittington and Moorefields Research Ethics Committee. All study participants gave informed written consent to participate in the study and the process was documented as per Good Clinical Practice (GCP) and MHRA guidelines. The participants were assigned randomly generated study numbers which were used to anonymise all data and samples, and analysis was carried out by blinded researchers.

### Patients and symptom collection
Adult patients presenting with lower urinary tract symptoms were recruited from incontinence clinics from October 2009 to October 2012 and informed consent obtained. We compared urine samples from 75 healthy controls and 340 patients presenting with LUTS. The demographic data can be seen in Table 1. The control group consisted of 49 females and 26 males, with mean age 38.2 yrs (95% CI 34.5 - 41.8). Within the LUTS group there were 314 females and 26 males, with a mean age of 58.6 yrs (95% CI 56.8 - 60.4). All patients completed detailed validated LUTS questionnaires covering 38 symptoms, including frequency, nocturia, urgency, incontinence episodes, symptoms relating to storage function, voiding problems, stress urinary incontinence and pain, which were recorded on a bespoke clinical database. Control subjects completed questionnaires thereby confirming absence of symptoms. There are popular, validated symptom scores such as the ICIQ series [19] which are suitable as intervention outcome measures because changes in individual scores can be normalised for group comparisons. However, adjectival scaling such as 'bother', when deployed in cross-sectional, descriptive work, is vulnerable to semantic interpretation differences, and considerable error may occur [20]. To avoid this, we used validated scales that measure symptoms dichotomously and achieve scaling by counting the contexts in which symptoms occur. These are effective measures for cross-sectional observation studies [21-23].

### Midstream urine (MSU) collection
Samples were obtained by the midstream clean-catch method. Patients were given detailed instruction on how to collect a meticulous midstream urine sample and avoid perineal contamination. This included use of an antiseptic wipe to clean the genital area prior to voiding and use of a

**Table 1 Demographic data**

| | Controls | | | | LUTS patients | | | |
|---|---|---|---|---|---|---|---|---|
| Gender male | N = 26 | | | | N = 26 | | | |
| Gender female | N = 49 | | | | N = 314 | | | |
| No pyuria | N = 58 (female = 35, male = 23) | | | | N = 100 (female = 92, male = 8) | | | |
| Any pyuria | N = 17 (female = 14, male = 3) | | | | N = 240 (female = 222, male = 18) | | | |
| | **Mean** | | **Std deviation (sd)** | | **Mean** | | **Std deviation (sd)** | |
| Age (years) | 38.2 | | 15.8 | | 58.6 | | 16.6 | |
| | **Mean** | **Median** | **sd** | **Quartile range** | **Mean** | **Median** | **sd** | **Quartile range** |
| 24 hour frequency | 6.2 | 6.2 | 6.0 to 7.0 | 6.0 to 7.0 | 9.2 | 8.0 | 8.0 to 10.0 | 6.0 to 11.0 |
| 24 hour incontinence | 0 | 0 | 0.0 to 0.0 | 0.0 to 0.0 | 0.8 | 0.5 | 0.5 to 1.2 | 0.0 to 1.0 |
| Number of urgency symptoms | 0 | 0 | 0.0 to 0.0 | 0.0 to 0.0 | 2.8 | 2.0 | 2.0 to 3.6 | 0.0 to 4.0 |
| Number of pain symptoms | 0 | 0 | 0.0 to 0.0 | 0.0 to 0.0 | 0.4 | 0.0 | 0.2 to 0.6 | 0.0 to 0.0 |
| Number of stress inc symptoms | 0 | 0 | 0.0 to 0.0 | 0.0 to 0.0 | 0.3 | 0.0 | 0.08 to 0.5 | 0.0 to 0.0 |
| Number of voiding symptoms | 0 | 0 | 0.0 to 0.0 | 0.0 to 0.0 | 1.4 | 0.0 | 1.0 to 1.8 | 0.0 to 2.0 |
| Number of LUTS | 0 | 0 | 0.0 to 0.0 | 0.0 to 0.0 | 5.0 | 3.5 | 4.0 to 6.0 | 1.0 to 6.0 |

sterile large flexible container introduced to collect the urine mid-flow and removed before completion of voiding.

### Routine urine culture

The urine was cultured using the Kass [7] threshold for significance which is the standard method of analysis in UK-NHS practice. A 1 μl loop of urine was plated on a chromogenic agar plate and incubated at 37°C for 24 hours. Cultures were reported as positive if there was bacterial growth of a single urinary pathogen of greater than $10^5$ cfu ml$^{-1}$, negative bacterial growth if less than $10^5$ cfu ml$^{-1}$ and reported as mixed growth if there was more than one uropathogen with total growth greater than $10^5$ cfu ml$^{-1}$. Although $10^5$ cfu ml$^{-1}$ threshold is known to be inadequate [6,3,24], we included it in this study because it such a ubiquitous gold standard.

### Microscopic leucocyte count

A fresh aliquot of urine was examined by microscopy. 10 μl of urine was loaded into a Neubauer haemocytometer counting chamber [25] and examined by light microscopy (magnification x200) for leucocytes.

### Blinding

Microscopy and ATP analysis were performed by researchers blinded to the details or symptoms of the participants. Samples presented for analysis were identified only by a randomly generated four-digit study number.

### ATP analysis

Samples were processed using Sigma-Aldrich Adenosine 5′-triphosphate (ATP) Bioluminescent Assay Kit, at an approximate cost of £250, which is able to detect concentrations of $2 \times 10^{-12}$ to $8 \times 10^{-5}$ mol/L. Urine samples stored at -80°C and -20°C were thawed in a water bath in room temperature (23°C) and processed according to the manufacturer's instructions. Reagents were prepared as per the manufacturer's recommendation with measures included to prevent degradation. The standard assay kit (SigmaAldrich; Missouri, USA) applied a bioluminescent reaction involving the breakdown of luciferin by luciferase, which requires ATP. The average luminescence recorded, in relative light units (RLU), was proportional to the concentration of ATP. This was converted to ATP moles ml$^{-1}$ using a standard curve.

### Evaluation of the effect of time on urinary ATP

Urine samples used to assess stability of ATP over time were stored at room temperature (23°C). Aliquots were taken at 0 hours (immediately), 12 hours, 24 hours, 48 hours, 168 hours and frozen at -80°C.

### Evaluation of the effect of storage temperature on urinary ATP

The literature tends to recommend storage at -80°C; however, this is not convenient for many clinical services. The effects of freezing at -80°C and -20°C were therefore studied. 2 ml aliquots of fresh urine were taken from each participant. One aliquot was frozen immediately after microscopy and stored at -80°C and another at -20°C.

### Evaluation of the use of boric acid preservative on urinary ATP

We studied the effects of boric acid preservation on decay of urinary ATP. 10mls of urine was introduced into pre-prepared boric acid tubes (Becton Dickinson Vacutainer® C & S Preservative Urine Tubes for Culture and Sensitivity) and stored at room temperature. Aliquots were taken at

0 hours (immediately), 12 hours, 24 hours, 48 hours, 168 hours and frozen at -80°C.

### Evaluation of the effect of centrifugation on urinary ATP
Urinary ATP may originate from several sources including bacteria, urothelial cells and white cells. Therefore, we sought to discover whether centrifuging the urine alters the assay result, either by removing cells from the supernatant, or by lysing cells in the process [26]. An aliquot of urine was spun at 620 g for 5 minutes and the supernatant was frozen at -80°C.

All of the urine aliquots for the clinical experiments were frozen immediately at -80°C. These samples were processed for urinary ATP between eight to twelve weeks after collection and storage. The frozen urine aliquots were thawed to room temperature (23°C) using a water bath and then immediately analysed using the standard luciferin-luciferase assay and protocol, which was described earlier.

### Statistics
We used multivariate linear regression analyses to scrutinise the $log_{10}$ ATP as the response variable using two models. In the first, the explanatory variables were gender (0 = female, 1 = male); age; average 24-hour frequency; average 24-hour incontinence; number of stress incontinence symptoms, pain symptoms, voiding symptoms and OAB symptoms; the presence or absence of any pyuria (0 = none, 1 = any pyuria); and the MSU culture result (0 = negative, 1 = positive). In the second model we looked more closely at the effect of the degree of pyuria. Pyuria was grouped as zero pyuria, pyuria 1-9 or pyuria $\geq$10, subgroups which are currently used by most clinicians, and these were referenced to control samples. The sample had 83% power to detect a .04 increment in $R^2$ if ten predictor variables were included in the regression model with alpha = 0.05. In the laboratory experimental series, paired data was collected and hence we used different statistical analysis methods to the clinical experiment. We used the paired t-test to analyse the difference in $log_{10}$ ATP between paired samples stored at -20°C and -80°C; paired samples stored with and without boric acid; and paired samples centrifuged or uncentrifuged. The diagnostic potential of urinary $log_{10}$ ATP was assessed by ROC plots using Positive MSU at $10^5$ cfu ml$^{-1}$ of a pure isolate of a known urinary pathogen; pyuria $\geq$ 10 wbc $\mu l^{-1}$ and pyuria > 0 wbc $\mu l^{-1}$.

### Results
We compared urine samples from 75 healthy controls and 340 patients presenting with LUTS. The demographic data can be seen in Table 1. The patients cohort was grouped in the first model; with pyuria ($\geq$1 wbc $\mu l^{-1}$) or without pyuria (0 wbc $\mu l^{-1}$). For the second model we

used categorical scaling so that we compared pyuria 1-9 wbc $\mu l^{-1}$ (n = 120) and pyuria $\geq$10 wbc $\mu l^{-1}$ (n = 120) with a baseline factor of zero pyuria (0 wbc $\mu l^{-1}$). Of those with LUTS, 33.3% had only OAB symptoms, 4.1% had pain alone, 3.7% had only stress incontinence and 13.2% had only voiding dysfunction. Patients had a median of 3.5 LUTS (quartile range 1 to 6). The overlap of symptoms is illustrated in Figure 1.

$Log_{10}$ transformation of ATP changed the skewness from 4.2 to -0.3 and kurtosis from 27.5 to 1.1. The results of the two regression analyses are shown in Table 2. It can be seen that female gender was associated with higher predictions of the $log_{10}$ ATP. However given the small number of males and predominance of female patients, which is a reflection of this condition, limited discriminatory power precludes extrapolation. Voiding symptoms were also predictive of higher $log_{10}$ ATP. Interestingly, voiding symptoms in both sexes have been reported to be associated with inflammatory disease of the lower urinary tract [22]. A positive culture result predicted lower $log_{10}$ ATP. The first regression model shows that the presence of any pyuria was not predictive of higher $log_{10}$ ATP. The second regression model demonstrates that a pyuria $\geq$10 wbc $\mu l^{-1}$ was predictive of a higher $log_{10}$ ATP; however, lower levels of pyuria 1-9 wbc $\mu l^{-1}$ were not. These data do demonstrate that urinary ATP is elevated in association with inflammation but that urinary ATP lacks the discriminating properties at lower levels of pyuria, which are necessary for a useful clinical surrogate marker. This is illustrated by the ROC analysis which showed an area under the curve of 0.6 for a positive culture; 0.5 for pyuria > 0 wbc $\mu l^{-1}$ and 0.6 for pyuria $\geq$ 10 wbc $\mu l^{-1}$ (Figure 2). These data imply that there is no useful diagnostic role for this assay. The regression analyses showed that, age, average 24-hour frequency, average 24-hour incontinence, the number of urgency, stress incontinence, and pain symptoms provided no substantial explanation of the variance of urinary $log_{10}$ ATP.

### Urinary ATP decay over time
A subgroup of 20, randomly selected patient samples was used to plot the urinary ATP concentration in samples at differing time points after collection; 0 hours, 12 hours, 24 hours, 48 hours, 168 hours. Aliquots were taken at each point and frozen at -80°C and stored for assays in batches. The ATP concentration fell with time with the rate of decline very dependent on the initial concentration, as illustrated in Figure 3, where the time course of each sample is plotted.

### Urinary ATP and effect of storage with boric acid preservative
Figure 4 shows box plots of the $log_{10}$ ATP concentration at each time point comparing the effect of boric acid.

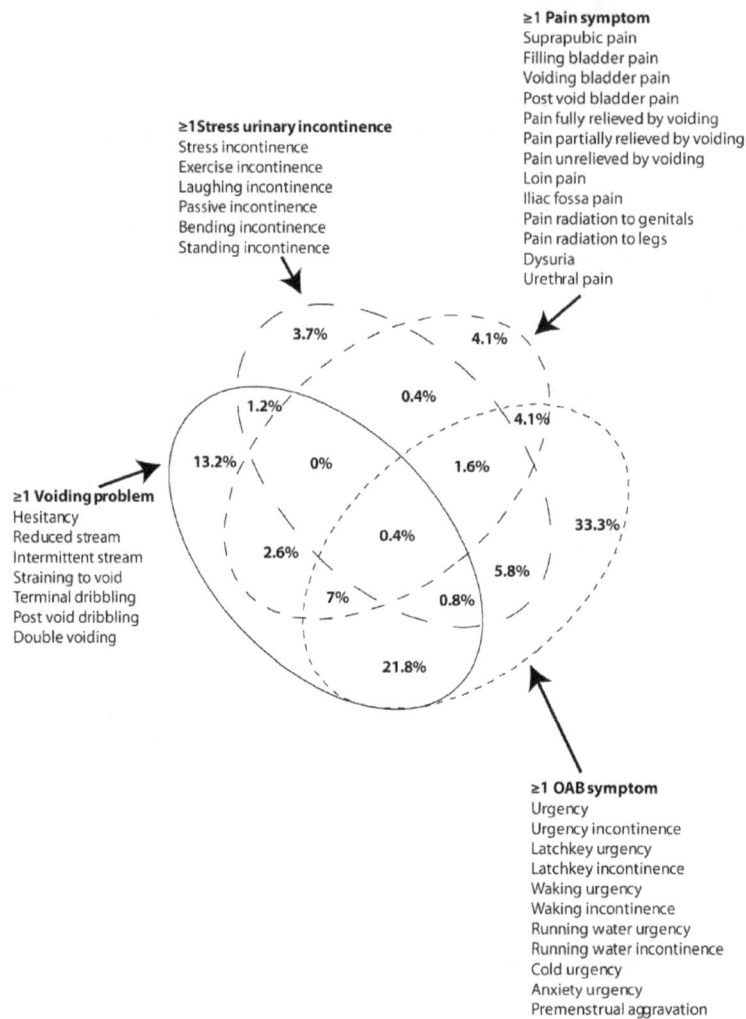

**Figure 1 Venn diagram of symptom analysis.** A four-way Venn diagram illustrating the overlap of symptom amongst the patients studied. The ellipses circumscribe patients who had one or more symptoms in the particular subset. The diagram is not scaled to the size of sets.

An analysis of 20 paired samples at 24-hours demonstrated the significance of this difference: mean $\log_{10}$ ATP (moles) in samples stored without boric acid was -6.3 $\log_{10}$ moles and in samples stored at with boric acid was -6.5 $\log_{10}$ moles (95% CI difference 0.15 to 0.29, t = 6.2, p < .001). (*Put significance at end of paragraph as you did for the following paragraphs*) These data show that boric acid caused loss of ATP.

### Urinary ATP and effect of storage temperature
Comparison of 30 paired samples of urine stored at -20°C and -80°C showed no significant difference in ATP concentration: mean $\log_{10}$ ATP (moles) in samples stored at -20°C was -6.7 $\log_{10}$ moles and in samples stored at -80°C was -6.8 $\log_{10}$ moles (95% CI difference -0.09 to +0.01, t = -1.7, p = .1). Thus storage at -20°C for 8 weeks would seem reasonable.

### Urinary ATP and effect of centrifugation
Comparison of 30 paired samples of urine unspun and spun showed that the supernatant urine had a slightly lower level of ATP: mean $\log_{10}$ ATP (moles $ml^{-1}$) in uncentrifuged samples = -6.9 $\log_{10}$ moles and in the supernatant after centrifuge mean = -6.8 $\log_{10}$ moles (95% CI difference 0.03 to 0.1, t = 3.5, p = .002). Whilst statistically different, this is a very small difference and of little clinical significance.

### Discussion
ATP has been proposed as a potential clinical marker of infection for both acute and chronic LUTS [10,27]. To avoid premature use, when assessing the diagnostic potential of test, it is important to assess first whether the measure explains the symptoms and other manifestations of the disease of interest [28]. The data published

**Table 2 Output from regression analysis**

Model 1 pyuria described by dichotomy

| | B coefficient | p | 95% confidence interval for B | |
| | | | Lower bound | Upper bound |
| --- | --- | --- | --- | --- |
| (Constant) | -8.026 | .000 | -8.400 | -7.652 |
| Age | .004 | .197 | -.002 | .009 |
| **Gender 0 = female, 1 = male** | **-.537** | **.001** | **-.865** | **-.209** |
| **MSU 0 = negative 1 = positive** | **-.346** | **.004** | **-.582** | **-.110** |
| Average 24-hour frequency | -.004 | .743 | -.026 | .019 |
| Average 24-hour incontinence | -.001 | .990 | -.092 | .090 |
| Number of stress incontinence symptoms | -.065 | .179 | -.161 | .030 |
| **Number of voiding symptoms** | **.124** | **.000** | **.061** | **.187** |
| Number of pain symptoms | .082 | .382 | -.103 | .267 |
| Number of urgency symptoms | -.030 | .163 | -.072 | .012 |
| Pyuria 0 = none 1 = any | .157 | .107 | -.034 | .349 |

Model 2 pyuria described by ordinal scale

| | B coefficient | p | 95% confidence interval for B | |
| | | | Lower bound | Upper bound |
| --- | --- | --- | --- | --- |
| (Constant) | -8.058 | .000 | -8.431 | -7.685 |
| Age | .002 | .404 | -.003 | .008 |
| **Gender 0 = female, 1 = male** | **-.522** | **.002** | **-.845** | **-.199** |
| **MSU 0 = negative 1 = positive** | **-.406** | **.001** | **-.642** | **-.171** |
| Average 24-hour frequency | -.002 | .878 | -.024 | .021 |
| Average 24-hour incontinence | -.024 | .607 | -.114 | .067 |
| Number of stress incontinence symptoms | -.060 | .210 | -.154 | .034 |
| **Number of voiding symptoms** | **.106** | **.001** | **.043** | **.169** |
| Number of pain symptoms | .085 | .356 | -.096 | .266 |
| Number of urgency symptoms | -.024 | .257 | -.066 | .018 |
| Pyuria1 to 9 wbc $\mu l^{-1}$ | .207 | .059 | -.008 | .422 |
| **Pyuria $\geq$ 10 wbc $\mu l^{-1}$** | **.432** | **.000** | **.203** | **.662** |

Dependent variable is urinary $\log_{10}$ ATP concentration

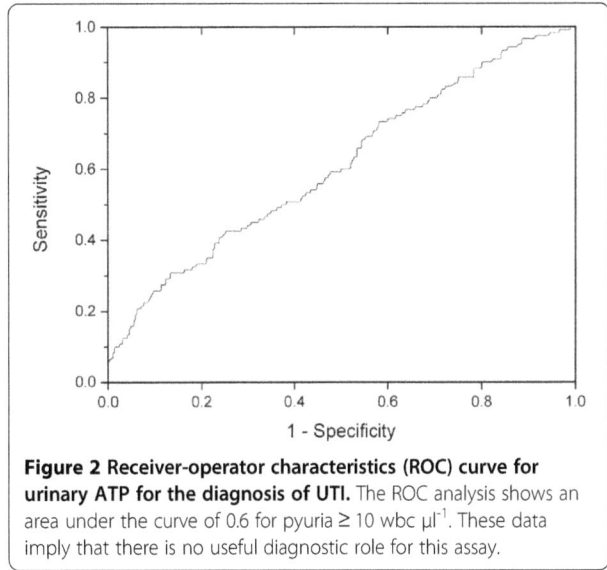

**Figure 2** Receiver-operator characteristics (ROC) curve for urinary ATP for the diagnosis of UTI. The ROC analysis shows an area under the curve of 0.6 for pyuria $\geq$ 10 wbc $\mu l^{-1}$. These data imply that there is no useful diagnostic role for this assay.

ATP. However, this signal was not a discriminating marker for low levels of lower urinary tract inflammation (pyuria 1-9 wbc $\mu l^{-1}$) as shown by our second regression model, and it is in these clinical circumstances that there is greatest need for novel clinical surrogate markers. It has been shown that low-level pyuria [26], voiding symptoms [22], overactive bladder symptoms [24] and pain symptoms [23] all correlate with urinary infection. Only voiding symptoms explained a small amount of the variance in ATP. These findings are therefore discouraging.

Counter-intuitively, urinary ATP was lower, given a positive urine culture. This unexpected result may reflect

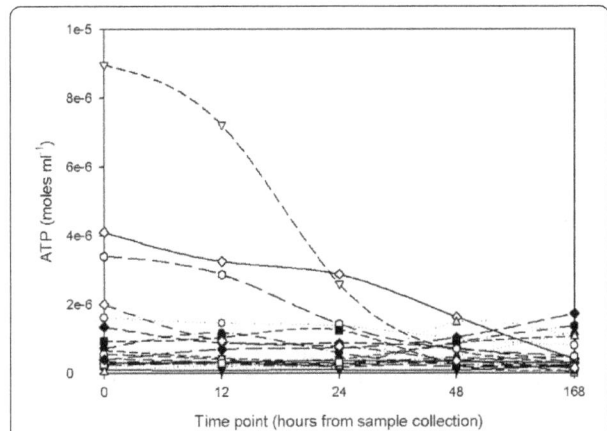

**Figure 3 The ATP decay curves for a subset of 20 urine samples.** The rate of decay is substrate concentration dependent; such that a sample with a higher ATP concentration shows a more marked decay. It is therefore important to assay or freeze immediately after collection of the urine specimen to preserve the ATP signal.

here demonstrate that urinary ATP does not offer any additional benefit to tests currently used in screening for infection in patients presenting with LUTS, and therefore does not show promise for future development of a diagnostic test for this particular group. This observation is confirmed in the ROC curves that explore sensitivity and specificity properties.

Our results demonstrate that patients with LUTS and any pyuria do not manifest a significantly raised urine ATP concentration. It is only when there is pyuria of greater than 10 wbc $\mu l^{-1}$, which is a currently used marker of urinary infection, that there is a significantly raised urinary

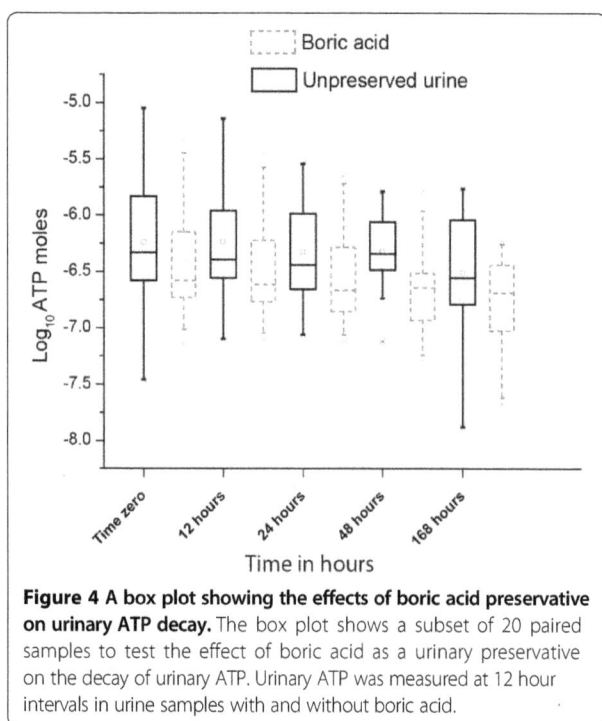

**Figure 4 A box plot showing the effects of boric acid preservative on urinary ATP decay.** The box plot shows a subset of 20 paired samples to test the effect of boric acid as a urinary preservative on the decay of urinary ATP. Urinary ATP was measured at 12 hour intervals in urine samples with and without boric acid.

the fact that there were so few positive cultures (16.9%) that there weren't enough data to draw meaningful conclusions. Increased microbial dephosphorylation of ATP to adenosine, which we did not assay, may also be a contributing factor. In addition, the urinary ATP reflects the urinary microbial biomass directly post void and there may be significant variation in the urinary biomass at the time of culture secondary to transportation and processing delay.

There was an unbalanced sample size with fewer control participants with a lower average age, and this reflects the common difficulty of finding older subjects without any urinary tract symptoms. The controls in this experiment were all asymptomatic. We did control for these differences in the analysis but would nevertheless wish to avoid wide inferential generalisations. The essence of this study was to scrutinise the discriminating properties amongst patients. The recruitment field was also predominantly female which may explain the gender difference. The small numbers of males were nevertheless included in the analysis as the model was sufficiently powered for this variable, which required ≥20 for each independent variable. The sample was powerful enough to detect the influence of voiding symptoms, pyuria and culture, despite the wide variance. Urinary ATP concentrations proved independent of age and the number and nature of LUTS symptoms, other than voiding symptoms. The association with voiding symptoms was not surprising because in patients with chronic LUTS,

these have been reported to be correlated with pyuria in both genders, in clear contrast to OAB and pain symptoms [22].

We found that urinary ATP could not pick out low levels of inflammation (pyuria 1-9 wbc $\mu l^{-1}$) when used alone, a situation where clinicians need most help. Current dipstick methods and direct urinary microscopy are able to identify pyuria when it is abundant [26], so urinary ATP would offer no additional advantage. There can be little doubt that ATP plays a very significant role in the pathophysiology of urinary tract disease [29,30] but it would seem that this does not translate into a useful role as a clinical test when used alone.

The laboratory experimental series showed that urine samples should be processed immediately or frozen and stored at below -20°C. We demonstrated significant urinary ATP decay with time when samples were left at room temperature, with the rate being substrate dependent. We also found that storage of urine at -20°C is adequate and this therefore allows for wider use of standard freezers as opposed to the specialised -80°C devices. The centrifuge studies examined the effect of the removing cellular material. The supernatant showed marginally lower levels of ATP. This could be attributed to increased ATPase activity from burst cells or it may have resulted from delayed freezing, allowing additional time for enzyme activity. Additionally, centrifugation results in the removal of biomass and hence this may explain the lower levels of urinary ATP. This marginal difference, though statistically significant, may not be clinically significant; nevertheless, centrifuging of urine prior to freezing or analysis is an additional labour worth avoiding. Boric acid proved counterproductive and so should not be used as a preservative.

**Conclusion**

In summary these data discourage the idea that urinary ATP should be developed as a clinical surrogate test for UTI in patients presenting with LUTS. This assay does not appear more effective than markers used in current clinical practice [3,26]. However, abundant urinary ATP is certainly evident amongst patients with lower urinary tract symptoms and dysfunction and these data do encourage continued interest in the pharmacology and pathophysiology of purinergic functions in the bladder. For those committed to these avenues of discovery, we provide valuable data on human sample processing, storage and assay.

In conclusion, urinary ATP does not improve on the use of microscopy as a surrogate marker of urinary tract infection in patients presenting with LUTS and is therefore not a promising clinical diagnostic marker. We need to continue to explore other potential markers that can be used to screen LUTS patients for UTI, particularly applicable to those that have lower levels of pyuria, where significant disease may currently be overlooked [26]. The relevance of measuring ATP to study the pathophysiology of the lower urinary tract is still very evident and in that context urine is a useful biological sample.

## Abbreviations
ATP: Adenosine-5'-triphosphate; CFU: Colony forming units; LUTS: Lower urinary tract symptoms; MSU: Midstream urine; UPEC: Uropathogenic E. coli; UTI: Urinary tract infection.

## Competing interests
The authors declare that they have no competing interests.

## Authors' contributions
Authors KG, HH, SS, AK, RK, JH and JML have made substantial contributions to the conception and design of this experiment, acquisition of data including microscopy, urine culture and carrying out ATP assays, drafting and revising the manuscript. Authors KG, GB, MDI and JML have made substantial contributions to the analysis and interpretation of the data, drafting and revising the manuscript. All authors read and approved the final manuscript.

## Acknowledgements
The authors would like to thank Miss L Brackenridge, Miss L Collins, and Dr S Swamy for their help with recruitment. In addition the authors would like to thank Mr T Brenton, Miss C Jones, Miss L Chung and Miss A Jeykumar for their help with sample collection and processing.

## Author details
[1]Division of Medicine, University College London, Archway Campus, London, UK. [2]Department of Statistics, University College London, London, UK. [3]Medway School of Pharmacy, The Universities of Kent and Greenwich at Medway, Chatham, Kent, UK. [4]Research Department of Clinical Medicine, Division of Medicine, University College London, Wolfson House, 2 – 10 Stephenson Way, NW1 2HE London, UK.

## References
1. Coyne KS, Sexton CC, Thompson CL, Milsom I, Irwin D, Kopp ZS, et al. The prevalence of lower urinary tract symptoms (LUTS) in the USA, the UK and Sweden: results from the Epidemiology of LUTS (EpiLUTS) study. B J UInt. 2009;104(3):352–60.
2. Staskin D, Kelleher C, Bosch R, Cotterill N, Emmanuel A, Yoshida M, et al. Initial Assessment of Urinary and Faecal Incontinence in Adult Male and Female Patients. In: Abrams P, Cardozo L, Khoury S, Wein A, editors. 4th International Conusltation on Incontinence. International Conusltation on Incontinence, vol. 1. Paris: Health Publications Ltd; 2009. p. 333–62.
3. Khasriya R, Khan S, Lunawat R, Bishara S, Bignal J, Malone-Lee M, et al. The Inadequacy of Urinary Dipstick and Microscopy as Surrogate Markers of Urinary Tract Infection in Urological Outpatients With Lower Urinary Tract Symptoms Without Acute Frequency and Dysuria. J Urol. 2010;183(5):1843–7.
4. Deville WL, Yzermans JC, van Duijn NP, Bezemer PD, van der Windt DA, Bouter LM. The urine dipstick test useful to rule out infections. A meta-analysis of the accuracy. BMC Urol. 2004;4:4.
5. Gorelick MH, Shaw KN. Screening tests for urinary tract infection in children: A meta-analysis. Pediatrics. 1999;104(5):e54.
6. Stamm WE, Counts GW, Running KR, Fihn S, Turck M, Holmes KK. Diagnosis of coliform infection in acutely dysuric women. N Engl J Med. 1982;307(8):463–8.
7. Kass EH. Bacteriuria and the diagnosis of infection in the urinary tract. Arch Intern Med. 1957;100:709–14.
8. Siegman-Igra Y. The significance of urine culture with mixed flora. Curr Opin Nephrol Hypertens. 1994;3(6):656–9. PubMed PMID: 7881993. Epub 1994/11/01. eng.
9. Hurlbut 3rd TA, Littenberg B. The diagnostic accuracy of rapid dipstick tests to predict urinary tract infection. Am J Clin Pathol. 1991;96(5):582–8. PubMed PMID: 1951183. Epub 1991/11/01. eng.
10. Burnstock G. Therapeutic potential of purinergic signalling for diseases of the urinary tract. BJU Int. 2011;107(2):192–204. PubMed PMID: 21208364.

11. Van der Wijk T, De Jonge HR, Tilly BC. Osmotic cell swelling-induced ATP release mediates the activation of extracellular signal-regulated protein kinase (Erk)-1/2 but not the activation of osmo-sensitive anion channels. Biochem J. 1999;343(Pt 3):579–86. PubMed PMID: 10527936. Pubmed Central PMCID: 1220589. Epub 1999/10/21. eng.
12. van der Weyden L, Conigrave AD, Morris MB. Signal transduction and white cell maturation via extracellular ATP and the P2Y11 receptor. Immunol Cell Biol. 2000;78(4):369–74. PubMed PMID: 10947861. Epub 2000/08/18. eng.
13. Lundin A, Hallander H, Kallner A, Lundin UK, Osterberg E. Bacteriuria testing by the ATP method as an integral part in the diagnosis and therapy of urinary tract infection (UTI). J Biolumin Chemilumin. 1989;4(1):381–9. PubMed PMID: 2801224, Epub 1989/07/01. eng.
14. Save S, Persson K. Extracellular ATP and P2Y receptor activation induce a proinflammatory host response in the human urinary tract. Infect Immun. 2010;78(8):3609–15.
15. Hanberger H, Nilsson LE, Kihlstrom E, Maller R. Postantibiotic effect of beta-lactam antibiotics on Escherichia coli evaluated by bioluminescence assay of bacterial ATP. Antimicrob Agents Chemother. 1990;34(1):102–6. PubMed PMID: 2183707, Pubmed Central PMCID: 171528. Epub 1990/01/01. eng.
16. Poulis JA, de Pijper M, Mossel DA, Dekkers PP. Assessment of cleaning and disinfection in the food industry with the rapid ATP-bioluminescence technique combined with the tissue fluid contamination test and a conventional microbiological method. Int J Food Microbiol. 1993;20(2):109–16. PubMed PMID: 8268054. Epub 1993/11/01. eng.
17. Meers PD, Chow CK. Bacteriostatic and bactericidal actions of boric acid against bacteria and fungi commonly found in urine. J Clin Pathol. 1990;43(6):484–7.
18. Khan S, Chandhyoke N, Bishara S, Mahmood W, Khasriya RK, Lunawat R, et al. The Preservation of Pyuria in Urine Samples with Boric Acid. Int Urogynecol J. 2009;20:S132–S3.
19. Avery K, Donovan J, Peters TJ, Shaw C, Gotoh M, Abrams P. ICIQ: a brief and robust measure for evaluating the symptoms and impact of urinary incontinence. Neurourol Urodyn. 2004;23(4):322–30.
20. Heuer RJ. Center for the Study of Intelligence (U.S.). Psychology of intelligence analysis. New York: Novinka Books; 2006. xii, 216 p. p.
21. Al Buheissi S, Khasriya R, Maraj BH, Malone-Lee J. A simple validated scale to measure urgency. J Urol. 2008;179(3):1000–5.
22. Gill K, Kupelian A, Brackenridge L, Horsley H, Sathiananthamoorthy S, Malone-Lee J. Surprising symptoms indicating urinary tract infection. International Continence Society Meeting 2011. Glasgow: International Continence Society; 2011.
23. Kupelian A, Chaliha C, Gill K, Brackenridge L, Horsley H, Malone-Lee J. Pain symptoms as part of the OAB complex. Int Urogynecol J. 2009;22 Suppl 1:189–90.
24. Khasriya R, Sathiananthamoorthy S, Ismail S, Kelsey M, Wilson M, Rohn JL, et al. Spectrum of bacterial colonization associated with urothelial cells from patients with chronic lower urinary tract symptoms. J Clin Microbiol. 2013;51(7):2054–62.
25. McGinley M, Wong LL, McBride JH, Rodgerson DO. Comparison of various methods for the enumeration of blood cells in urine. J Clin Lab Anal. 1992;6(6):359–61.
26. Kupelian AS, Horsley H, Khasriya R, Amussah RT, Badiani R, Courtney AM, et al. Discrediting microscopic pyuria and leucocyte esterase as diagnostic surrogates for infection in patients with lower urinary tract symptoms: results from a clinical and laboratory evaluation. BJU International. 2013;112(2):231–8.
27. Osterberg E, Hallander HO, Kallner A, Lundin A, Aberg H. Evaluation of the adenosine triphosphate test in the diagnosis of urinary tract infection. European journal of clinical microbiology & infectious diseases: official publication of the European Society of Clinical Microbiology. 1991. Feb;10(2):70-3. PubMed PMID: 1864277.
28. Crawford ED, Rove KO, Trabulsi EJ, Qian J, Drewnowska KP, Kaminetsky JC, et al. Diagnostic performance of PCA3 to detect prostate cancer in men with increased prostate specific antigen: a prospective study of 1,962 cases. J Urol. 2012;188(5):1726–31. PubMed PMID: 22998901.
29. Burnstock G, Cocks T, Kasakov L, Wong HK. Direct evidence for ATP release from non-adrenergic, non-cholinergic ("purinergic") nerves in the guinea-pig taenia coli and bladder. Eur J Pharmacol. 1978;49(2):145–9. PubMed PMID: 658131. Epub 1978/05/15. eng.

# 5

# A new surgical technique for concealed penis using an advanced musculocutaneous scrotal flap

Dong-Seok Han, Hoon Jang, Chang-Shik Youn and Seung-Mo Yuk*

## Abstract

**Background:** Until recently, no single, universally accepted surgical method has existed for all types of concealed penis repairs. We describe a new surgical technique for repairing concealed penis by using an advanced musculocutaneous scrotal flap.

**Methods:** From January 2010 to June 2014, we evaluated 12 patients (12–40 years old) with concealed penises who were surgically treated with an advanced musculocutaneous scrotal flap technique after degloving through a ventral approach. All the patients were scheduled for regular follow-up at 6, 12, and 24 weeks postoperatively. The satisfaction grade for penile size, morphology, and voiding status were evaluated using a questionnaire preoperatively and at all of the follow-ups. Information regarding complications was obtained during the postoperative hospital stay and at all follow-ups.

**Results:** The patients' satisfaction grades, which included the penile size, morphology, and voiding status, improved postoperatively compared to those preoperatively. All patients had penile lymphedema postoperatively; however, this disappeared within 6 weeks. There were no complications such as skin necrosis and contracture, voiding difficulty, or erectile dysfunction.

**Conclusions:** Our advanced musculocutaneous scrotal flap technique for concealed penis repair is technically easy and safe. In addition, it provides a good cosmetic appearance, functional outcomes and excellent postoperative satisfaction grades. Lastly, it seems applicable in any type of concealed penis, including cases in which the ventral skin defect is difficult to cover.

**Keywords:** Penis, Scrotum, Lymphedema

## Background

Concealed penis (CP) is a congenital abnormality in which the penis is concealed within the subcutaneous tissue [1]. Specifically, the penis appears to be fused to the scrotum, and the penile shaft is entrapped within the subcutaneous tissue.

CP can cause phimosis, balanitis, difficulties with hygiene and voiding, and embarrassment among peers. Since most cases of CP do not spontaneously resolve, surgical correction is recommended, except in cases where CP is secondary to excessive suprapubic or prepubic fat.

In the surgical correction of CP, covering the penile skin defect is a major challenge, but is also the most important part of the procedure. By performing the surgical procedure through a ventral approach, the ventral skin defect is created; therefore, any skin available for covering the ventral defect is deficient in most cases. Covering the ventral skin defect is dependent on the appearance of the penis and whether there is enough elongation without tension during penile erection. Sufficient coverage of the ventral skin defect results in successful, functional, and cosmetic outcomes.

Numerous surgical techniques for correcting CP have been described. However, until recently, no single, universally accepted surgical method has existed for all CP repairs. Occasionally, the skin defect cannot be covered following previous surgical intervention. Therefore, new surgical techniques are warranted to achieve better cosmetic and functional outcomes.

* Correspondence: doctor6@hanmail.net
The Catholic University of Korea, Daejeon Saint Mary's Hospital, 64, Daeheung-ro, Jung-gu, Daejeon 301-723, Republic of Korea

We discuss using the advanced musculocutaneous scrotal flap for covering the ventral skin defect in the correction of CP, and we evaluated the patients' surgical outcomes.

## Methods

### Subjects

From January 2010 to June 2014, we evaluated 12 cases of CPs that were surgically treated using the advanced musculocutaneous scrotal flap technique after degloving through a ventral approach.

During the preoperative examinations, all patients had the initial appearance of a short penis with a minimal penile shaft skin, and the normal penile shaft was palpated and visualized while applying pressure on both sides of the shaft base.

All patients enrolled in this study did not have appropriate penile skin coverage, according to the methodologies of Sugita et al. [2] and Kim et al. [3] Patients were scheduled for regular follow-up visits at 6, 12, and 24 weeks postoperatively. Data on patients' age, operative times, postoperative complications, and satisfaction were collected, and retrospective analysis was performed.

### Evaluation of patients' satisfaction and postoperative complications

We administered a questionnaire on penile size, morphology, and voiding status to evaluate the patients' satisfaction. The degree of satisfaction was determined on a scale of 1–5 using the following description: grade 1, very unsatisfactory; grade 2, unsatisfactory; grade 3, neither satisfactory nor unsatisfactory; grade 4, satisfactory; and grade 5, very satisfactory. The questionnaire was administered at all follow-ups. Information regarding the complications was obtained during the patients' postoperative hospital stay and at all follow-ups.

### Surgical technique

The patient was anesthetized using general endotracheal anesthesia and was positioned supine on the operating table. An incision was made along the ventral midline just proximal to the corona down to the penoscrotal junction in order to create a slit in the phimotic ring of the prepuce (Fig. 1a), and the glans were completely exposed. A diamond-shaped ventral skin defect was created (Fig. 1b), and a circumferential skin incision was made between each side of the diamond-shaped skin defect. Then the penile shaft was completely degloved. Dissection was performed proximally along the Buck's fascia frees the penis from its deep tetherings to the penile base. Subsequently, the penile shaft became elongated, and the ventral skin defect became increased (Fig. 1c). If it was not possible to cover the ventral skin defect using the redundant dorsal skin according to the

methodologies by Sugita et al. [2] and Kim et al., [3] we proceeded with the advanced musculocutaneous scrotal flap technique. We marked and incised two paramedian lines, which extended from the defect to the scrotum and two triangles with bases slightly shorter than the length of the defect (Fig. 1d). After excising both triangles, we mobilized the flap and advanced it over the defect. We confirmed that the skin defect was completely covered, and there was no tension in the suture lines (Fig. 1e).

The dermal tissue at the penopubic junction was sutured to Buck's fascia at the 11–1 o'clock position, and another dermal tissue flap at the penoscrotal junction was sutured to the fascia at the 5–7 o'clock position. Lastly, interrupted sutures with 5-zero polyglycolic acid were placed (Fig. 1f). No urethral catheter was left, and antibiotic ointment was applied with a dressing.

### Statistical analysis

All statistical analyses were performed using SPSS, version 20.0 for Windows (SPSS Inc., Chicago, IL, USA). The Friedman test was used to compare the changes between the pre- and postoperative satisfaction grades to the time after operation. A p-value <0.05 was considered statistically significant.

### Ethical statement

The study was approved by the Catholic Medical Center Office of Human Research Protection Program of the Catholic University of Korea (DC13OISI0083), and written informed consent was obtained from the patients for participation in this study. For participants aged 16 years, or younger, written consent was obtained for their parents or legal guardian. Written informed consent was also obtained from the patient (s) for publication of any accompanying images.

## Results

The mean age of the patients who underwent operation was 19.9 years (range, 12–40 years), and the mean follow-up period was 27.4 months (range, 10–46 months). The patients' satisfaction grades, including the penile size, morphology, and voiding status, were improved postoperatively compared to those preoperatively. These improvements became clearer after 6 weeks and lasted after 24 weeks of follow-up (Table 1).

All patients had penile lymphedema postoperatively (Fig. 1g); however, it disappeared within 6 weeks (Fig. 1h). Additionally, postoperative wound infection occurred in one patient, and it was resolved by performing daily sterile dressings and administering oral antibiotics for 2 weeks.

There were no complications such as skin necrosis, tissue contracture, voiding difficulty, or erectile dysfunction.

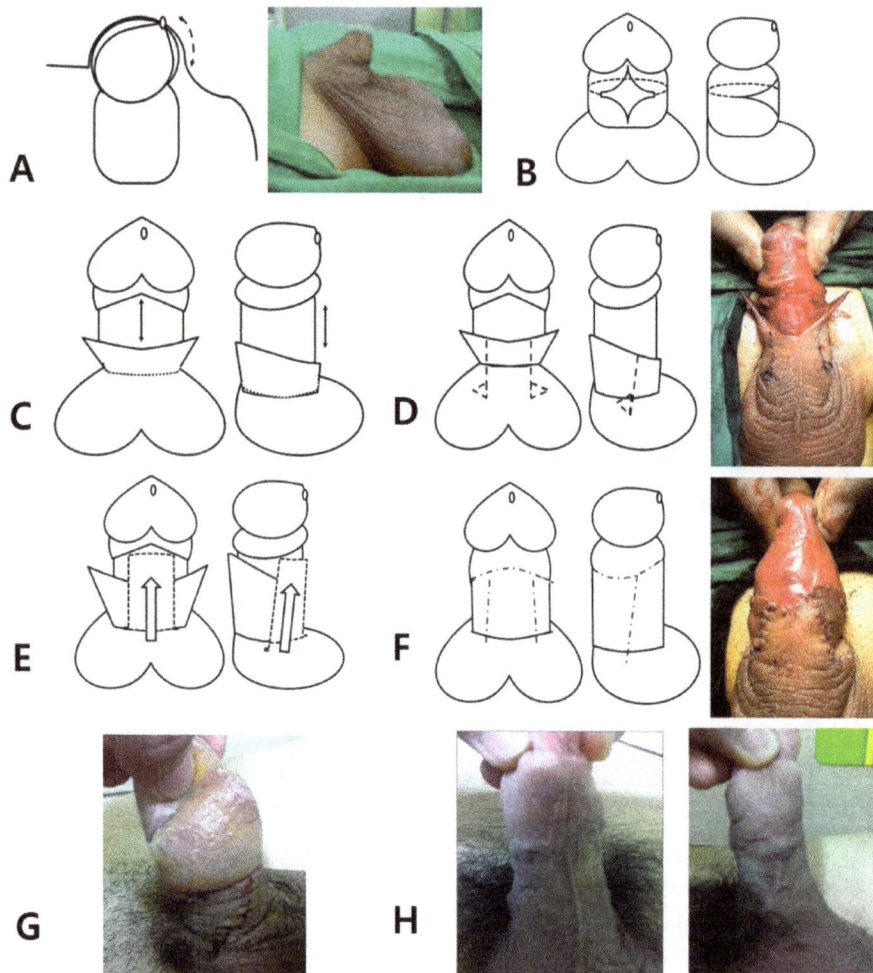

**Fig. 1** The advanced musculocutaneous scrotal flap technique procedures for correcting concealed penis: **a**) the ventral vertical incision (dotted line); **b**) the fully exposed glans, creation of the diamond-shaped skin defect, and an additional circumferential incision (dotted line); **c**) penile elongation with complete degloving; **d**) the paramedial vertical incision (dotted line) with triangles; **e**) scrotal flap advancement; **f**) the interrupted suture; **g**) postoperative lymphedema; and **h**) the final features of the penis. Written informed consent was also obtained from the patient (s) for publication of any accompanying images

In one patient, temporary discoloration developed on the distal end of the dorsal skin, which was not a part of the advanced musculocutaneous scrotal flap; however, this resolved spontaneously after 2 weeks.

## Discussion

CP results from a combination of deficient penile skin, poor attachment of the penile skin to the deeper layers at the base of the penis, dartos tethering, and sometimes excessive suprapubic fat [4]. It appears that a skin defect of the penile shaft is due to abnormal attachment of the dartos muscle to the corporal bodies during penile development. These abnormal fibromuscular attachments result in tethering of the penile shaft skin to the abdominal wall, which prevents normal skin development [4].

To correct CP, numerous surgical techniques have been described with various surgical outcomes. During

the surgical correction of CP, there are four important steps to follow: [5] 1) the penis must be mobilized/elongated by completely degloving it at its base; 2) the dermis and dartos fascia must be secured to the deeper fascia; 3) the penopubic and penoscrotal angles must be restored; and 4) the preputial skin must be re-established to provide skin cover. A deficiency in the penile shaft skin usually occurs because of lack of skin development.

In various surgical techniques for correcting CP, Wollin et al. [6] introduced a surgical method via a ventral approach in 1990. Among the surgical techniques using the ventral approach, the methodologies by Sugita et al. [2] and Kim et al. [3] are useful in correcting CP. The major difference between these method is which skin flap is used for the penile skin defect. In Sugita et al.'s method, the Byars flap is transpositioned using an

**Table 1** Patients' demographics, satisfaction grade, and surgical complications

| Mean age (years) | 19.86 ± 12.63 (range, 12–41) | | | | | |
|---|---|---|---|---|---|---|
| Operative time (mins) | 130.08 ± 3.54 | | | | | |
| Mean follow up (months) | 27.44 ± 12.63 | | | | | |
| | Patient satisfaction grade | | | | | |
| | Pre-OP | Post-Op | 6 weeks | 12 weeks | 24 weeks | p-value |
| Penile size | 1.42 ± 0.51 | 3.66 ± 0.49 | 4.75 ± 0.45 | 4.67 ± 0.49 | 4.75 ± 0.45 | 0.000 |
| Penile morphology | 1.33 ± 0.49 | 3.91 ± 0.29 | 4.67 ± 0.49 | 4.42 ± 0.51 | 4.41 ± 0.51 | 0.000 |
| Voiding status | 1.83 ± 0.72 | 4.00 ± 0.43 | 4.41 ± 0.52 | 4.45 ± 0.52 | 4.41 ± 0.51 | 0.000 |
| | Complications (n) | | | | | |
| | Post-Op | | 6 weeks | 12 weeks | 24 weeks | |
| Lymphedema | 12 | | 0 | 0 | 0 | |
| Skin necrosis | 0 | | 0 | 0 | 0 | |
| Tissue contracture | 0 | | 0 | 0 | 0 | |
| Wound infection | 1 | | 0 | 0 | 0 | |

Pre-op, preoperatively; Post-op, postoperatively

inverted T-shaped incision on the distal dorsal prepuce, which is used for covering the ventral skin defect. In Kim et al.'s method, the Byars flap is transpositioned using a longitudinal incision on the proximal dorsal prepuce, which is used for covering the ventral skin defect.

However, there is an important pre-condition in their surgical procedures. For functional and cosmetic success, it is imperative to have a sufficient length of the dorsal prepuce to cover the ventral skin defect, because the shaft skin defect occurs after penile degloving and elongation. If there is excessive penile elongation, the ventral skin defect will not be covered by Sugita et al. and Kim et al.'s methods. Therefore, in a case where the dorsal prepuce is insufficient or limited for penile lengthening, it is necessary to use a new method to cover the ventral skin defect.

We used an advanced musculocutaneous scrotal flap for covering the ventral skin defect after penile degloving through a ventral approach during the surgical correction of CP. The scrotum has three blood supplies (i.e., anterolaterally, the superficial and deep external pudendal arteries; posteriorly, the perineal branches of the internal pudendal arteries and deep layer; and the cremasteric branch of the inferior epigastric arteries and branches of the testicular arteries) [7]. Additionally, the scrotum has more tissue elasticity. Therefore, scrotal flaps have been used to cover the ventral surface of the penis after urethroplasty [8–10]. In addition, scrotal advancement [10] and transposition [11] flaps have been used to cover the base of the denuded penis. Advantages of scrotal flaps include the ease and rapidity with which they can be elevated, the fact that they are directly adjacent to the penis, and that the scrotal donor site can be closed primarily without difficulty [12].

In our surgical method, the dorsal penile skin defect that occurred during penile elongation was covered by the dorsal prepuce. Therefore, the ventral skin defect was covered by our advanced musculocutaneous scrotal flap. It was sufficient to cover the defect using the dorsal penile skin, because the dorsal prepuce was not used for the Byars flap transposition. There was no size limitation in covering the ventral skin defect by using our advanced musculocutaneous scrotal flap because of its better tissue elasticity and abundant blood supply. Furthermore, the definite penoscrotal junction can be made using an artificial triangle excision, which has a better cosmetic result.

Although CP can cause hygiene problems, voiding difficulties, and embarrassment among peers, it is not a life-threatening disease. Therefore, the success or failure of the operation was decided based on the satisfaction of the patients and their families, and their satisfaction was based on the functional and cosmetic outcomes. Previous studies have shown that patients and families are generally satisfied with the surgical results [2, 13] and would recommend the surgery to a friend whose child had a similar condition [3].

Our surgical method showed a satisfaction rate that was comparable to findings from previous studies on penile size, morphology, and voiding status. However, there was a difference between previous reports and our study. In our study, the median age at surgery was higher (19.9 years) than that of previous reports, including Sugita et al. (33 months) [2] and Kim et al. (4.7 years) [3]. During the interviews with patients and their families, we found that the patient's parents lacked the medical knowledge on CP. Therefore, they visited the hospital only when the patient recognized his penis abnormality compared to others, and appealed to their parents about this difference. Additionally, adult patients found it difficult to visit the hospital because of their sexual humiliation associated with hygiene problems, abnormal penile appearance, and embarrassment. Although the median age at surgery was higher than that of previous reports, we evaluated the postoperative satisfaction directly from most of the patients, not from their parents and families.

The mean follow-up period was 27.44 months, and patient satisfaction improved postoperatively compared to that preoperatively in our study. This improvement became more definite after 6 weeks and lasted after 24 weeks of follow-up. We thought that a more improved satisfaction after 6 weeks compared to the postoperative state would be a result of a definite penile appearance after resolving penile lymphedema.

Postoperative complications associated with the correction of CP such as lymphedema [14–16], skin necrosis, and tissue contracture were reported [2]. After performing our surgical method, postoperative lymphedema occurred in all patients and it seemed to be caused by circumferential dissection during complete degloving along Buck's fascia. However, it resolved spontaneously by 6 weeks postoperatively. Additionally, there was no skin necrosis and tissue contracture. We thought that this result was based on the abundant blood supply and elasticity of the advanced musculocutaneous scrotal flap.

There are some disadvantages to our surgical method. First, most patients mentioned the differences in the skin properties and the scrotal hair bearing on the penile shaft. However, these changes to the penile shaft skin were limited to the part of the entire penile shaft, and most of the patients considered this condition to be a tolerable inconvenience, compared to satisfactory surgical results, such as a normalized penile appearance, increased penis size, and restoration of sexual self-confidence. Second, a bilateral incision scar was made in our surgical method. However, it was not considered to be serious according to the patients' satisfaction.

## Conclusions

Our advanced musculocutaneous scrotal flap technique for correcting CP is technically easy and safe. Our surgical method provided patients with a good cosmetic appearance, functional outcomes, and excellent postoperative satisfaction grades. Additionally, it seems applicable in any type of CP, including cases in which covering the ventral skin defect is difficult.

**Competing interests**
The authors declare that they have no competing interests, including financial.

**Authors' contributions**
HJ and SMY performed the advanced musculocutaneous scrotal flap technique for correcting concealed penis, and they drafted the manuscript. CSY performed the statistical analyses and participated in drafting the manuscript. DSH supervised the operations and participated in drafting the manuscript. All the authors read and approved the final manuscript.

**Acknowledgements**
We thank Min-Sung Kim and Man-Su Kim who helped in the operation and acquisition of data.

**References**
1. Maizels M, Zaontz M, Donovan J, Bushnick PN, Firlit CF. Surgical correction of the buried penis: description of a classification system and a technique to correct the disorder. J Urol. 1986;136(1 Pt 2):268–71.
2. Sugita Y, Ueoka K, Tagkagi S, Hisamatsu E, Yoshino K, Tanikaze S. A new technique of concealed penis repair. J Urol. 2009;182(4 Suppl):1751–4.
3. Kim JJ, Lee DG, Park KH, Baek M. A novel technique of concealed penis repair. Eur J Pediatr Surg. 2014;24((2):158–62. Zeitschrift fur Kinderchirurgie.
4. Herndon CD, Casale AJ, Cain MP, Rink RC. Long-term outcome of the surgical treatment of concealed penis. J Urol. 2003;170(4 Pt 2):1695–7. discussion 1697.
5. Srinivasan AK, Palmer LS, Palmer JS. Inconspicuous penis. TheScientificWorldJOURNAL. 2011;11:2559–64.
6. Wollin M, Duffy PG, Malone PS, Ransley PG. Buried penis. A novel approach. Br J Urol. 1990;65(1):97–100.
7. Robert B, Richard R. Complication of Urologic Surgery. Philadelphia: W.B.Saunders Co.; 1990.
8. Cecil AB. Hypospadias and epispadias; diagnosis and treatment. Pediatr Clin N Am. 1955;711–728.
9. Smith DR. Surgical treatment of hypospadias. J Urol. 1955;73(2):329–34.
10. Robinson DW, Stephenson KL, Padgett EC. Loss of coverage of the penis, scrotum and urethra. Plast Reconstr Surg. 1946;1:58–68.
11. Horton CE, McCraw JB, Devine Jr CJ, Devine PC. Secondary reconstruction of the genital area. Urol Clin North Am. 1977;4(1):133–41.
12. Horton CE KI. Local skin Flaps of the Penis. In: Strauch BVL, Hall-Findlay EJ, Lee BT, editors. Grabb's Encyclopeia of Flaps. 3rd ed. Philadelphia: Lippincott Williams & Wilkins; 2009. p. 1216–25. a WOLTERS KLUWER business.
13. Donahoe PK, Keating MA. Preputial unfurling to correct the buried penis. J Pediatr Surg. 1986;21(12):1055–7.
14. Lee T, Suh HJ, Han JU. Correcting congenital concealed penis: new pediatric surgical technique. Urology. 2005;65(4):789–92.
15. Frenkl TL, Agarwal S, Caldamone AA. Results of a simplified technique for buried penis repair. J Urol. 2004;171(2 Pt 1):826–8.
16. Borsellino A, Spagnoli A, Vallasciani S, Martini L, Ferro F. Surgical approach to concealed penis: technical refinements and outcome. Urology. 2007;69(6):1195–8.

# Chronic bacterial prostatitis: efficacy of short-lasting antibiotic therapy with prulifloxacin (Unidrox®) in association with saw palmetto extract, lactobacillus sporogens and arbutin (Lactorepens®)

Gian Maria Busetto[1,3]*, Riccardo Giovannone[1], Matteo Ferro[2], Stefano Tricarico[1], Francesco Del Giudice[1], Deliu Victor Matei[2], Ottavio De Cobelli[2], Vincenzo Gentile[1] and Ettore De Berardinis[1]

## Abstract

**Background:** Bacterial prostatitis (BP) is a common condition accounting responsible for about 5-10% of all prostatitis cases; chronic bacterial prostatitis (CBP) classified as type II, are less common but is a condition that significantly hampers the quality of life, (QoL) because not only is it a physical condition but also a psychological distress. Commonly patients are treated with antibiotics alone, and in particular fluoroquinolones are suggested by the European Urology guidelines. This approach, although recommended, may not be enough. Thus, a multimodal approach to the prolonged antibiotic therapy may be helpful.

**Methods:** 210 patients affected by chronic bacterial prostatitis were enrolled in the study. All patients were positive to Meares-Stamey test and symptoms duration was > 3 months. The purpose of the study was to evaluate the efficacy of a long lasting therapy with a fluoroquinolone in association with a nutraceutical supplement (prulifloxacin 600 mg for 21 days and an association of Serenoa repens 320 mg, Lactobacillus Sporogens 200 mg, Arbutin 100 mg for 30 days). Patients were randomized in two groups (A and B) receiving respectively antibiotic alone and an association of antibiotic plus supplement.

**Results:** Biological recurrence at 2 months in Group A was observed in 21 patients (27.6%) and in Group B in 6 patients (7.8%). Uropathogens found at the first follow-up were for the majority Gram – (E. coli and Enterobacter spp.). A statistically significant difference was found at the time of the follow-up between Group A and B in the NIH-CPSI questionnaire score, symptoms evidence and serum PSA.

**Conclusions:** Broad band, short-lasting antibiotic therapy in association with a nutritional supplement (serenoa repens, lactobacillus sporogens and arbutin) show better control and recurrence rate on patients affected by chronic bacterial prostatitits in comparison with antibiotic treatment alone.

* Correspondence: gianmaria.busetto@uniroma1.it
[1]Department of Urology, Sapienza Rome University, Rome, Italy
[3]Policlinico Umberto I, Sapienza Rome University, viale del Policlinico, 155, 00161 Rome, Italy
Full list of author information is available at the end of the article

## Background

Bacterial prostatitis (BP) is a common condition in which an infective origin is accepted, and accounts for about 5-10% of all prostatitis cases [1]. This is one of the most common reasons for younger men to consult with a urologist. Regarding duration of symptoms, we describe two main types: acute and chronic. In particular, when chronic, symptoms last more than 3 months and in agreement with the National Institute of Health (NIH) chronic bacterial prostatitis (CBP) is classified as type II. Even if in many cases the aetiology is known, in others there are only these symptoms: pelvic area pain and lower urinary tract symptoms (LUTS). Chronic prostatitis is a condition that significantly hampers the quality of life (QoL) of the majority of patients affected, because it is not only a physical condition but also a psychological distress. The impact of CBP is similar to those patients who had a myocardial infarction, unstable angina or Crohn's disease [2]. Pathophysiology of CBP at the moment remains unknown although some mechanisms of actions, like infectious, immunological, neurological, endocrine and psychological, have been postulated [3]. Commonly patients are treated with antibiotics alone as recommended by the European Urology guidelines. In particular, for chronic bacterial prostatitis, fluoroquinolones, thanks to their favourable pharmacokinetic properties, prostate penetration, bioavailability and excellent activity against typical/atypical pathogens together with a good safety profile, are considered drugs of choice. The use of fluoroquinolones, a broad-spectrum antibiotic, is strengthened by the well-known evidence that CBP is commonly caused by Gram-negative bacteria such as Escherichia coli, and also by the recent consideration of some authors that reported an emerging prevalence of Gram-positive and atypical bacteria together with anaerobes [4,5]. Usually high-doses and a long-lasting therapy are preferred because only low-molecular-weight and lipid-soluble drugs, not tightly connected to plasma proteins, are able to penetrate the epithelial membrane, even considering reported side-effects (gastrointestinal disorders and development of antibiotics resistance) [6-8]. This approach, although recommended, may not be enough, considering patients' and urologists' high rate of dissatisfaction. Furthermore, given the overlapping of lower urinary tract symptoms, antibiotics alone could be inadequate. The main purpose of the therapy is to eradicate uropathogens without forgetting to relieve symptoms that mainly act on QoL. Considering the heterogeneous nature of chronic prostatitis and recurrence rate of this disorder, a multimodal approach to the prolonged antibiotic therapy may be helpful for the solution of the problem at hand. The use of plant-derived products is reaching popularity in North America and Europe and is often one of the treatments of choice for chronic conditions [9]. Main advantages of such a therapy are unique mechanisms of action, response against LUTS, low side-effects profile, low cost and high level of acceptance by patients. Main disadvantages are unknown drug interactions and meaningless labels [9]. Serenoa Repens, saw palmetto extract, is the most commonly used phyto-therapy in urology and has an action against type I-II 5-α-reductase (conversion of testosterone in dihydrotestosterone), anti-inflammatory effect by inhibition of arachidonic acid metabolites and also an anti-edematous effect [10]. Arbutin, the active principle of bearberry, is an antioxidant agent with an anti-inflammatory action through lypopolisaccharide induced production of NO and expression of iNOS and COX-2 [11]. The use of probiotics, in particular lactobacillus sporogens, is a good alternative for the treatment and prevention of urinary tract infection (UTI) through different mechanisms including attachment to the uroepithelial cells and direct antimicrobial activity [12]. Lactobacillus is an important part of the normal flora, which is commonly found in the mouth cavity, gastrointestinal tract and genitourinary tract. Reduction in number of lactobacillus increases the risk of UTI [13].

In the article we report results of an association therapy with third generation fluoroquinolone (prulifloxacin 600 mg) and nutraceutical supplement (Serenoa repens 320 mg, Lactobacillus Sporogens 200 mg, Arbutin 100 mg) in the treatment of chronic bacterial prostatitis.

## Methods

From January 2012 to December 2012 a total of 210 patients with an average age of 36.6 (19–54) were enrolled in the study. In particular all of the patients were affected by chronic bacterial prostatitis and in accordance with the definition of the disease were positive to the Meares-Stamey test and symptoms duration was > 3 months (dysuria, pelvic pain and/or discomfort). The Meares-Stamey test, also known as 4-glass test, is the standard method of assessing inflammation and presence of bacteria in the lower urinary tract of men presenting CBP. The test has been performed on each patient before and after the therapy. The Meares-Stamey evaluation allows the collection of four samples: first voided urine (VB1) that represents urethra, mid-stream urine (VB2) that represents bladder, expressed prostatic secretion (EPS) and post-prostatic massage urine (VB3) that represent the prostate. It is considered positive when we have urophathogen colony-forming units (CFU)/mL $\geq 10^3$.

The NIH-Chronic Prostatitis Symptom Index (NIH-CPSI) is a questionnaire with 13 questions developed to evaluate symptoms and quality of life in men with chronic prostatitis/chronic pelvic pain syndrome (CP/CPPS). Every question has a score differing by the answer, and the questionnaire has a total score ranging from 0 to 43. The score is divided by three subscales: pain (score range 0–21),

**Table 1 Patients characteristics**

|  | Group A | Group B |
|---|---|---|
| No. of patients* | 76 | 77 |
| Median age (±S.D.) (years)* | 35.9 (6.2) | 37.1 (6.5) |
| *Sexual bahaviour (%)* |  |  |
| Only 1 partner* | 50 (65.8) | 52 (67.5) |
| 2 or more partners* | 26 (34.2) | 25 (32.5) |
| *Contraceptive method (%)* |  |  |
| No contraceptive** | 28 (36.7) | 31 (40.3) |
| Condom* | 9 (11.8) | 9 (11.7) |
| Coitus interruptus** | 39 (51.3) | 37 (48.1) |
| *Urinary symptoms (%)* |  |  |
| Burning* | 65 (85.6) | 65 (84.4) |
| Tenesmus* | 24 (31.6) | 26 (33.8) |
| Pain** | 40 (52.6) | 34 (44.2) |
| Urgency** | 40 (52.6) | 32 (41.6) |
| Frequency** | 46 (60.5) | 55 (71.4) |
| Beginning of CBP (months)* | 15.9 | 17.4 |

*not-statistically significant difference between Group A and B.
**statistically significant difference between Group A and B.

**Table 2 Uropathogens characteristics and disease recurrences**

|  | Group A | Group B |
|---|---|---|
| *Uropathogens (baseline) (%)* |  |  |
| Gram negative | 41 (53.9) | 39 (50.6) |
| Escherichia coli | 33 (80.5) | 33 (84.6) |
| Proteus mirabilis | 3 (7.3) | 1 (2.6) |
| Klebsiella spp. | 7 (17.1) | 5 (12.8) |
| Serratta spp. | 2 (4.88) | 4 (10.3) |
| Pseudomonas aeruginosa | 0 (0) | 0 (0) |
| Enterobacter spp. | 20 (48.8) | 15 (38.5) |
| Gram positive | 35 (46.1) | 38 (49.4) |
| Enterococcus spp. | 25 (71.4) | 27 (71) |
| Staphylococcus saprophyticus | 10 (28.6) | 10 (26.3) |
| Staphylococcus epidermidis | 2 (5.7) | 4 (10.5) |
| Staphylococcus aureus | 1 (2.8) | 0 (0) |
| Streptococcus B group | 6 (17.1) | 4 (10.5) |
| Recurrences (2 months) (%) | 21 (27.6) | 6 (7.8) |
| *Uropathogens (2 months) (%)* |  |  |
| Gram negative | 21 (95.4) | 6 (100) |
| Escherichia coli | 17 (81) | 4 (66.7) |
| Proteus mirabilis | 0 (0) | 0 (0) |
| Klebsiella spp. | 2 (9.5) | 1 (16.7) |
| Serratta spp. | 0 (0) | 0 (0) |
| Pseudomonas aeruginosa | 0 (0) | 0 (0) |
| Enterobacter spp. | 2 (9.5) | 1 (16.7) |
| Gram positive | 1 (4.5) | 0 (0) |
| Enterococcus spp. | 1 (100) | 0 (0) |
| Staphylococcus saprophyticus | 0 (0) | 0 (0) |
| Staphylococcus epidermidis | 0 (0) | 0 (0) |
| Staphylococcus aureus | 0 (0) | 0 (0) |
| Streptococcus B group | 0 (0) | 0 (0) |

urinary symptoms (score range 0–10) and quality of life (QoL) (score range 0–12). The pain subscale includes six items scoring from 0 to 1, one scoring from 0 to 5 and one scoring from 0 to 10. The urinary subscale consists of two items, both of them scored from 0 to 3. The QoL subscale includes further two items scored from 0 to 3, and one scored from 0 to 6. The sum of all single scores is the total score. The reason every item has a different maximum score is because they have a different potential. NIH-CPSI characteristics are: good reliability, validity, and responsiveness to change. It has been used in many large-scale trials regarding CP/CPPS as the primary outcome variable [14]. Exclusion criteria of the study were: positivity to Chlamydia trachomatis, Ureaplasma urealiticum, Mycoplasma, Neisseria gonorrhoeae, herpes simplex viruses (HSV 1/2) and human papillomavirus (HPV); age less than 18 years; history of neurological disease, urinary stones or cancer; allergy to fluoroquinolones; refusal to sign the informed consent; incomplete follow-up time. Taking into account the aforementioned criteria, 57 patients were excluded. The purpose of the study was to evaluate the efficacy of a short lasting therapy with a fluoroquinolone, recommended as first choice in this disease, in association with a nutraceutical supplement. In particular prulifloxacin, a third generation fluoroquinolone, has demonstrated to be not-inferior to levofloxacin in the treatment of urinary tract infections [15]. Treatment schedule was based on oral prulifloxacin 600 mg (Unidrox®) 1 tablet daily for 21 days and an association of Serenoa repens 320 mg, Lactobacillus Sporogens 200 mg,

Arbutin 100 mg (Lactorepens®) 1 tablet daily for 30 days. All eligible patients signed an informed consent to participate in the study and everyone, before the beginning of the treatment, underwent medical history, urological examination, Meares-Stamey test, PSA evaluation and compiled the NIH-CPSI questionnaire (Italian version). In order to exclude the presence of other urological disease simulating a prostatitis, every patients had a bladder and prostate ultrasound and compiled a voiding diary. At 2 months, 4 months and at 6 months from the start of the therapy a follow-up examination was scheduled, and in particular every patient underwent the same tests as at the beginning of the treatment. Randomization was carried out using a double-blind ratio of 1:1. Patients were divided in two groups: Group A (76 patients) receiving antibiotic alone and Group B (77 patients) receiving an association of antibiotic and supplement. Outcomes of the study were: clinical resolution of the disease and relief of the symptoms. Clinical resolution was defined as being asymptomatic for a minimum of 1 month, and clinical failure as the persistence of symptoms together with clinical signs (Meares-Stamey positivity) after treatment or after the suspension of the therapy. Regarding symptoms evaluation, we used the NIH-CPSI subscale (urinary symptoms - score range 0–10) and we defined asymptomatic a patient with a score of 0. Furthermore, spontaneously reported adverse events or those noted by the investigator were recorded during the whole study period.

Statistical analysis was carried out with BMDP statistical software, version 7 (Statistical Solutions, Saugus, MA) and SPSS (Chicago, IL, version 15.00 for Windows). Statistical significance was achieved if the p-value was <0.05. All reported P-values are two-sided.

The ethical committee approval (Sapienza Rome University - Department of Gynecological-Obstetric Sciences and Urological Sciences - Ethical Committee) was obtained and all treatments applied are part of routine standard care. The study was conducted in line with European Urology and Good Clinical Practice guidelines, with ethical principles laid down in the latest version of the Declaration of Helsinki. Every patient signed an informed consent to participate in the study.

## Results

Including an initial population of 210 patients and considering the exclusion criteria, 57 patients have been excluded. In particular, 21 patients were positive to Chlamydia trachomatis/Ureaplasma urealiticum, 10 patients positive to Mycoplasma and 8 positive to HPV (2 patients Chlamydia together with Mycoplasma). Furthermore,

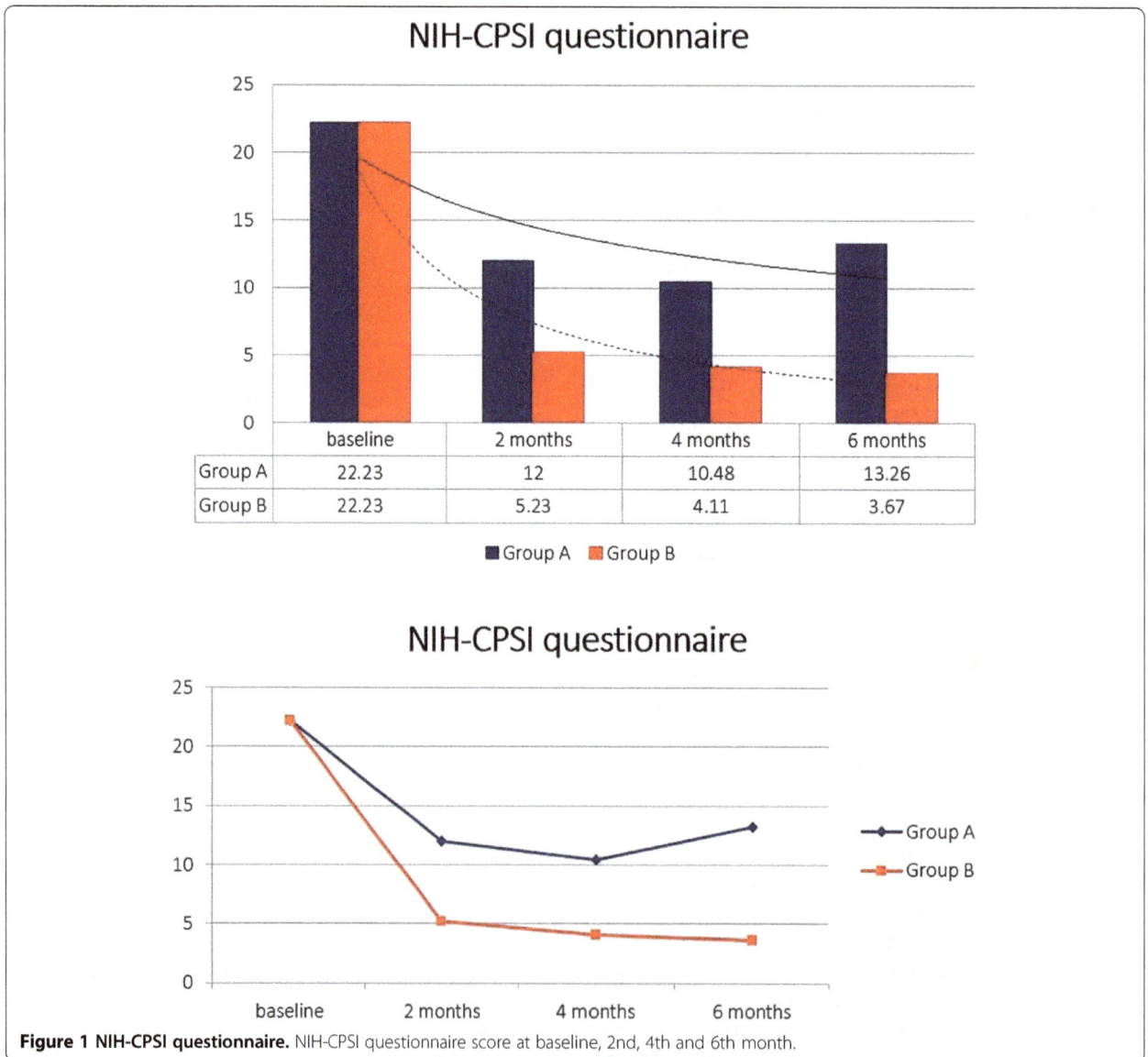

**Figure 1 NIH-CPSI questionnaire.** NIH-CPSI questionnaire score at baseline, 2nd, 4th and 6th month.

7 patients were positive for urinary stones and only one referred an allergy to fluoroquinolones. The follow-up time of 6 months was not reached by 10 patients. Patients' characteristics are listed in Table 1. In our study, in total, 153 patients have been enrolled. Mean age of patients was $36.6 \pm 6.4$ and median symptom time was 16.4 months (4–24). Considering uropathogens found in the Meares-Stamey test, there was a balance between Gram-positive and Gram-negative bacteria: 73 (47.7%) Gram + and 80 (52.3%) Gram − (Table 2). Biological recurrence at 2 months (positivity of Meares-Stamey test) in Group A was observed in 21 patients (27.6%) and in Group B in 6 patients (7.8%). Uropathogens found at the first follow-up were for the majority Gram − (E. coli and Enterobacter spp.) and are listed in Table 2. Patients with recurrence, in accordance with antibiogram, received an alternative antibiotic therapy without uptake of any supplement. Looking at the NIH-CPSI questionnaire before the therapy (baseline) we reported a score of $22.23 \pm 5.55$. All patients compiled the questionnaire after 2 months, 4 months and 6 months from the beginning of the therapy and results are as follows: Group A $12.00 \pm 4.34$, Group B $5.23 \pm 2.76$ at 2 months; Group A $10.48 \pm 4.14$, Group B $4.11 \pm 2.32$ at 4 months; Group A $13.26 \pm 4.88$, Group B $3.67 \pm 1.98$ at 6 months (Figure 1). Data regarding the NIH-CPSI questionnaire divided in the 3 subscales are listed in Table 3. Furthermore, the difference between the Groups is always statistically significant with a p value at 2, 4 and 6 months always < 0.001. Serum median PSA at baseline was $2.4 \pm 1.8$ ng/ml. PSA values after the therapy were: Group A $1.8 \pm 1.2$, Group B $1.4 \pm 0.9$ at 2 months; Group A $1.8 \pm 1.2$, Group B $1.5 \pm 0.9$ at 4 months; Group A $1.9 \pm 1.2$, Group B $1.7 \pm 1.0$ at 6 months (Figure 2). After the therapy the difference between the groups isn't statistically significant with a p value at 2, 4 and 6 months always > 0.05. Symptoms related to CBP have been reported by 15 patients (19.7%) in Group A and 7 patients (9%) in Group B at 2 months, 18 patients in Group A (23.7%) and 7 patients (9%) in Group B at 4 months, 20 patients (26.3%) in Group A and 5 patients (6.5%) in Group B at 6 months (Figure 3). Symptoms reported by the patients are: burning, tenesmus, urgency, frequency, post voiding dribble and micturition with pain. During the follow-up time all the symptoms improved in both groups with a difference at 2, 4 and 6 months not always statistically significant; in particular, the difference, is significant only at 4 and 6 months with a p value respectively of 0.012 and < 0.001. All included patients received therapy properly without any dose/tablet variation and with a compliance of 100%. No side effects were reported with either therapy scheme (antibiotic vs antibiotic + compound). Only patients with a biological recurrence received an additional antibiotic course in accordance with antibiogram.

**Table 3 NIH-CPSI questionnaire results**

| | Group A | Group B |
|---|---|---|
| *Symptoms score (NIH-CPSI questionnaire 0–43) (±S.D.)* | | |
| Baseline | $21.85 \pm 5.23$ | $22.56 \pm 5.78$ |
| 2 months | $12.00 \pm 4.34$ | $5.23 \pm 2.76$ |
| 4 months | $10.48 \pm 4.14$ | $4.11 \pm 2.32$ |
| 6 months | $13.26 \pm 4.88$ | $3.67 \pm 1.98$ |
| *Pain score (NIH-CPSI questionnaire 0–21) (±S.D.)* | | |
| Baseline | $11.65 \pm 3.23$ | $12.00 \pm 2.78$ |
| 2 months | $6.20 \pm 2.35$ | $2.13 \pm 1.90$ |
| 4 months | $5.82 \pm 2.10$ | $1.65 \pm 1.17$ |
| 6 months | $8.06 \pm 2.81$ | $1.25 \pm 0.99$ |
| *Urinary score (NIH-CPSI questionnaire 0–10) (±S.D.)* | | |
| Baseline | $4.65 \pm 2.11$ | $4.26 \pm 2.28$ |
| 2 months | $2.35 \pm 1.35$ | $1.34 \pm 0.89$ |
| 4 months | $2.10 \pm 1.15$ | $1.11 \pm 0.89$ |
| 6 months | $2.65 \pm 1.44$ | $1.01 \pm 0.76$ |
| *Symptoms (%)* | | |
| Baseline | 76 (100) | 77 (100) |
| 2 months | 15 (19.7) | 7 (9) |
| 4 months | 18 (23.7) | 7 (9) |
| 6 months | 20 (26.3) | 5 (6.5) |
| *QoL (NIH-CPSI questionnaire 0–12) (±S.D.)* | | |
| Baseline | $5.76 \pm 2.44$ | $5.66 \pm 2.39$ |
| 2 months | $2.89 \pm 1.68$ | $1.85 \pm 1.00$ |
| 4 months | $2.60 \pm 1.43$ | $1.66 \pm 0.95$ |
| 6 months | $3.09 \pm 1.74$ | $1.40 \pm 0.94$ |

## Discussion

Chronic bacterial prostatitis (CBP) type II, although its prevalence is low, is a frustrating condition for patients because it is characterized by a high impact on quality of life (QoL) and also by a frequent recurrence rate [16,17]. This condition represents a challenge for urologists and, to date, the optimal management remains controversial and the only recommended treatment is antibiotic therapy and surgery in those limited cases with severe complications [18,19]. Other treatments, commonly adopted, are anti-inflammatory drugs, α-blockers, phytotherapy and alternative therapies such as biofeedback, psychotherapy and acupuncture [20]. Long-lasting therapy with fluoriquinolones antibiotics is one of the best treatments in patients with CBP because of a pharmacokinetic favourable profile and in particular ciprofloxacin and levofloxacin are recommended. The latter also has a favourable action against Gram + pathogens. Prulifloxacin, a third generation fluoroquinolone, has been approved for the

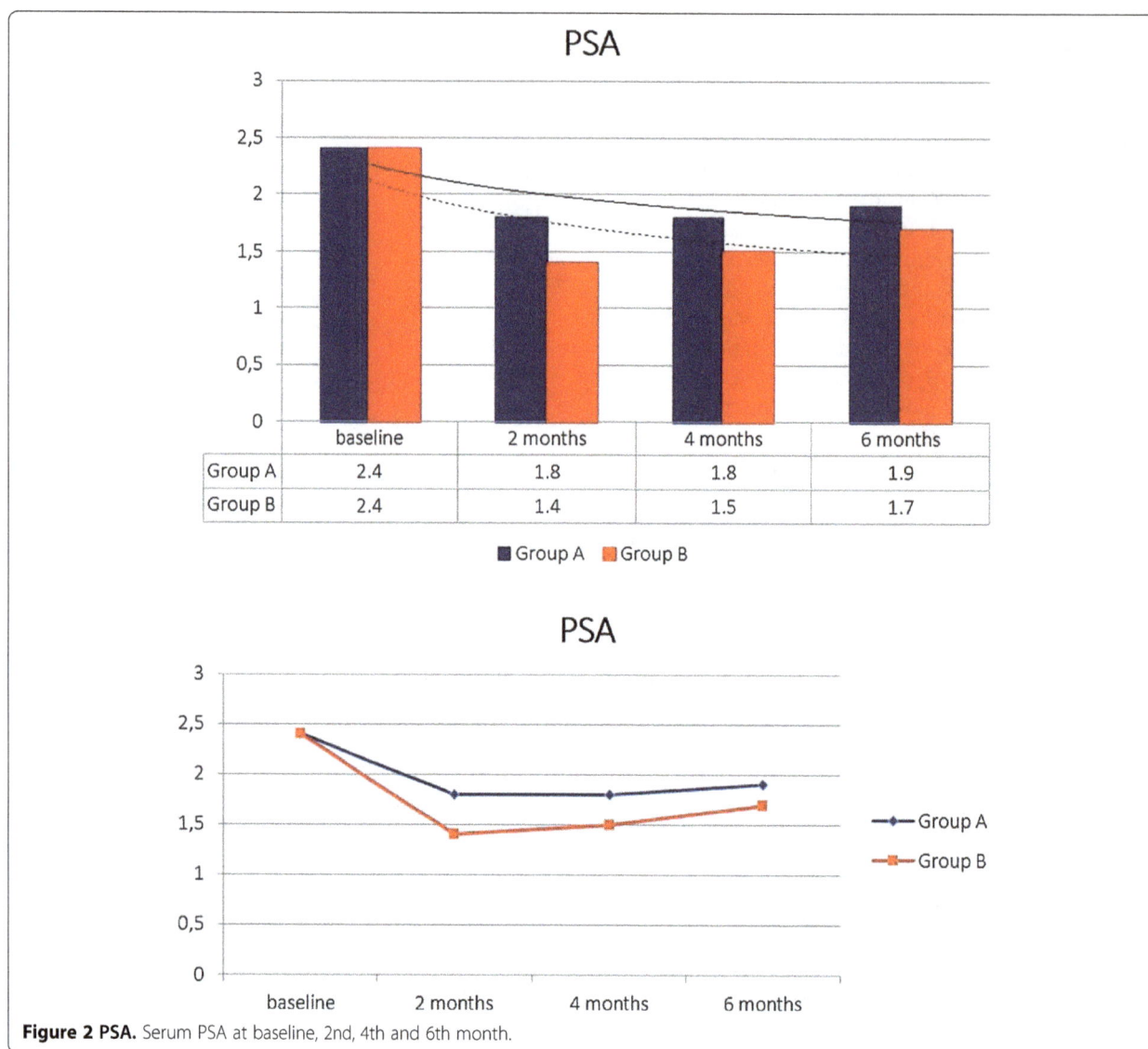

**Figure 2 PSA.** Serum PSA at baseline, 2nd, 4th and 6th month.

treatment of lower urinary tract infection. Furthermore, it has demonstrated its ability to better penetrate into prostatic tissue compared to other quinolones, thus confirming a potential therapeutic role in the treatment of bacterial prostatic infections [21]. Giannarini et al., comparing a 4-weeks course of prulifoxacin in comparison with levofloxacin in the treatment of chronic bacterial prostatitis, report, at 6 months, a microbiological eradication of 72.73% and 71.11%, repectively, and a reduction in the NIH-CPSI of 10.75 and 10.73. The authors conclude that prulifloxacin is at last as effective and safe as levofloxacin [15]. Serenoa repens, saw palmetto extract, the most widely used supplement for lower urinary tracts (LUTS), and in particular for prostatic infection and inflammation, has a multimodal effect that is explained with a set of different mechanisms of action: selective antagonism of the link between dihydrotestosterone and androgen receptor;

inhibition of 5-alpha-reductase, involved in the transformation of testosterone to its biologically active metabolite, that stimulates cell proliferation and hypertrophy of the prostate tissue; anti-inflammatory and anti-oedema effect, demonstrated by reduced capillary permeability induced by histamine; anti-estrogenic effect given by decline in estrogen receptors, which seems to potentiate the action of hormones in the development of BHP [22,23]. Unlike 5-α-reductase inhibitors (5-ARI), a selective competitive inhibitors of α-reductase type II that is more specific for prostate, serenoa repens isn't selective and acts against both types (type I and II). Cai et al., comparing the usage of prulifloxacin alone with plurifloxacin in association with serenoa repens, urtica dioica, quercitin and curcumin in the treatment of chronic bacterial prostatitis type II, report a statistically significant difference in QoL and symptoms (absence of symptoms: 27% vs 89.6%) [17].

Chronic bacterial prostatitis: efficacy of short-lasting antibiotic therapy with prulifloxacin (Unidrox®)...

39

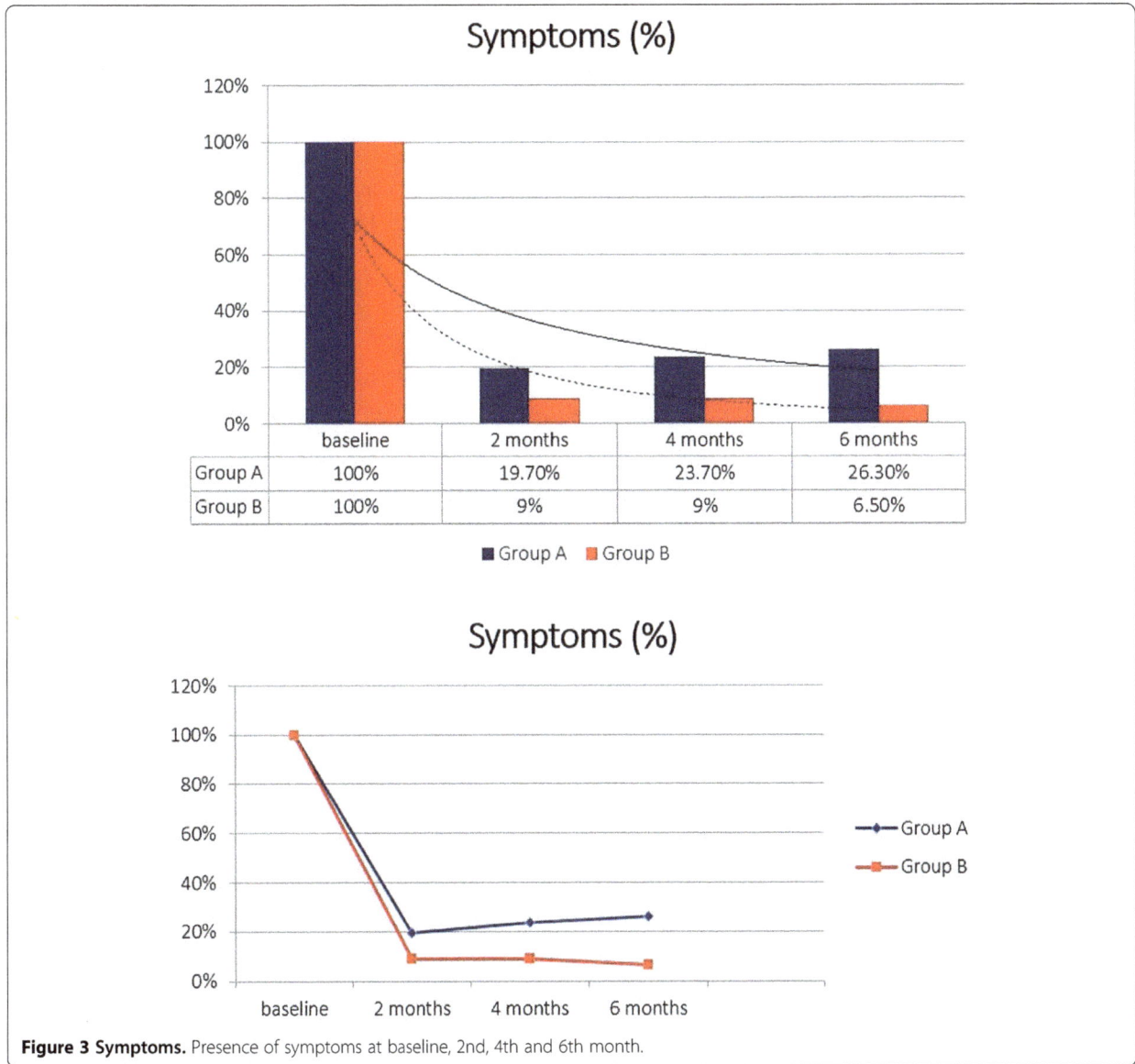

**Figure 3 Symptoms.** Presence of symptoms at baseline, 2nd, 4th and 6th month.

| | baseline | 2 months | 4 months | 6 months |
|---|---|---|---|---|
| Group A | 100% | 19.70% | 23.70% | 26.30% |
| Group B | 100% | 9% | 9% | 6.50% |

Probiotics are important to reduce gastrointestinal side-effects caused by the prolonged use of broad-band antibiotics. Considering that pathogens found in the prostate often derive from intestinal bacterial overgrowth, it is important to remark the role of probiotics in maintaining a regular intestinal bacterial flora [24]. Some authors have postulated that urethral dysbacteriosis is one of the primary causes of CP, further contributing to its recidivity and refractoriness [12]. In particular, when this condition occurs, the urethral microflora infects the prostate through prostatic reflux of urine into prostatic ducts causing bacterial prostatitis and inflammation [25]. Overused and overprescribed antibiotics are usually the cause of urethral dysbacteriosis while probiotics are considered a viable potential alternative for treating and preventing prostatitis and all urinary tract infections.

Probiotics, with different mechanisms of action, have the ability to attach to uroepithelial cells and obtain direct antimicrobial activity [26]. The reason we suggest using probiotics in association with a long-course antibiotic is to rebalance intestinal bacterial flora and to avoid any urinary tract dysbacteriosis and to prevent UTI recurrences [12]. One of the limits of many studies on chronic prostatitis is that they focus only on infection eradication instead of symptoms improvement. Inflammation, together with neuromuscular spasm, is often the most important cause of chronic prostatitis symptoms [27]. Arbutin, a glycoside extracted from bearberry plant, is a traditional supplement for treating UTI mainly because of its anti-inflammatory effect due to antioxidant capability dispatched on lypopo-lisaccharide, induced production of NO and expression of iNOS and COX-2 [11].

Our study has been drawn to evaluate the efficacy of a short-course, broad band antibiotic therapy (21 days of prulifloxacin 600 mg) to eradicate pathogens in patients with CBP and to evaluate if an association with a supplement (30 days of serenoa repens 320 mg, lactobacillus sporogens 200 mg and arbutin 100 mg) is able to prevent recurrences and improve symptoms in those patients with this particularly frustrating condition. To evaluate the outcomes, patients, divided in two different groups (A and B), have been submitted to different therapies: antibiotic or antibiotic plus supplement. Looking at the results we can notice, with a statistically significant difference, that patients treated with the association of compounds obtain better effects as demonstrated with the NIH-CPSI questionnaire. Analysing first, second and third follow-up, patients in Group A obtain an improvement at 2 and 4 months while there is a decrease in results at the 6th month. Patients in Group B obtain better results in comparison with Group A, and furthermore the NIH-CPSI score continues to also decrease at the 6th month follow-up. Symptoms, probably the most invalidating condition for the patients, have been reported by patients in Group A to improve only at 2nd month follow-up while at 4th and 6th month there is a turnaround. Patients in Group B continued to report benefits till the end of follow-up time. Reported symptoms together with the NIH-CPSI questionnaire score are better in all patients treated with antibiotic plus supplement, confirming more stable and long-standing results in QoL that is always the main target of CBP patients. Prostatic specific antigen (PSA) decreases in both groups with a lower value in Group B probably because of the effect of serenoa repens that acts on type I-II 5-$\alpha$-reductase, inhibiting testosterone conversion to its active metabolite. With regards to this, it is important to remark that the prostate specific antigen does not always increase during a prostatitis and does not seem to be systematically correlated to prostate inflammation [28]; this is the most important reason why it isn't a good parameter to show a therapy's response. Finally we found a difference between Group A and B in uropathogens eradication; in particular we have a recurrence rate at 2 months of 27.6% and 7.8%, respectively. Pathogens found during follow-up are often different from pathogens found at baseline. We think that the main reason is because repeated cycles of antibiotic therapy are never able to prevent bacteria relapsing [29] and this is why we can improve results by adding compounds to antibiotic therapy alone. In particular, results, show that association therapy obtains better results in avoiding the majority of recurrences and prolonging the recurrence-free time.

Limitations of the study are: small number of patients, not randomized double-blind placebo controlled trial, impossibility to attribute to single components of the compound the action, antibiotic therapy duration scientifically debated, and difficulty to evaluate if the results in the patients with recurrence have been altered by different antibiotic administered in accordance with antibiogram.

## Conclusions
In summary, a broad band, short-lasting antibiotic therapy in association with a nutritional supplement (serenoa repens, lactobacillus sporogens and arbutin) show better control and recurrence rates on patients affected by chronic bacterial prostatitis, in comparison with compared to antibiotic treatment alone.

### Competing interests
The authors declare that they have no competing interests.

### Authors' contributions
GMB analysed data and drafted the manuscript. RG acquired data. MF participated in interpretation of data. ST and FDG gave their contribution in acquiring data. ODC and VG critically revised the manuscript. EDB participated in the conception and design of the study. All authors read and approved the final manuscript.

### Acknowledgements
We are very thanks to Jennifer Partridge (Dallas, TX – USA) for making significant language revision of the article. The authors haven't received any source of funding.

### Author details
[1]Department of Urology, Sapienza Rome University, Rome, Italy. [2]Department of Urology, European Oncology Institute, Milan, Italy. [3]Policlinico Umberto I, Sapienza Rome University, viale del Policlinico, 155, 00161 Rome, Italy.

### References
1. Pontari MA: **Chronic prostatitis/chronic pelvic pain syndrome.** *Urol Clin North Am* 2008, **35**:81–89.
2. Wenninger K, Heiman JR, Rothman I, Berghuis JP, Berger RE: **Sickness impact of chronic nonbacterial prostatitis and its correlates.** *J Urol* 1996, **155**:965–968.
3. Pontari MA, Ruggieri MR: **Mechanisms in prostatitis/chronic pelvic pain syndrome.** *J Urol* 2008, **179**:S61–S67.
4. Mazzoli S: **Conventional bacteriology in prostatitis patients: microbiological bias, problems and epidemiology on 1686 microbial isolates.** *Arch Ital Urol Androl* 2007, **79**:71–75.
5. Nickel JC, Xiang J: **Clinical significance of nontraditional bacterial uropathogens in the management of chronic prostatitis.** *J Urol* 2008, **179**:1391–1395.
6. Bjerklund Johansen TE, Grüneberg RN, Guibert J, Bjerklund Johansen TE, Grüneberg RN, Guibert J, Hofstetter A, Lobel B, Naber KG, Palou Redorta J, van Cangh PJ: **The role of antibiotics in the treatment of chronic prostatitis: a consensus statement.** *Eur Urol* 1998, **34**(6):457–466.
7. Naber KG: **Antimicrobial treatment of bacterial prostatitis.** *Eur Urol* 2003, **43**(Suppl 2):23–26.
8. Stamey TA, Meares EM, Winningham DG: **Chronic bacterial prostatitis and diffusion of drugs into prostatic fluid.** *J Urol* 1970, **103**:187–194.
9. Shoskes DA: **Phytotherapy in chronic prostatitis.** *Urology* 2002, **60**(Suppl 6A):35–37.
10. Kaplan SA, Volpe MA, Te AE: **A prospective, 1-year trial using saw palmetto versus finasteride in the treatment of category III prostatitis/chronic pelvic pain syndrome.** *J Urol* 2004, **171**:284–288.
11. Lee HJ, KIM KW: **Anti-inflammatory effects of arbutin in lypopolysaccharide-stimulated BV2 microglial cells.** *Inflamm Res* 2012, **61**(8):817–825.
12. Liu L, Yang J, Lu F: **Urethral dysbacteriosis as an underlying, primary cause of chronic prostatitis: potential implications for probiotic therapy.** *Med Hypotheses* 2009, **73**:741–743.

13. Amdekar S, Singh V, Singh DD: **Probiotic therapy: immunomodulating approach toward urinary tract infection.** *Curr Microbiol* 2011, **63**(5):484–490.

14. Probert KJ, Alexander RB, Nickel JC, Kusek JW, Litwin MS, Landis JR, Nyberg LM, Schaeffer AJ, Chronic Prostatitis Collaborative Research Network: **Design of a multicenter randomized clinical trial for chronic prostatitis/chronic pelvic pain syndrome.** *Urology* 2002, **59**(6):870–876.

15. Giannarini G, Mogorovich A, Valent F, Morelli G, De Maria M, Manassero F, Barbone F, Selli C: **Prulifloxacin versul levofloxacin in the treatment of chronic bacterial prostatitis: a prospective, randomized, double-blind trial.** *J Chemother* 2007, **19**(3):304–308.

16. Magri V, Trinchieri A, Pozzi G, Restelli A, Garlaschi MC, Torresani E, Zirpoli P, Marras E, Perletti G: **Efficacy of repeated cyclesnof combination therapy for the eradication of infecting organisms in chronic bacterial prostatitis.** *Int J Antimicrob Agents* 2007, **29**:549–556.

17. Cai T, Mazzoli S, Bechi A, Addonisio P, Mondaini N, Pagliai RC, Bartoletti R: **Serenoa repens associated with Urtica dioica (ProstaMEV) and curcumin and quercitin (FlogMEV) extracts are able to improve the efficacy of prulifloxacin in bacterial prostatitis patients: results from a prospective randomised study.** *Int J Antimicrob Agents* 2009, **33**(6):549–553.

18. Schaeffer AJ, Weidner W, Barbalias GA: **Summary consensus statement: diagnosis and management of chronic prostatitis/chronic pelvic pain syndrome.** *Eur Urol* 2003, **3**(Suppl 2):1–4.

19. Thakkinstian A, Attia J, Anothaisintawee T, Nickel JC: **α-blockers, antibiotics and anti-inflammatories have a role in the management of chronic prostatitis/chronic pelvic pain syndrome.** *BJU Int* 2012, **110**(7):1014–1022.

20. Shoskes DA: **Phytotherapy and other alternative forms of care for the patients with prostatitis.** *Curr Urol Rep* 2002, **3**:330.

21. Giberti C, Gallo F, Rosignoli MT, Ruggieri A, Barattè S, Picollo R, Dionisio P: **Penetration of orally administered prulifloxacin into human prostate tissue.** *Clin Drug Investig* 2009, **29**(1):27–34.

22. Wilt TJ, Ishani A, Stark G, MacDonald R, Lau J, Mulrow C: **Saw palmetto extracts for treatment of benign prostatic hyperplasia: a systematic review.** *JAMA* 1998, **280**(18):1604–1609.

23. Di Silverio F, Monti S, Sciarra A, Varasano PA, Martini C, Lanzara S, D'Eramo G, Di Nicola S, Toscano V: **Effects of long-term treatment with Serenoa repens (Permixon) on the concentrations and regional distribution of androgens and epidermal growth factor in benign prostatic hyperplasia.** *Prostate* 1998, **37**(2):77–83.

24. Weinstock LB, Geng B, Brandes SB: **Chronic prostatitis and small intestinal bacterial overgrowth: effect of rifaximin.** *Can J Urol* 2011, **18**(4):5826–5830.

25. Kirby RS, Lowe D, Bultitude MI, Shuttleworth KE: **Intra-prostatic urinary reflux: an aetiological factor in abacterial prostatitis.** *Br J Urol* 1982, **54**:729–731.

26. Fraga M, Scavone P, Zunino P: **Preventive and therapeutic administration of an indigenous Lactobacillus sp. Strain against Proteus mirabilis ascending urinary tract infection in a mouse model.** *Antoine Ven Leeuwenhoek* 2005, **88**:25–34.

27. Shoskes DA, Hakim L, Ghoniem G, Jackson CL: **Long-term results of multimodal therapy for chronic prostatitis/chronic pelvic pain syndrome.** *J Urol* 2003, **169**(4):1406–1410.

28. Bruyere F, Amine LM: **PSA interest and prostatitis: literature review.** *Prog Urol* 2013, **23**(16):1377–1381.

29. Magri V, Trinchieri A, Ceriani I, Marras E, Perletti G: **Eradication of unusual pathogens by combination pharmacological tharapy is parallel by improvement of signs and symptoms of chronic prostatitis syndrome.** *Arch Ital Urol Androl* 2007, **79**:93–98.

# 7

# High pressure balloon dilation for vesicourethral anastomotic strictures after radical prostatectomy

Gen Ishii[1][*], Takehito Naruoka[2], Kanako Kasai[1], Kenichi Hata[1], Hiroshi Omono[1], Masayasu Suzuki[1], Takahiro Kimura[2] and Shin Egawa[2]

## Abstract

**Background:** Vesicourethral anastomotic stricture (VAS) is a rare but serious complication following radical prostatectomy (RP), and various types of managements for VAS have been proposed. We investigated the efficacy of transurethral balloon dilation in the management of VAS after RP.

**Methods:** A total of 128 consecutive patients underwent open RP at our hospital between 2008 and 2013; of these, 10 patients (7.8 %) developed VAS. Transurethral balloon dilation was performed in all 10 patients, using a high pressure balloon catheter under fluoroscopic and endoscopic guidance. Follow-up endoscopy was performed, and patients in whom the stricture had recurred underwent repeat dilation. We retrospectively evaluated the management of VAS and short-term efficacy of high pressure balloon dilation.

**Results:** The mean time from RP to diagnosis of VAS was 9 months (2–40 months); eight patients (80 %) were diagnosed within 6 months of RP. Balloon dilation of VAS was technically successful in all patients, and no perioperative complications were recorded. The median follow-up after balloon dilation was 24 months (7–67 months). There was no recurrence of VAS in eight patients (80 %) after the first balloon dilation, and all patients were controlled within the twice.

**Conclusion:** High pressure balloon dilation is a highly effective and minimally invasive procedure for treating VAS.

**Keywords:** Balloon dilation, Vesicourethral anastomotic stricture, Prostatectomy

## Background

Vesicourethral anastomotic stricture (VAS) is one of the most common complications after radical prostatectomy (RP), with rates ranging from 0.48-32 % [1, 2]. The development of a VAS can cause severe voiding dysfunction and result in significant deterioration of the patients' quality of life.

Factors predisposed to the development of a VAS are not well understood, but they are reported to be related to prior transurethral resection of the prostate (TURP), the oncologic outcome, excessive blood loss, anastomotic ischemia, or urinary extravasation at the site of the VAS [3, 4]. Surgical techniques, including the suturing procedure and choice of bladder neck reconstruction, or bladder neck preservation, are also considered important factors [5].

There are various methods for managing a VAS, including simple or balloon dilation; cold knife incision, electrocautery incision or resection, and laser treatment. Among these options, cold knife incision is one of the most commonly used techniques, although optimal treatment remains controversial. While balloon dilation has also been used for managing VAS, previous studies have indicated that the outcomes of balloon dilation were poor, compared to those of alternative treatment modalities [6, 7]. We used the X Force® U30 balloon dilation catheter (Bard Medical Division), which can inflate up to 30 standard atmosphere (ATM). It provides sufficient dilation against even a severe VAS compared to conventional catheters. Therefore in this study, we assessed the efficacy of performing high

* Correspondence: ishiigen@gmail.com
[1] Atsugi City Hospital, 1-16-36 Mizuhiki, zip 243-8588 Atsugi City, Kanagawa, Japan
Full list of author information is available at the end of the article

pressure balloon dilation of VASs that occur in patients following RP.

## Methods

The study was approved by Atsugi City Hospital's review board, and written informed consent was obtained from all patients. Data from 128 consecutive patients who had undergone open RP for clinically localized prostate cancer were enrolled between 2008 and 2013. Patients who complained of voiding difficulties (n = 10, 7.8 %) subsequently developed a VAS, and the presence of which was confirmed endoscopically in all cases (Fig. 1). All patients were treated with transurethral balloon dilation for VAS.

At the time of open RP, bladder reconstruction and eversion of the bladder mucosa had been performed as routine techniques, and vesicourethral anastomosis was performed using four interrupted sutures. Descriptive characteristics of the study population are shown in Table 1. In two cases, TURP was performed prior to RP. The median blood loss during RP was 1,387 mL, and five patients (50 %) had excessive bleeding (>1.5 L). Prolonged urinary leakage at the site of anastomosis occurred in 1 case. All the patients could void with a decent stream at the time of urethral catheter removal. None of the patients had suspected local recurrence of prostate cancer, but two who had extra prostatic extension (EPE) with resection margin (RM) received adjuvant radiotherapy for the prostate region.

Transurethral balloon dilation was performed under regional anesthesia. We used a high pressure balloon catheter, the X Force®, which consists of a 6-French (Fr) open lumen, blunt-tip catheter, and 6-cm long balloon that inflates fully to 30 Fr at a maximum inflation pressure of 30 ATM. A 10-mL Eagle inflation device was also used.

After confirming the presence of VAS via endoscopy, a guide wire was inserted beyond the stricture under fluoroscopic guidance. The guide wire was inserted into the bladder before the dilation catheter was advanced over the guide wire into the bladder. The dilation catheter was positioned in the middle of the VAS, overlapping the normal urethra and likely including the external urethral sphincter. The balloon was inflated to 30 ATM pressure for 5 minutes, using pure contrast medium so that dilation of the VAS could be visualized (Fig. 2). Balloon dilation was performed three times with an interval period of 1 minute. After the procedure, a transurethral 16-Fr Foley catheter was placed until the following day.

Follow-up was performed via endoscopy. In patients with recurrent stricture, a second dilation procedure was performed. Recurrence of the stricture and the incidence

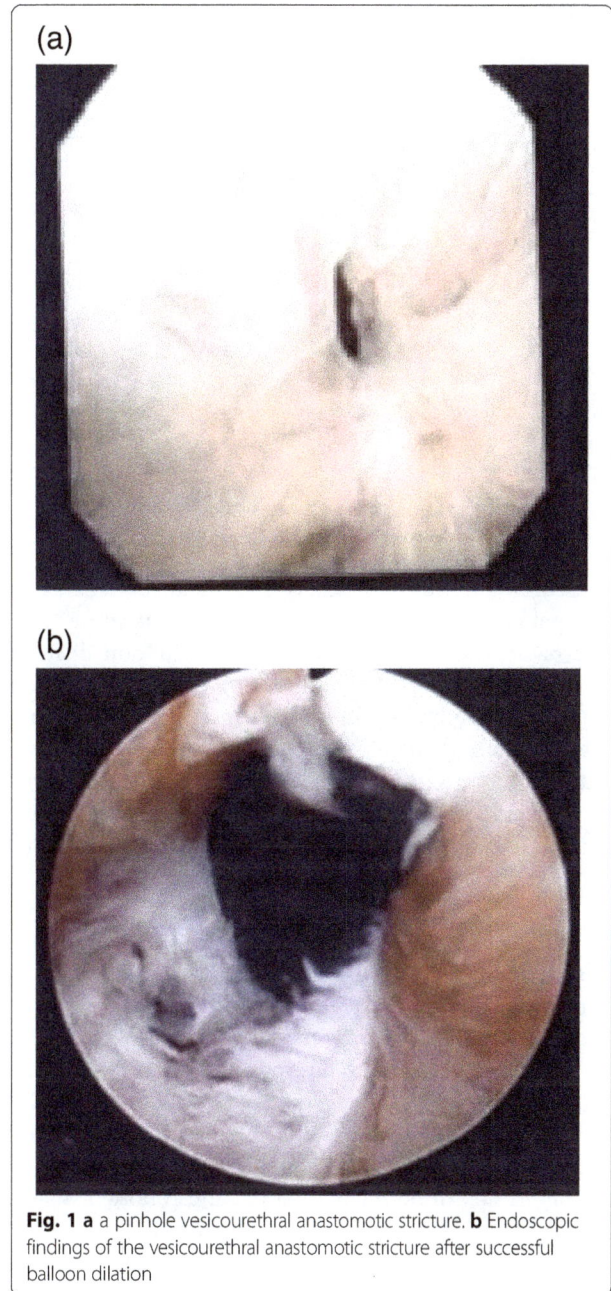

**Fig. 1 a** a pinhole vesicourethral anastomotic stricture. **b** Endoscopic findings of the vesicourethral anastomotic stricture after successful balloon dilation

of complications, particularly incontinence, were evaluated retrospectively.

## Results

The mean time from RP to the diagnosis of VAS was 9 months (range, 2–40 months) (Table 2), and eight patients (80 %) were diagnosed within 6 months after RP. Balloon dilation of VAS was technically successful in all patients, and no perioperative complications were recorded. All the patients were able to void spontaneously after the transurethral catheter was removed.

**Table 1** Demographic characters of patients with vesicourethral strictures (VAS) after radical prostatectomy (RP)

| | |
|---|---|
| No. of Patient | 10 |
| Age (median) | 70 (61–75) |
| Prior TURP | 2 |
| Gleason score | |
| 6 | 3 |
| 7 | 6 |
| unknown | 1 |
| EPE | 2 |
| RM | 2 |
| Blood loss at the time of RP (median) | 1387 (775–3780) |
| Adjuvant radiotherapy | 2 |

Urinary continence before balloon dilation was controlled by only using a safety pad in all patients, but one patient complained about having to use more than one pads. The median follow-up after balloon dilation was 24 months (7–67 months). Eight patients (80 %) were successfully treated, without recurrence, following the first balloon dilation procedure. In the remaining 2 patients, recurrence of the stricture necessitated a repeat balloon dilation procedure, which was performed within 6 months of the initial dilation. No patient required > 2 balloon dilations.

## Discussion

Worldwide, open RP is performed as a standard procedure for organ-confined prostate cancer. VAS is one of the most common complications after open RP, although rates of VAS development vary widely [1, 2]. Occasionally, VAS can be associated with severe voiding dysfunction, and consequently a deterioration in quality of life. In both laparoscopic and robotic assisted laparoscopic RP, there are lower incidences of VAS, in the ranging from 0–3 % [8–10]. While there is no definitive cause of VAS, it has been suggested that the suturing technique is the most important preventative aspect [10].

Numerous approaches are available for the managing VAS, and much has been published on the various procedures (Table 3). Simple dilation using catheters or bougies is often performed as the initial treatment modality; however, this is associated with high recurrence rates. Cold knife incision is the most commonly performed invasive procedure, with high success rates [7, 11]. More recently, new modalities using bipolar electrocautery or the holmium YAG laser have been reported with acceptable efficacies [12, 13].

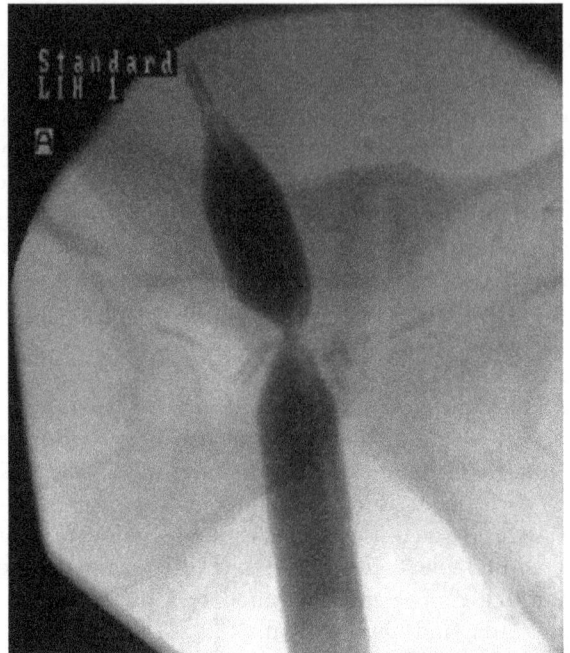

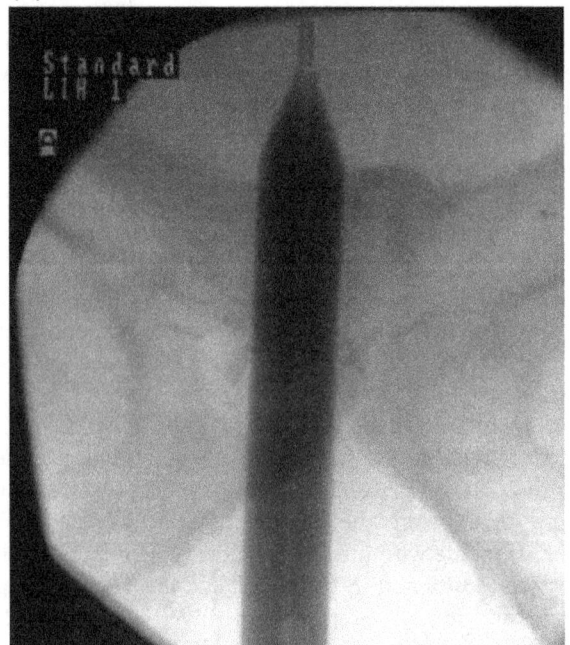

**Fig. 2 a** Fluoroscopic image demonstrates the concentric deformity in the balloon at the site of the vesicourethral anastomotic stricture. **b** No deformity is noted in the balloon after dilation with high pressure inflation

Transurethral balloon dilation is an established method of treatment for urethral stricture. The radial application of forces dilates the stricture, while avoiding

**Table 2** Time from radical prostatectomy to stricture and the outcomes following high pressure balloon dilation

| Patient | VAS occurrence after RP (months) | No. of Stricture recurrences | Time to the first recurrence (months) | Follow up | Recurrence at the time of the last follow up | No. of pad (/day) pre dilation | No. of pads (/day) post dilation |
|---|---|---|---|---|---|---|---|
| 1 | 6 | 1 | 5 | 67 | - | 1 | 5 |
| 2 | 6 | 1 | 3 | 53 | - | 0 | 0 |
| 3 | 3 | - | - | 31 | - | 0 | 0 |
| 4 | 3 | - | - | 31 | - | 0 | 0 |
| 5 | 3 | - | - | 27 | - | 1 | 1 |
| 6 | 4 | - | - | 20 | - | 1 | 1 |
| 7 | 40 | - | - | 16 | - | 1 | 1 |
| 8 | 4 | - | - | 14 | - | 1 | 1 |
| 9 | 2 | - | - | 22 | - | 0 | 0 |
| 10 | 22 | - | - | 7 | - | 0 | 0 |

the potentially traumatic shearing forces associated with sequential rigid dilation. Although transurethral balloon dilation has been performed for VAS previously, there are limited data regarding the outcomes in comparison to other modalities. Ramchandani et al. reported a recurrence rate of 41 %. In their series, the balloon of the dilation catheter did not expand completely [6].

We used a new urethral balloon catheter that achieves sufficient dilation against a more severe VAS using high pressure of up to 30 ATM. However, it is unclear whether a higher pressure of balloon dilation is more effective than conventional balloon dilation.

In the present study, balloon dilation was associated with a high success rate (80 %), and recurrent strictures could be controlled by performing repeated balloon dilation. However no patients required further treatment. Such findings are comparable to those associated with cold knife incision, which is considered the standard management for VAS.

Transurethral balloon dilation is simpler and less invasive than cold knife incision. Balloon dilation also has the advantage of a lower risk of urethral vascular injury. There is a wide range of complications associated with cold knife incision. Perineal hematoma and urethral hemorrhage are the most common complications ranging up to 20 % [15], and also de novo incontinence as a result of VAS has an incidence of 75 % [7].

However, no complications were reported in our study, except for worsened urinary incontinence in one patient (10 %).

Although our study was limited by the small number of patients and relatively short follow-up duration, dilation using this new high pressure balloon catheter appears to be an effective and minimally invasive treatment for VAS.

## Conclusion

Although balloon dilation for VAS has been performed previously, it was believed to have a low efficacy. We demonstrated excellent short-term results by using this new catheter, which can be inflated to a higher pressure than standard balloon catheters. High pressure balloon dilation appears to be a viable option for the managing VAS secondary to RP.

**Table 3** Managing vesicourethral anastomotic strictures (VAS) following radical prostatectomy reported in the literature

| | management | cases | Recurrence rate | Follow up (month) |
|---|---|---|---|---|
| Giannarini et al., [7] | Cold knife incision | 43 | 26.0 % | 12 |
| Popken et al., [14] | Electricautery resection | 15 | 53.3 % | 12-72 |
| Brodak et al., [12] | Bipolar resection | 22 | 9.0 % | 14-72 |
| Lagerveld et al., [13] | Holmium YAG laser | 10 | 0 % | 3-29 |
| Ramchandani et al., [6] | Conventional balloon dilation | 27 | 41.0 % | 1-84 |
| Present study | High pressure balloon dilation | 10 | 20.0 % | 7-67 |

## Abbreviations

VAS: Vesicourethral anastomotic stricture; RP: Radical prostatectomy; ATM: Atmosphere; TURP: Transurethral resection of the prostate; EPE: Extra prostatic extension; RM: Resection margin.

## Competing interests

The authors declare that they have no competing interests.

## Authors' contributions

GI, KH and MS have made conception, design and analysis of data. GI, TN, KK, and HO have made acquisition of data. TK and SE reviewed the manuscript critically. All authors approved the final version of the manuscript.

## Acknowledgements

No sources of funding have to be declared.

## Author details

[1]Atsugi City Hospital, 1-16-36 Mizuhiki, zip 243-8588 Atsugi City, Kanagawa, Japan.
[2]Jikei University School of Medicine, 3-25-8 Nishishinbashi minato-ku, zip 105-8461 Tokyo, Japan.

## References

1. Besarani D, Amoroso P, Kirby R. Bladder neck contracture after radical retropubic prostatectomy. BJU Int. 2004;94:1245–7.
2. Augustin H, Pummer K, Daghofer F, Habermann H, Primus G, Hubmer G. Patient self-reporting questionnaire on urological morbidity and bother after radical retropubic prostatectomy. Eur Urol. 2002;42(2):112–7.
3. Berlin JW, Ramchandani P, Banner MP, Pollack HM, Nodine CF, Wein AJ. Voiding cystourethrography after radical prostatectomy: Normal finding and correlation between contrast extravasation and anastomotic strictures. AJR Am J Roentgenol. 1994;162:87–91.
4. Surya BV, Provet J, Johanson K-E, Brown J. Anastomotic strictures following radical prostatectomy: Risk factors and management. J Urol. 1990;143:755–8.
5. Shelfo SW, Obek C, Soloway MS. Update on bladder neck preservation during radical retropubic prostatectomy: Impact on pathologic outcome, anastomotic strictures, and incontinence. Urol. 1998;51:73–8.
6. Ramchandani P, Banner MP, Berlin JW, Dannebaum MS, Wein AJ. Vesicourethral anastomotic strictures after radical prostatectomy: efficacy of transurethral balloon dilation. Radiology. 1994;193(2):345–9.
7. Giannarini G, Manassero F, Mogorovich A. Cold-knife incision of anastomotic strictures after radical retropubic prostatectomy with bladder neck preservation: Efficacy and impact on urinary continence status. Eur Urol. 2008;54:647–56.
8. Msezane LP, Reynolds WS, Gofrit ON, Shalhav AL, Zagaja GP, Zorn KC. Bladder neck contracture after robot-assisted laparoscopic radical prostatectomy: evaluation of incidence, risk factors, and impact on urinary function. J Endourol. 2008;22:97–104.
9. Guillonneau B, Vallancien G. Laparoscopic radical prostatectomy: the Montsouris experience. J Urol. 2000;163:418–22.
10. Webb DR, Sethi K, Gee K. An analysis of the causes of bladder neck contracture after open and robot-assisted laparoscopic radical prostatectomy. BJU Int. 2009;103:957–63.
11. Yukanin JP, Dalken BL, Cui H. Evaluation of cold knife urethrotomy for treatment of anastomotic stricture after radical retropubic prostatectomy. J Urol. 2001;165:1545–8.
12. Brodak M, Kosina J, Pacovsky J, Navrati P, Holub L. Bipolar transurethral resection of anastomotic strictures after radical prostatectomy. J Endourol. 2010;24:1477–81.
13. Lagerveld BW, Laguna MP, Debruyne FM, De La Rosette JJ. Holmium YAG laser for treatment of strictures of vesicourethral anastomosis after radical prostatectomy. J Endourol. 2005;19:497–501.
14. Popken G, Sommerkamp H, Schultze-Seemann W, Wetterauer U, Katzenwadal A. Anastomotic stricture after radical prostatectomy. Incidence, findings and treatment. Eur Urol. 1998;33(4):382–6.
15. Naudé AM, Heyns CF. What is the place of internal urethrotomy in the treatment of urethral stricture disease? Nat Clin Pract Urol. 2005;2(11):538–45.

# 8

# Evaluating the safety of intraoperative instillation of intravesical chemotherapy at the time of nephroureterectomy

Michael A. Moriarty, Matthew A. Uhlman[†], Megan T. Bing, Michael A. O'Donnell, James A. Brown, Chad R. Tracy, Sundeep Deorah, Kenneth G. Nepple and Amit Gupta[*]

## Abstract

**Background:** Urothelial carcinoma (UC) is a common cancer affecting many patients in the United States. Nephroureterectomy remains the gold standard for the treatment of high grade upper tract disease or low grade tumors that are not amenable to endoscopic management. Recent reports have shown a decrease in UC recurrence in patients who underwent nephroureterectomy and who had Mitomycin C (MMC) instilled into the bladder at the time of catheter removal. At our institution instillation of intravesical MMC at the time of nephroureterectomy has been common for more than 10 years. Given the recent data, we sought to formally describe our experience with and evaluate the safety of intravesical instillation of cytotoxic chemotherapy at the time of nephroureterectomy.

**Methods:** We retrospectively reviewed 51 patients who underwent intraoperative intravesical instillation of cytotoxic chemotherapy (MMC ($n = 48$) or adriamycin ($n = 3$)) at the time of nephroureterectomy (2000–2012). The procedure was performed in a similar fashion by 8 different surgeons from the same institution, with drainage of the bladder prior to management of the bladder cuff. Patient characteristics and perioperative data including complications out to 90 days after surgery were collected. Perioperative complications for all patients were graded using the modified Clavien-Dindo classification.

**Results:** Twenty-four men and 27 women underwent intraoperative intravesical instillation of cytotoxic chemotherapy at the time of nephroureterectomy. Median age at the time of operation was 74 years (range 48–88). Median dwell time was 60 min. Twenty three patients had a total of 45 perioperative complications. The majority (36/45) were Clavien grades I and II. No patients experienced any intraoperative or postoperative complications attributable to MMC or Adriamycin instillation.

**Conclusion:** Intraoperative intravesical instillation of cytotoxic chemotherapy at the time of nephroureterectomy is safe and feasible. Multicenter trials to study the efficacy of early cytotoxic chemotherapy administration to prevent recurrence of bladder urothelial carcinoma following nephroureterectomy are warranted.

**Keywords:** Carcinoma, Intravesical chemotherapy, Intraoperative mitomycin C, Nephroureterectomy, Urothelial carcinoma

* Correspondence: amit-gupta-1@uiowa.edu
†Equal contributors
Department of Urology, University of Iowa, 200 Hawkins Drive, 3RCP, Iowa City, IA 52242, USA

## Background

Urothelial carcinoma of the bladder is the sixth most common cancer affecting patients in the United States [1]. The majority of urothelial carcinomas are found in the bladder, but upper tract disease accounts for approximately 5–10 % of urothelial carcinomas [2, 3]. Nephroureterectomy is the standard treatment for high grade upper tract disease or low grade tumors that are not amenable to endoscopic management [4]. However, the recurrence rate for urothelial carcinoma in the bladder is still high, with reports ranging from 25 % to nearly 70 % [5–11]. While some recurrence may be due to a field effect, it has been hypothesized that recurrence in the bladder may be due to implantation of sloughed neoplastic cells from the upper tract. This hypothesis is supported by several molecular studies showing matching molecular markers and DNA sequence changes in upper tract primaries and subsequent recurrences in the lower tract [12–16].

Strategies have been developed to prevent recurrence of urothelial carcinoma. Early during nephroureterectomy the ureter can be clipped to prevent tumor migration with kidney manipulation. Additionally, intravesical therapy has been utilized [10, 11]. Intravesical instillation of mitomycin C (MMC) after transurethral resection of bladder tumor (TURBT) has been shown to reduce recurrence of urothelial carcinoma in the bladder in several studies and is the current standard of care in the USA and Europe [17, 18]. More recently, 2 randomized studies have looked at the effect of intravesical MMC instillation on urothelial carcinoma recurrence in the bladder following nephroureterectomy. The ODMIT-C trial, a multicenter randomized trial, demonstrated a decrease in bladder recurrence in patients who received a single dose of intravesical MMC at various times postoperatively prior to catheter removal [10]. Another smaller randomized controlled study showed similar decreases in recurrence with a 30-min intravesical instillation of pirarubicin (THP) performed within 48 h after nephroureterectomy [11]. In that study, the 36 patients who received THP and were analyzed for recurrences had a lower risk of bladder recurrence in comparison to the non-treatment group.

A common theme between these studies was that instillation of the cytotoxic agent was performed days to weeks following surgery. This delay in instillation was due to concerns for spillage into the surgical field if given intraoperatively or extravasation of the cytotoxic agent from the bladder if given postoperatively before the bladder has healed. However, it is known that following bladder tumor resection MMC is most effective in preventing tumor implantation if given within 6 h of surgery [19, 20]. Hence, it is possible that intraoperative use of MMC at time of nephroureterectomy may be better than delayed instillation. To our knowledge, due to lack of safety data, no studies to date have examined the efficacy of intravesical instillation of MMC at the time of nephroureterectomy. This safety data would be critically relevant in the design of future prospective studies that evaluate earlier administration of intravesical chemotherapy.

## Methods

The University of Iowa Institutional Review Board approved this study prior to the retrospective identification and reviewing of patient records and has therefore been performed in accordance with the ethical standards laid down in the 1964 Declaration of Helsinki and its later amendments.

After receiving approval from the Institutional Review Board, we retrospectively identified and reviewed the records for 51 patients from 2000 to 2012 who had undergone nephroureterectomy and had received intravesical MMC or Adriamycin. Signed informed consent was obtained on all patients prior to surgery and included consent for instillation of MMC or Adriamycin. Given the retrospective nature of the study, it was determined that no additional informed consent was required to examine data. Adriamycin was utilized when MMC was in short supply nationally, which occurred sporadically from 2008 through 2012. Use of cytotoxic intravesical chemotherapy was based on surgeon preference.

For each patient, a two-way catheter was sterilely inserted into the bladder on the operative field at the beginning of the surgical procedure. After the bladder had been completely drained, MMC (40 mg MMC in 40 ml sterile water) was instilled into the bladder and the catheter was clamped. During times of MMC shortage, three patients received intraoperative intravesical Adriamycin (50 mg in 50 ml saline). The catheter was typically left clamped for one to two hours. Kidney and ureteral dissection were performed prior to bladder incision. Intraoperatively, we always attempted to clip or ligate the ureter distal to the cancer site as soon as possible. After one to two hours of dwell time, the catheter was unclamped and the cytotoxic chemotherapy was allowed to drain passively, well before the bladder was opened for distal ureterectomy. The catheter bag was then disposed as cytotoxic waste. The bladder was occasionally irrigated with saline at surgeon discretion. The technique of distal ureteral dissection was left to the discretion of the surgeon. They included cystotomy with an intravesical bladder cuff, extravesical incision of the ureter with a bladder cuff, distal ureterectomy and extravesical dissection of the ureter with an intramural ureterectomy. The majority of cases (30/51) were performed with an extravesical excision of the ureter with a bladder cuff.

Patient charts were reviewed and demographic and clinical data were carefully reviewed. Intraoperative and postoperative complications up to 90 days after surgery were recorded. All patients were seen at least twice within 90 days post operatively. Complications were graded according to the modified Clavien-Dindo grading system [21, 22], which scores deviations in normal postoperative care based on severity.

## Results

We identified 51 patients who received intraoperative intravesical chemotherapy during the study period. Demographic and clinical information presented in Table 1. The majority of patients (36/51) presented with gross hematuria and were smokers (39/51), with a median smoking history of 20 pack years. Median age at time of nephroureterectomy was 74 years. Twenty-eight of the 51 patients had a history of prior bladder cancer.

The median dwell time for the cytotoxic intravesical chemotherapy was 60 min (range 45–120 min). Both contained a dye such that any extravesical spillage could be identified at the time of surgery. There were no intraoperative complications related to MMC or Adriamycin instillation. Eight patients had intraoperative complications: ureteral transection prior to ureterectomy (1), incomplete bladder closure (1), bowel injury requiring resection (1), acute blood loss requiring transfusion (3), and iliac vein injury requiring repair (1). Intraoperative spillage of MMC into the surgical field was not experienced in any of the surgeries.

Postoperatively, there were a total of 45 complications in 23 patients (Table 2). Twenty-two patients had 0 complications, 7 had 1 complication, 11 had 2 complications, 4 had 3 complications and 1 had 4 complications. The majority of the complications were Clavien grades 1 or 2 (35/45). Grades 3 and 4 postoperative complications included one occurrence each of watershed cerebral infarct, myocardial infarction, respiratory failure requiring ventilation, foley catheter occlusion with clots requiring irrigation, reoperation due to bleeding, acute renal failure requiring dialysis, SICU transfer due to septic shock and urinoma requiring drain placement. There were no complications resulting in prolonged or chronic disability. Notably, the patient who experienced a bladder leak requiring drain placement had no symptoms or signs of peritonitis. No patients experienced any postoperative complications directly attributable to MMC or Adriamycin instillation such as severe or chronic pelvic pain or chemical peritonitis. The median length of stay was 4.0 days (range 2–21 days).

## Discussion

Intravesical MMC has been a standard of care for the treatment of bladder cancer for over 30 years. As an extension of that use, physicians at various centers have

**Table 1** Demographic and clinical characteristics of study patients

| Variable | | Number |
|---|---|---|
| Patient Sex | | |
| | Male | 24 |
| | Female | 27 |
| Median Age, yrs (range) | | 74 (48–88) |
| Smoking status | | |
| | Smoker (Current or Past) | 39 |
| | Non-smoker | 12 |
| Pathological Stage after Nephroureterectomy | | |
| | Ta | 14 |
| | Tis | 2 |
| | T1 | 13 |
| | T2 | 7 |
| | T3 | 15 |
| Pathologic Grade after Nephroureterectomy | | |
| | LG | 16 |
| | HG | 34 |
| | Not Reported | 1 |
| Distal Ureter Handling | | |
| | Cystotomy with intravesical bladder cuff | 9 |
| | Extravesical incision of ureter with bladder cuff | 30 |
| | Distal ureterectomy | 9 |
| | Extravesical dissection of ureter with intramural ureterectomy | 3 |

**Table 2** Severity of post-operative complications

| | | |
|---|---|---|
| Total number of complications | | 45 |
| Complications due to MMC Instillation | | 0 |
| Complication Severity | | |
| | Clavien Grade | |
| | I | 20 |
| | II | 16 |
| | IIIa | 2 |
| | IIIb | 1 |
| | IV-a | 5 |
| | IV-b | 1 |
| | V | 0 |

also administered it intravesically at the onset of performing radical cystectomy or nephro-ureterectomy and then draining the bladder roughly 60 min later, prior to more formal bladder manipulation. This has been our standard clinical practice for more than 15 years and as such was incorporated into our standard operative consent. It was only later that we realized this practice was not uniformly applied elsewhere and, as such, we obtained appropriate IRB approval to perform this retrospective study.

In this study of 51 patients, intraoperative instillation of intravesical cytotoxic therapy at the time of nephroureterectomy was found to be safe. None of the patients experienced any adverse events directly attributable to MMC instillation either intraoperatively or postoperatively. This study provides safety data in support of a prospective trial designed to assess the efficacy of earlier intravesical chemotherapy in the prevention of bladder tumors after nephroureterectomy. Recent studies have found that without the administration of adjuvant postoperative intravesical therapy, the bladder urothelial carcinoma recurrence rate is approximately 25–70 % [10, 11] at median follow-up of 12–45 months. Two randomized studies have shown that in patients with upper tract urothelial carcinoma, postoperative intravesical instillation of a single dose of a cytotoxic agent such as MMC or THP decreases recurrence of bladder urothelial carcinoma. However, in these studies the intravesical cytotoxic agent was administered 2 days to a few weeks after the nephroureterectomy. The ODMIT-C trial was a multicenter phase III study that randomized 284 patients to MMC and control [10]. MMC was administered a median of 7 days after nephroureterectomy, at the time of catheter removal. At one year, there was a 10 % absolute and 40 % relative decrease in the risk of recurrence in the bladder with instillation of MMC. Ito et al. conducted a randomized phase II trial of single-dose intravesical instillation of THP that was administered within 48 h of surgery [11]. This trial randomized 77 patients and found an absolute decrease of 14.9 % and

25.3 % at one and two years, respectively. Interestingly, in both studies the absolute incidence of bladder tumors in the treatment arm was about 16 %, with a number needed to treat of 9 in the ODMIT trial. For patients with bladder urothelial carcinoma, studies have shown the instillation of MMC reduces recurrence rates when administered within 6 h of surgery, but not when it is instilled greater than 24 h after surgery [23–25]. In fact, one randomized controlled trial demonstrated that pre-TURBT electromotive instillation of MMC was superior to post-TURBT MMC. [26].

Hence, it is entirely plausible that the efficacy of MMC in preventing recurrence of the urothelial carcinoma in the bladder may be higher if MMC is administered during or immediately after nephroureterectomy rather than several days later.

Immediate postoperative instillation of MMC in the bladder after TURBT has been shown to be safe even in the setting of tumor resection and some element of continued bleeding, so it is not surprising that our experience with instillation and immediate drainage was not associated with any adverse effects.

In the ODMIT-C trial, the timing of instillation was delayed due to concern for extravasation of MMC into the pelvis from the bladder [10]. Within the THP monotherapy study group trial, administration of intravesical chemotherapy was within 48 h of surgery [11]. The group did not mention the reason for choosing this particular time for instillation, but did note that the bladder cuff resection was performed in an open fashion so as to assure the wall was tightly sutured. In theory, this timing of administration might have decreased the efficacy of these agents.

Despite evidence from these 2 randomized studies [10], postoperative intravesical instillation of MMC at the time of catheter removal has not become standard practice. The reasons for this lack of dissemination and implementation are not known and are likely multi-factorial. Even after TURBT, when safety and efficacy rates are known to be high, the utilization of a single postoperative dose of mitomycin has been reported to be as low as 38 % [27]. One contributing factor may be that intravesical instillation is not built into the workflow of the typical postoperative course, and in many cases may require the patient to return to the clinic after hospital discharge. When patients return for follow-up and catheter removal, the clinic encounter is likely to be focused on the patient's symptoms and discussion of the pathology report, prognosis and treatment plan. Additional barriers such as the need for timely coordination with the pharmacy, biohazard precautions and the requirement for specialized nursing may make the administration of MMC less likely. Therefore, it is plausible that by standardizing the administration of MMC intraoperatively and engaging the urologic team directly, it may increase the probability of patients receiving this therapy.

At our institution, a number of physicians (8 over the last 12 years) have instilled cytotoxic chemotherapy in the bladder at the time of nephroureterectomy. To the best of our knowledge, we are the first to report on the safety of this approach. Our experience with 51 patients has been a highly positive one. All patients tolerated the instillation without issue and no intra or postoperative complications related to cytotoxic chemotherapy occurred. A larger prospective study would provide greater reliability on the safety of this approach as well as more reliable data in regard to its efficacy, which theoretically could be better than the previously described randomized studies.

There are number of limitations that should be addressed. Our review included data from 51 patients who underwent nephroureterectomy from 2000 to 2012 and included 28 patients who had a prior history of bladder cancer. As such, time to recurrence of bladder cancer is not meaningful and efficacy cannot be studied in this cohort. Additionally, a retrospective review of complications may underestimate the number of complications that occurred; however, our data are comparable to a number of previous reports and highlight the relatively low but significant percentage of Clavien grades 3 and 4 complications. Second, the handling of the distal ureter was left to the discretion of the surgereon, though the majority of cases (30/51) involved an extravesical excision of the ureter along with a bladder cuff. Next, there are currently no data on the efficacy of intraoperative intravesical cytotoxic chemotherapy for upper tract urothelial carcinoma, though extrapolation from TURBT data may be appropriate. This does, however, highlight an important reminder from our study – the rarity of upper tract urothelial carcinoma and the inherent difficulty in studying a rare disease. The majority of our patients had a prior history of bladder cancer, whereas to study the efficacy of an intravesical agent, a cohort of patients without prior bladder cancer is needed. Thus, given the rarity of the disease, and our findings demonstrating that intraoperative instillation of intravesical cytotoxic chemotherapy is safe, multicenter prospective trials are needed to determine whether this approach is effective in preventing recurrence of urothelial carcinoma in the bladder following nephroureterectomy. This data provides important preliminary safety data in support of such a trial.

## Conclusion

Intraoperative, intravesical instillation of cytotoxic chemotherapy at the time of nephroureterectomy is safe and feasible. Multicenter clinical trials to study the efficacy of this approach to prevent recurrence of bladder urothelial carcinoma are warranted.

## Abbreviations

UC: Urothelial Carcinoma; MMC: Mitomycin C; TURBT: Transurethral resection of bladder tumor; THP: Pirarubicin.

## Competing interests

The authors declare that they have no competing interests.

## Author's contributions

MM participated in project design and development, data collection/management, and manuscript writing/editing. MU participated in project design and development, data collection/management, data analysis, and manuscript writing/editing. MB participated in project design and development, and manuscript writing/editing. MO participated in project design and development, and manuscript writing/editing. JB participated in project design and development, and manuscript writing/editing. CT participated in project design and development, and manuscript writing/editing. SD participated in project design and development, and manuscript writing/editing. KN participated in project design and development, and manuscript writing/editing. AG participated in project design and development, data collection/management, data analysis, and manuscript writing/editing. All authors read, edited and approved the final version of the manuscript.

## Acknowledgements

We would like to acknowledge Dr. Surena F Matin (Dept. of Urology, MD Anderson Cancer Center, Houston, TX) for his critical insight and suggetions in refining the manuscript. No authors received any external funding for the present study.

## References

1. Howlader N, Noone AM, Krapcho M, et al. SEER Cancer Statistics Review, 1975-2010, National Cancer Institute. Bethesda, MD, http://seer.cancer.gov/csr/1975_2010/, based on November 2012 SEER data submission, posted to the SEER web site, April 2013. Accessed May 10, 2013.
2. Raman JD, Messer J, Sielatycki JA, Hollenbeak CS. Incidence and survival of patients with carcinoma of the ureter and renal pelvis in the USA, 1973–2005. BJU Int. 2011;107:1059–64.
3. Siegel R, Naishadham D, Jemal A. Cancer statistics, 2013. CA Cancer J Clin. 2013;63:11–30.
4. Roupret M, Babjuk M, Comperat E, et al. European guidelines on upper tract urothelial carcinomas: 2013 update. Eur Urol. 2013;63:1059–71.
5. Terakawa T, Miyake H, Muramaki M, Takenaka A, Hara I, Fujisawa M. Risk factors for intravesical recurrence after surgical management of transitional cell carcinoma of the upper urinary tract. Urology. 2008;71:123–7.
6. Racioppi M, D'Addessi A, Alcini A, Destito A, Alcini E. Clinical review of 100 consecutive surgically treated patients with upper urinary tract transitional tumours. Br J Urol. 1997;80:707–11.
7. Matsui Y, Utsunomiya N, Ichioka K, et al. Risk factors for subsequent development of bladder cancer after primary transitional cell carcinoma of the upper urinary tract. Urology. 2005;65:279–83.
8. Raman JD, Ng CK, Boorjian SA, Vaughan Jr ED, Sosa RE, Scherr DS. Bladder cancer after managing upper urinary tract transitional cell carcinoma: predictive factors and pathology. BJU Int. 2005;96:1031–5.
9. Cha EK, Shariat SF, Kormaksson M, et al. Predicting clinical outcomes after radical nephroureterectomy for upper tract urothelial carcinoma. Eur Urol. 2012;61:818–25.
10. O'Brien T, Ray E, Singh R, Coker B, Beard R. British association of urological surgeons section of O. Prevention of bladder tumours after nephroureterectomy for primary upper urinary tract urothelial carcinoma: a prospective, multicentre, randomised clinical trial of a single postoperative Intravesical dose of mitomycin C (the ODMIT-C trial). Eur Urol. 2011;60:703–10.
11. Ito A, Shintaku I, Satoh M, et al. Prospective randomized phase II trial of a single early Intravesical instillation of pirarubicin (THP) in the prevention of bladder recurrence after nephroureterectomy for upper urinary tract urothelial carcinoma: the THP Monotherapy study group trial. J Clin Oncol. 2013;31:1422–7.
12. Lunec J, Challen C, Wright C, Mellon K, Neal DE. c-erbB-2 amplification and identical p53 mutations in concomitant transitional carcinomas of renal pelvis and urinary bladder. Lancet. 1992;339:439–40.
13. Habuchi T, Takahashi R, Yamada H, Kakehi Y, Sugiyama T, Yoshida O. Metachronous multifocal development of urothelial cancers by intraluminal seeding. Lancet. 1993;342:1087–8.

14. Sidransky D, Frost P, Von Eschenbach A, Oyasu R, Preisinger AC, Vogelstein B. Clonal origin bladder cancer. N Engl J Med. 1992;326:737–40.

15. Li M, Cannizzaro LA. Identical clonal origin of synchronous and metachronous low- grade, noninvasive papillary transitional cell carcinomas of the urinary tract. Hum Pathol. 1999;30:1197–200.

16. Fadl-Elmula I, Gorunova L, Mandahl N, et al. Cytogenetic monoclonality in multifocal uroepithelial carcinomas: evidence of intraluminal tumour seeding. Br J Cancer. 1999;81:6–12.

17. Perlis N ZA, Beyene J, Finelli A, Fleshner NE, and Kulkarni GS. Immediate Post–Transurethral Resection of Bladder Tumor Intravesical Chemotherapy Prevents Non– Muscle-invasive Bladder Cancer Recurrences: An Updated Meta-analysis on 2548 Patients and Quality-of-Evidence Review. Eur Urol. 2013;64(3):421–30.

18. Sylvester RJ, Oosterlinck W, van der Meijden AP. A single immediate postoperative instillation of chemotherapy decreases the risk of recurrence in patients with stage Ta T1 bladder cancer: a meta-analysis of published results of randomized clinical trials. J Urol. 2004;171:2186–90. quiz 435.

19. Tolley DA, Parmar MK, Grigor KM, et al. The effect of intravesical mitomycin C on recurrence of newly diagnosed superficial bladder cancer: a further report with 7 years of follow up. J Urol. 1996;155:1233–8.

20. Mostafid AH, Rajkumar RG, Stewart AB, Singh R. Immediate administration of intravesical mitomycin C after tumour resection for superficial bladder cancer. BJU Int. 2006;97:509–12.

21. Dindo D, Demartines N, Clavien PA. Classification of surgical complications: a new proposal with evaluation in a cohort of 6336 patients and results of a survey. Ann Surg. 2004;240:205–13.

22. Clavien PA, Sanabria JR, Strasberg SM. Proposed classification of complications of surgery with examples of utility in cholecystectomy. Surgery. 1992;111:518–26.

23. Sekine H, Fukui I, Yamada T, Ohwada F, Yokokawa M, Ohshima H. Intravesical mitomycin C and doxorubicin sequential therapy for carcinoma in situ of the bladder: a longer followup result. J Urol. 1994;151:27–30.

24. Solsona E, Iborra I, Ricos JV, Monros JL, Casanova J, Dumont R. Effectiveness of a single immediate mitomycin C instillation in patients with low risk superficial bladder cancer:short and long-term followup. J Urol. 1999;161:1120–3.

25. Duque JL, Loughlin KR. An overview of the treatment of superficial bladder cancer. Intravesical chemotherapy. Urol Clin North Am. 2000;27:125–35.

26. Di Stasi SM, Valenti M, Verri C, et al. Electromotive instillation of mitomycin immediately before transurethral resection for patients with primary urothelial non- muscle invasive bladder cancer: a randomised controlled trial. Lancet Oncol. 2011;12(9):871–9.

27. Barocas DA, Liu A, Burks FN, et al. Practice-based collaboration to improve the use of immediate intravesical therapy after resection for non-muscle-invasive bladder cancer. J Urol. 2013;190(6):2011–6.

# 9

# Utility of copeptin and standard inflammatory markers in the diagnostics of upper and lower urinary tract infections

Anna Masajtis-Zagajewska, Ilona Kurnatowska, Malgorzata Wajdlich and Michal Nowicki[*]

## Abstract

**Background:** A new serum marker of inflammation copeptin (CPP) a stable C-terminal pro-vasopressin was assessed along with conventional markers such as C-reactive protein (CRP), procalcitonin (PCT) and IL-6 to discriminate between lower and upper bacterial urinary tract infections (UTI).

**Methods:** Study population comprised 45 patients including 13 with lower UTI (L-UTI) and 32 with upper UTI (U-UTI) and 24 healthy controls. Serum markers, blood cultures and urine cultures were assessed before commencing antibiotic treatment and repeated 24, 48 h and 7 days thereafter. Receiver operating curves (ROC) were plotted to assess a diagnostic utility of different inflammatory markers.

**Results:** Before antibiotic therapy all inflammatory markers including serum CPP ($2821.1 \pm 1072.4$ pg/ml vs. $223.8 \pm 109.3$ pg/ml; $p < 0.05$) were higher in UTI than in controls. CPP was not different between L- and U-UTI ($2253 \pm 1323$ pg/ml vs $3051 \pm 1178$ pg/ml; $p = 0.70$) despite significant differences in hsCRP ($2.09 \pm 1.7$ mg/dl vs $127.3 \pm 62.4$ mg/dl; $p < 0.001$), PCT ($0.05 \pm 0$ vs $5.02 \pm 0.03$ ng/ml $p < 0.001$) and IL-6 ($22.5 \pm 1.6$ vs $84.8 \pm 67$ pg/ml $p < 0.001$). For U-UTI the areas under the ROC curves were 1.0 for both hsCRP and CPP, 0.94 for PCT and 0.7 for IL-6 and for L-UTI 0.571, 1, 0.505 and 0.73, respectively. After 7 days of treatment all markers decreased in parallel to clinical response.

**Conclusion:** Although elevated serum copeptin may become a marker of UTI it seems to be inferior compared to traditional serum inflammation markers for differentiation of bacterial infections involving upper and lower urinary tract.

**Keywords:** Copeptin, Urinary tract infection, Biomarker

## Background

Bacterial urinary tract infection (UTI) is the most common infection across all age groups. Although the part of the urinary tract involved, i.e., low or upper UTI needs to be quickly established this is not always possible if based on clinical symptoms only. Typically, clinical symptoms of lower (L-UTI) are dysuria, frequent and difficult or painful urination. In most cases clinical symptoms of upper UTI (U-UTI) are dominated by fever and side pain [1]. In the latter an accurate diagnosis and early treatment is crucial due to a risk of urosepsis and long-term consequences including chronic kidney disease

[2, 3]. The duration of therapy recommended for L-UTI is shorter compared to a complicated UTI that involves the kidneys [4]. Thus there is a need to quickly and reliably identify the biomarkers which could be used not only for diagnostic purposes but also to determine the severity and location of the infection inside the urinary tract.

Arginine vasopressin (AVP) is one of the key hormones of cardio-vascular homeostasis and is an important part of an endocrine stress response resulting in a release of adrenal steroids [5]. Despite its dominant role in cardio-vascular disease, the measurement and diagnostic application of vasopressin have never been found useful in clinical practice due to methodological problems caused by its short half-life, functional interactions with platelets in serum and small molecular size [6, 7].

Copeptin (CPP), is a 39-amino acid glycosylated peptide [8]. Vasopressin and copeptin are derived from the same precursor protein – pre-pro-vasopressin, composed of 164

* Correspondence: nefro@wp.pl
Department of Nephrology, Hypertension and Kidney Transplantation, University Hospital and Education Centre of the Medical University of Lodz, Pomorska 251, 92-213 Lodz, Poland

amino acids and consisting of single proteins: vasopressin, neurophysin II and copeptin [9]. Thus, copeptin is a C-terminal part of pro-vasopressin (CT-pro-AVP) and is released along with vasopressin. In contrast to vasopressin, copeptin is stable in serum or plasma in room temperature and it is relatively easy to measure [10, 11]. Several recent studies have investigated the usefulness of copeptin as a diagnostic and prognostic biomarker in several clinical conditions including the lower respiratory tract infections [12], septic shock [13], and stroke [14, 15]. To the best of our knowledge no study has systematically evaluated serum copeptin levels in both L-UTI and U-UTI. The study was carried out in order to assess the utility of a potential new serum inflammation marker copeptin in diagnosis of UTI compared to other inflammatory markers and to discriminate between lower and upper UTI.

## Methods
### Patients
The subjects for this single-center observational, prospective study were recruited from the patients manifesting symptoms of UTI who were consecutively admitted to our hospital from May 2011 through September 2012 and diagnosed with acute pyelonephritis, as well as among patients with symptoms of L-UTI who were treated in our outpatient department. The reference group included healthy subjects without any clinical and laboratory symptoms of infection. In all subjects from that group blood was taken to confirm that blood count and C-reactive protein level were within normal range. Also the urinalysis was carried out to confirm an absence of leukocyturia.

The diagnosis of UTI in the subjects from the study group was established on the basis of typical clinical symptoms and at least one positive urine culture. The inclusion criteria included the presence of acute symptoms like fever, flank pain (U-UTI) or pelvic pain (L-UTI), dysuria, urinary frequency and costo-vertebral angle tenderness (U-UTI), presence of pyuria. The exclusion criteria included the eGFR <30 ml/min/1.73 m$^3$, presence of any concomitant organ or systemic infection, any hospitalization or surgical procedure within last 3 months, history of renal transplant and any permanent complicating factors of urinary tract (including complete obstruction, suspected or confirmed prostatitis) which cannot be effectively treated during the therapy of the infection and ongoing or recent (within last 7 days) antibiotic therapy. The patients with negative urine bacterial cultures and male subjects with perineal or rectal pain and perineal tenderness during the physical examination were excluded.

The Ethics Committee of the Medical University of Lodz approved the study protocol. All the subjects provided a written informed consent.

### Biochemical parameters
The following biochemical parameters were obtained before commencing an antibiotic treatment and all measurements were repeated according to the fixed schedule after 24, 48 h and 7 days. They included complete blood count, C-reactive protein (hsCRP), procalcitonin (PCT), IL-6, serum sodium, potassium, creatinine and serum copeptin. Urine and blood cultures were assessed on admission and after seven days of antibiotic therapy.

Circulating levels of copeptin were measured using a commercial ELISA kit from USCN Life Science (Houston, USA). All other parameters were measured with standard laboratory automated methods.

### Statistical analysis
All results are expressed as means ± SD and as median +/− interquartile ratio (IQR). Data distribution was checked by Kolmogorov – Smirnov test. Within-group comparisons were performed using $t$-test or non-parametric Wilcoxon test. For categorical variables, chi-square test or Fisher exact test were used. The cutoff points of all markers to optimum performance for differentiating L-UTI and U-UTI were determined by plotting the Receiver Operating Characteristic (ROC) curves [16]. Statistical analysis was performed using Statistica for Windows (version 10PL, StatSoft, Tulsa, OK, USA).

## Results
No clinically relevant side effects prompting a change or withdrawal of antibiotic therapy were observed.

### Patients
The study group comprised 45 patients (31 female, 14 male, age 50 ± 20 years) including 13 with L-UTI (10 female, 3 male, age 61 ± 24 years) and 32 with U-UTI (21 female, 11 male, age 54 ± 11 years). From 49 patients that were initially screened 4 were later excluded because of negative urine cultures thus resulting in 45 patients taken into the final analysis. The reference group included 24 healthy subjects (17 female, 7 male, age mean 50 ± 20 years).

### Biochemical parameters
Table 1 shows the clinical and biochemical characteristics of the participants. Before the introduction of the antibiotic therapy in UTI patients serum inflammation markers such as: hsCRP (91.3 ± 86.5 mg/dl), PCT (3.7 ± 15.3 ng/ml) and IL-6 (66.8 ± 81.6 pg/ml) were all significantly higher than in healthy patients (3.5 ± 2.3 mg/dl, 0.06 ± 0.02 ng/ml and 3.1 ± 1.6 pg/ml, respectively, p < 0.05 for all comparisons. Serum copeptin levels were also significantly higher in patients with

**Table 1** Clinical and baseline biochemical characteristics of the study group with urinary tract infection (UTI) and control group

|  | UTI group (n = 45) | Control (n = 24) | P value |
|---|---|---|---|
| Sex |  |  |  |
| Men | 14 (31 %) | 7 (29 %) | NS |
| Women | 31 (69 %) | 17 (71 %) |  |
| Age (years) | 56 ± 10 | 50 ± 20 | NS |
|  | [64 (39)] | [48.5 (33)] |  |
| Creatinine (mg/dl) | 1.3 ± 0.3 | 1.0 ± 0.3 | NS |
|  | [1.2 (0.4)] | [1.0 (0.3)] |  |
| GFR (ml/min/1.73 m³) | 73.1 ± 22 | 84.2 ± 26 | NS |
|  | [72.6 (39.5)] | [91.9 (41.6)] |  |
| Leucocyte count (G/l) | 12.8 ± 6.7 | 6.4 ± 2.1 | <0.001 |
|  | [11.9 (6.9)] | [5.6 (3.3)] |  |
| hsCRP (mg/L) | 91.3 ± 86.5 | 3.5 ± 2.3 | <0.001 |
|  | [98.2 (132.5)] | [3.3 (2.5)] |  |
| Procalcitonin (ng/ml) | 3.7 ± 15.3 | 0.06 ± 0.02 | <0.001 |
|  | [0.12 (1.15)] | [0.05 (0)] |  |
| IL –6 (pg/ml) | 66.8 ± 81.6 | 3.1 ± 1.6 | <0.001 |
|  | [41.6 (92.3)] | [2.8 (2)] |  |
| Copeptin (pg/ml) | 2821 ± 1072 | 224 ± 109 | <0.001 |
|  | [874 (1527)] | [209 (141)] |  |

Results are expressed as mean ± SD [median (IQR)]

UTI than in the controls (2821 ± 1072 vs. 223 ± 109 pg/ml; p < 0.05).

There were significant differences in serum hsCRP, PCT and IL-6 between L-UTI and U-UTI, but no difference in serum copeptin was observed (Table 2). Table 3 shows the comparison of biochemical parameters assessed at the time of the admission to the hospital emergency room in patients with the diagnosis of U-UTI. Statistical significant differences of these parameters between study and reference group were observed. Table 4 shows the differences of serum inflammatory markers between L-UTI and reference group. Only IL-6 and CPP differed significantly between the groups.

On day 7 of antibiotic treatment, all serum markers including serum copeptin levels, with the exception of PCT, decreased significantly in patients with UTI along with the clinical response (Table 5). Copeptin levels did not completely return to normal range over the 7 days of treatment (2821 ± 1072 pg/ml on day 0 vs. 2003 ± 838 on day 7, p = 0.0001).

Receiver operating curves (ROC) were plotted to assess a diagnostic utility of inflammatory markers. As shown in Table 6 the biomarkers that best identified U-UTI were serum hsCRP and CPP followed by PCT and IL-6. In case of L-UTI the best performing biomarker was serum CPP followed by IL-6, hsCRP and PCT.

**Table 2** Comparison of biochemical parameters assessed at hospital admission in patients with diagnosis of lower and upper urinary tract infection (UTI)

|  | Lower UTI (n = 13) | Upper UTI (n = 32) | P value |
|---|---|---|---|
| Leucocyte count (G/l) | 8.6 ± 3.3 | 14.5 ± 5.9 | 0.005 |
|  | [7.4 (3.4)] | [12.7 (13.5)] |  |
| hsCRP (mg/L) | 2.9 ± 1.7 | 127.3 ± 62.4 | <0.001 |
|  | [2.28 (2.81)] | [132.5 (124.8)] |  |
| PCT (ng/ml) | 0.05 ± 0 | 5.2 ± 0.03 | <0.001 |
|  | [0.05 (0)] | [0.42 (0.9)] |  |
| IL –6 (pg/ml) | 22.5 ± 1.6 | 84.8 ± 67 | <0.001 |
|  | [5.8 (41.9)] | [57.9 (64.3)] |  |
| CPP (pg/ml) | 2253 ± 1323 | 3051 ± 1178 | Ns |
|  | [1757 (1403)] | [2929 (2986)] |  |

Results are expressed as mean ± SD [median (IQR)]

## Discussion

To date several studies have been conducted to confirm the hypothesis that copeptin, as a stress hormone, could also be a biomarker of several pathologic conditions including inflammation.

In our study a number of blood leucocytes, serum hsCRP, PCT, IL-6 and CPP significantly increased in patients with UTI compared to healthy subjects. However, trying to differentiate the patients with L-UTI from those with pyelonephritis serum copeptin unlike other inflammatory markers was not significantly different between these groups.

The value of the assessment of serum copeptin and other inflammatory markers in the diagnosis and differentiating between U- from L-UTI was also established by plotting the ROC curves. The area under the ROC

**Table 3** Comparison of biochemical parameters assessed at hospital admission in patients with diagnosis upper urinary tract infection (U-UTI) and control group

|  | Upper UTI (n = 32) | Control (n = 24) | P value |
|---|---|---|---|
| Leucocyte count (G/l) | 14.5 ± 5.9 | 6.43 ± 2.1 | <0.001 |
|  | [12.7 (13.5)] | [5.6 (3.3)] |  |
| hsCRP (mg/L) | 127.3 ± 62.4 | 3.5 ± 2.3 | <0.001 |
|  | [132.5 (124.8)] | [3.3 (2.5)] |  |
| PCT (ng/ml) | 5.2 ± 0.03 | 0.06 ± 0.02 | <0.001 |
|  | [0.42 (0.9)] | [0.05 (0)] |  |
| IL –6 (pg/ml) | 84.8 ± 67 | 3.1 ± 1.6 | <0.001 |
|  | [57.9 (64.3)] | [2.8 (2)] |  |
| CPP (pg/ml) | 3051 ± 1178 | 224 ± 109 | <0.001 |
|  | [2929 (2986)] | [209 (141)] |  |

Results are expressed as mean ± SD [median (IQR)]

**Table 4** Comparison of biochemical parameters assessed at hospital admission in patients with diagnosis lower urinary tract infection (L-UTI) and control group

|  | Lower UTI (n = 13) | Control (n = 24) | P value |
|---|---|---|---|
| Leucocyte count (G/l) | 8.6 ± 3.3 [7.4 (3.4)] | 6.43 ± 2.1 [5.6 (3.3)] | NS |
| hsCRP (mg/L) | 2.9 ± 1.7 [2.28 (2.81)] | 3.5 ± 2.3 [3.3 (2.5)] | NS |
| PCT (ng/ml) | 0.05 ± 0 [0.05 (0)] | 0.06 ± 0.02 [0.05 (0)] | NS |
| IL –6 (pg/ml) | 22.5 ± 1.6 [5.8 (41.9)] | 3.1 ± 1.6 [2.8 (2)] | <0.001 |
| CPP (pg/ml) | 2253 ± 1323 [1757 (1403)] | 224 ± 109 [209 (141)] | <0.001 |

Results are expressed as mean ± SD [median (IQR)]

curve of copeptin was equal in lower and upper urinary tract infection. It seems therefore that the measurement of serum copeptin seems to less clinically useful than the estimation of serum CRP and PCT to distinguish between L- and U-UTI.

Several earlier studies have investigated serum copeptin levels in different acute disorders. Serum copeptin was significantly higher in patients with lower respiratory system infection in comparison to healthy persons, with the highest level observed in patients with the community acquired pneumonia [12]. The patients with positive blood cultures had higher copeptin levels than patients with negative blood cultures. All our patients with UTI had positive urine cultures but negative blood cultures that did not allow the direct comparison of our results with the study of Muller et al. [12] that investigated the patients with more severe systemic infections.

Morgenthaler et al. assessed serum copeptin levels in patients with septic shock [13]. Increased copeptin was

observed at time of hospital admission, including patients with different severity of sepsis compared with healthy control. Mean baseline serum copeptin was higher in patients who survived sepsis in comparison to those who died. Fluri at al. [14] performed the study comparing inflammatory markers and copeptin levels in patients suffering from stroke as early predictors for the development of post-stroke infection [14]. Serum procalcitonin, hsCRP, copeptin and leukocyte number were assessed as well as markers of pneumonia, UTI and other systemic infections. In that study mean levels of copeptin, CRP and number of leukocytes in blood in patients with UTI were similar to those with pneumonia and other infections with the exception of procalcitonin level that was lower in the former. In the patients with L-UTI in our study, increased levels of copeptin and IL-6 were observed but no other serum markers significantly differed from control group. That was not the case in patient with pyelonephritis, in whom serum levels of all markers were significantly higher compared to controls. Fluri et al. [14] concluded that copeptin, procalcitonin, CRP and number of blood leukocytes were good serum inflammatory markers in pneumonia and UTI however he did not divide their patients into L- and U-UTI. They also postulated that a combination of markers, including copeptin may be more helpful when making the decision about introducing a prophylactic antibiotic in patients with high risk of infection [14].

Copeptin levels were also measured in several studies performed in non-infectious diseases. Rechlin and Muller assessed the dynamic changes of copeptin levels in myocardial infarction [15]. In patients with myocardial infraction, copeptin levels increased within 4 h after the first symptoms, while troponin T levels still remained within normal range. Serum copeptin levels later decreased while troponin remained increased for the following several hours. The different kinetics of these markers could be used in the diagnosis of myocardial

**Table 5** Leucocyte count, IL-6, CRP, PCT and CPP levels during the treatment of UTI

|  | Day 0 | Day 1 | Day 2 | Day 7 | P value |
|---|---|---|---|---|---|
| Leucocyte count [G/l] | 12.8 ± 6.7 [11.9 (6.9)] | 10.5 ± 5.7 [8.9 (5.4)] | 8.7 ± 3.9 [7.3 (4.5)] | 6.6 ± 1.8 [6.7 (2.3)] | <0.001 |
| IL-6 [pg/ml] | 66.8 ± 81.6 [41.6 (92.3)] | 70.6 ± 98.7 [22.9 (90.5)] | 49.3 ± 68.4 [12.6 (73.6)] | 34.4 ± 64.8 [8.7 (29.9)] | <0.001 |
| hsCRP [mg/dl] | 91.3 ± 86.5 [98.2 (132.5)] | 77.6 ± 77.8 [57.6 (121.9)] | 56.7 ± 72.7 [25.29 (84.12)] | 13.5 ± 16.9 [7.4 (11.2)] | <0.001 |
| PCT [ng/ml] | 3.7 ± 15.3 [0.12 (1.15)] | 1.8 ± 8.2 [0.08 (0.5)] | 1.1 ± 4.6 [0.05 (0.2)] | 0.4 ± 1.7 [0.05 (0.03)] | 0.11 |
| CPP [pg/ml] | 2821 ± 1072 [2874 (1527)] | 2309 ± 890 [2134 (934)] | 2290 ± 799 [2140 (891)] | 2003 ± 838 [1814 (1151)] | <0.001 |

Results are expressed as mean ± SD [median (IQR)]

**Table 6** Areas the receiver operating characteristics (ROC) curves, 95 % Confidence Intervals (95 % CI) and cutoff points of optimum performance for differentiating upper from lower urinary tract

|  | Area under the ROC curve Upper urinary tract infection | 95 % CI | Cutoff point | Area under the ROC curve Lower urinary tract infection | 95 % CI | Cutoff point |
|---|---|---|---|---|---|---|
| hsCRP [mg/dl] | 1 | 1.0 – 1.0 | 9.45 | 0.571 | 0.37 – 0.771 | 8.37 |
| PCT [ng/ml] | 0.94 | 0.845 – 0.993 | 0.07 | 0.505 | 0.185 – 0.575 | 0.15 |
| IL-6 [pg/ml] | 0.7 | 0.737 – 0.95 | 8.3 | 0.73 | 0.535 – 0.924 | 10.4 |
| CPP [pg/ml] | 1.0 | 1.0 – 1.0 | 1140 | 1.0 | 1.0 – 1.0 | 828 |

infraction. In our study we only assessed the changes of serum copeptin from the appearance of first symptoms of urinary tract infections to the day 7 of antibiotic treatment. Although high initial copeptin concentration was observed its decrease was slower compared to other inflammatory markers. Copeptin was still above normal at day 7 while the concentration of other inflammatory markers approached normal values at that time.

The potential biomarkers such as copeptin have to be always estimated in the context of a careful clinical assessment. Similar to many other biomarkers assessment of copeptin has certain limitations. There are possibly many factors which can lead to false – positive and false – negative serum copeptin results [16]. For example prednisone therapy increases copeptin concentration compared to healthy persons [17]. That was not the case in our patients since none was on steroids. Serum copeptin levels are also higher in patients with end-stage chronic kidney disease [18]. In our study however the patients with advanced kidney disease were excluded.

The use of new biochemical biomarkers that can simplify diagnostic and prognostic evaluation is not always economically feasible in particular since diagnostics and prognostics are customarily based on several different parameters. However, the usefulness of biomarkers is defined by the degree of their impact on clinical decision making and by adding subsequent information, apart from easily accessible data obtained from patients' physical examination [19]. Although serum copeptin could be a clinically useful inflammation marker in case of UTI, our results show that it seems to be inferior compared to traditional serum inflammation markers for the differentiation of infections involving upper and lower part of the urinary tract.

The main limitation of our exploratory research performed in a single center was a relatively small group of patients.

## Conclusion

Although elevated serum copeptin may become a marker of UTI it seems to be inferior compared to traditional serum inflammation markers for differentiation of infections involving upper and lower urinary tract.

**Abbreviations**
AVP: Arginine vasopressin; CPP: Copeptin; CT-proAVP: C-terminal part of provasopressin; hsCRP: C-reactive protein; L-UTI: Lower urinary tract infection; PCT: Procalcitonin; ROC: Receiver operating curves; UTI: Urinary tract infection; U-UTI: Upper urinary tract infection..

**Competing interests**
The authors declare that they have no competing interests.

**Authors' contributions**
AMZ participated in the conception and design of entire study, performed the data acquisition, helped to draft the manuscript and performed the statistical analysis. MW performed the data acquisition. MN participated in the conception and design of entire study and performed the statistical analysis. All authors read and approved the final manuscript.

**Acknowledgments**
The study was suported by a Medical University of Lodz, Poland grant No. 503/1-151-02/503-01

**References**
1. Sobel JD, Kaye D. Urinary tract infections. In: Mandel GL, Raphael Dolin JB, editors. Principles and Practice of Infectious Diseases. 2005. p. 875–901.
2. Vernon SJ, Coulthard MG, Lambert HJ, Keir MJ, Mathews JN. New renal scarring in children who at age 3 and 4 years had normal scans with dimercaptosuccinic acid: follow up study. BMJ. 1997;315:905–8.
3. Jacobson SH, Erlöf O, Ericsson CG, Lins LE, Tidgren B, Winberg J. Development of hypertension and uremia after pyelonephritis in childhood: 27 year follow up. Br Med J. 1989;299:703–6.
4. Lichtenberger P, Hooton TM. Complicated urinary tract infections. Curr Infect Dis Rep. 2008;10:499–504.
5. McEwen BS. Physiology and neurobiology of stress and adaptation: central role of the brain. Physiol Rev. 2007;87:873–904.
6. Petraglia F, Genazzani AD, Aguzzoli L, Gallinelli A, de Vita D, Caruso A, et al. Pulsatile flucuations of plasma-gonadotropin-releasing hormone and corticotropin-releasing factor levels in healthy pregnant women. Acta Obstet Gynecol Scand. 1994;73:284–9.
7. Evans MJ, Livesey JH, Eblis MJ, Handle TG. Effect of anticoagulants and storage temperatures on stability of plasma and serum hormones. Clin Biochem. 2001;34:107–12.
8. Holwerda DA. A glycopeptide from the posterior lobe of pig pituitaries. I. Isolation and characterization. Eur J Biochem. 1972;28:334–9.
9. Land H, Achutz G, Schmale H, Richter D. Nucleotide sequence of cloned cDNA encoding bovine arginine vasopressin-neurophysin II precursor. Nature. 1982;295:299–303.
10. Struck J, Morgenthaler NG, Bergmann A. Copeptin, a stable peptide derived from the vasopressin precursor, is elevated in serum of sepsis patients. Peptides. 2005;26:2500–4.
11. Morgenthaler NG, Struck J, Alonso C, Bergmann A. Assay for the measurement of copeptin, a stable peptide derived from the precursor of vasopressin. Clin Chem. 2006;52:112–9.

12. Muller B, Morgenthaler N, Stolz D, Schuetz P, Müller C, Bingisser R, et al. Circulating levels of copeptin, a novel biomarker, in lower respiratory tract infections. Eur J Clin Invest. 2007;37:145–52.
13. Morgenthaler NG, Muller B, Struck J, Bergmann A, Redl H, Christ-Crain M. Copeptin, a stable of the arginine vasopressin precursor, is elevated in hemorrhagic and septic shock. Shock. 2007;28:219–26.
14. Fluri F, Morgenthaler N, Mueller B, Christ-Crain M, Katan M. Copeptin, procalcitonin and routine inflammatory markers – predictors of infection after stroke. PLoS One 2012, 7: doi: 10.1371/journal.pone.0048309
15. Rechlin T, Hochholzer W, Stelzi C, Laule K, Freidank H, Morgenthaler NG, et al. Incremental value of Copeptin for rapid rule out of acute myocardial infarction. J Am Coll Cardiol. 2009;54:60–8.
16. Christ-Crain M, Muller B. Procalcitonin in bacterial infections – Hyde, hope, more or less? Swiss Med Wkly. 2005;135:451–60.
17. de Kruif MD, Lemaire LC, Giebelen IA, Struck J, Morgenthaler NG, Papassotiriou J, et al. The influence of corticosteroids on the release of novel biomarkers in human endotoxemia. Intensive Care Med. 2008;34:518–22.
18. Bhandari SS, Loke I, Davies JE, Squire IB, Struck J, Ng LL. Gender and renal function influence plasma levels of copeptin in healthy individuals. Clin Sci (Lond). 2009;116:257–63.
19. Marshall JC. Biomarkers of sepsis. Curr Infect Dis Rep. 2006;8:351–7.

# 10

# Tolterodine extended release in the treatment of male oab/storage luts

Mauro Gacci[1*], Giacomo Novara[2], Cosimo De Nunzio[3], Andrea Tubaro[3], Riccardo Schiavina[4], Eugenio Brunocilla[4], Arcangelo Sebastianelli[1], Matteo Salvi[1], Matthias Oelke[5], Stavros Gravas[6], Marco Carini[1] and Sergio Serni[1]

## Abstract

**Background:** Overactive bladder (OAB)/ storage lower urinary tract symptoms (LUTS) have a high prevalence affecting up to 90% of men over 80 years. The role of sufficient therapies appears crucial. In the present review, we analyzed the mechanism of action of tolterodine extended-release (ER) with the aim to clarify its efficacy and safety profile, as compared to other active treatments of OAB/storage LUTS.

**Methods:** A wide Medline search was performed including the combination of following words: "LUTS", "BPH", "OAB", "antimuscarinic", "tolterodine", "tolterodine ER". IPSS, IPSS storage sub-score and IPSS QoL (International Prostate Symptom Score) were the validated efficacy outcomes. In addition, the numbers of urgency episodes/24 h, urgency incontinence episodes/24 h, incontinence episodes/24 h and pad use were considered. We also evaluated the most common adverse events (AEs) reported for tolterodine ER.

**Results:** Of 128 retrieved articles, 109 were excluded. The efficacy and tolerability of tolterodine ER Vs. tolterodine IR have been evaluated in a multicenter, double-blind, randomized placebo controlled study in 1529 patients with OAB. A 71% mean reduction in urgency incontinence episodes was found in the tolterodine ER group compared to a 60% reduction in the tolterodine IR ($p < 0.05$). Few studies evaluated the clinical efficacy of α-blocker/tolterodine combination therapy. In patients with large prostates (prostate volume >29 cc) only the combination therapy significantly reduced 24-h voiding frequency (2.8 vs. 1.7 with tamsulosin, 1.4 with tolterodine, or 1.6 with placebo). A recent meta-analysis evaluating tolterodine in comparison with other antimuscarinic drugs demonstrated that tolterodine ER was significantly more effective than placebo in reducing micturition/24 h, urinary leakage episodes/24 h, urgency episodes/24 h, and urgency incontinence episodes/24 h. With regard to adverse events, tolterodine ER was associated with a good adverse event profile resulting in the third most favorable antimuscarinic. Antimuscarinic drugs are the mainstay of pharmacological therapy for OAB / storage LUTS; several studies have demonstrated that tolterodine ER is an effective and well tolerated formulation of this class of treatment.

**Conclusion:** Tolterodine ER resulted effective in reducing frequency urgency and nocturia and urinary leakage in male patients with OAB/storage LUTS. Dry mouth and constipation are the most frequently reported adverse events.

**Keywords:** Lower urinary tract symptoms, Overactive bladder, Storage LUTS, Tolterodine, Urge incontinence, Frequency, Nocturia

* Correspondence: maurogacci@yahoo.it
[1]Department of Urology, University of Florence, Careggi Hospital, Viale S. Luca – 50134, Florence, Italy
Full list of author information is available at the end of the article

## Background

Lower Urinary Tract Symptoms (LUTS) have a high prevalence affecting up to 90% of men over 80 years [1]. The term LUTS comprises a large group of symptoms usually divided into storage LUTS (daytime urinary frequency, nocturia, urgency, urinary incontinence), voiding LUTS (slow stream, splitting or spraying, intermittency, hesitancy, straining, terminal dribble), and post micturition LUTS (sensation of incomplete emptying, post-micturition dribble) [2].

In men, LUTS may be associated with benign prostatic obstruction (BPO) typically resulting from benign prostatic hyperplasia (BPH) or benign prostatic enlargement (BPE) [3]. Approximately half of men with histological BPH develop BPE but only 25–50% of these men have LUTS [4,5].

OAB and storage LUTS are defined as the presence of urinary urgency, usually accompanied by frequency and nocturia, with or without urinary incontinence, in absence of urinary tract infection or other urethro-vesical dysfunctions [2]. Storage LUTS are generally a chronic condition, with a prevalence ranging from 10% to 26% [6,7]. Male storage symptoms could be caused by bladder dysfunction (like detrusor overactivity or detrusor impaired contractility), BPO (often caused by BPE) or by a combination of both bladder dysfunction and BPO [8,9]. In that scenario, the role of targeted therapies appears crucial. In order to obtain clinical relief of storage LUTS, an extensive counseling of patients is mandatory to evaluate all the possible treatments and their expected results since the lack of efficacy and the presence of bothering adverse events (AEs) can reduce compliance.

Behavioral therapies should be offered as first line treatment for all patients with storage LUTS. Their goal is to relieve bladder symptoms by changing voiding habits (bladder training, delayed voiding) or by improving control of urge suppression and urethral occlusion (PFMT). Nevertheless the gold standards of pharmacological therapy are antimuscarinic agents such as oxybutynin, tolterodine, fesoterodine, darifenacin, solifenacin, or trospium [10].

Antimuscarinics (m-cholinoceptor antagonists) especially block specific receptors at the level of the bladder ($M_2$ and $M_3$ receptors on smooth muscle cells of the detrusor) in a more or less selective manner, thereby reducing involuntary bladder contractions or altering contraction thresholds. Antimuscarinics act mainly during the urinary storage phase and decrease the activity of afferent bladder nerves [11] resulting in decreased urgency and increased bladder capacity. However, muscarinic receptors are also found in other parts of the body, including the brain, heart, gut, salivary glands, and tear ducts. First marketed antimuscarinics were limited by adverse effects, resulting in poor patient compliance and discontinuation of treatment [12].

Oxybutynin was the first antimuscarinic agent, used since the mid-70s, for the treatment of overactive bladder (OAB)/bladder storage symptoms [13]. Oxybutynin immediate release (IR) has proven efficacy for the condition [14]. However, it has a significant incidence of peripheral anti-muscarinic adverse events such as dry mouth, constipation, tachycardia, paralysis of accommodation and central nervous system side effects (cognitive dysfunction or delirium), resulting in poor compliance and early discontinuation of therapy in a large number of patients [12,13].

More than fifteen years ago, tolterodine was developed with the aim of obtaining a better efficacy/adverse event profile and improving the compliance of patients compared to other antimuscarinic drugs. It is lesser lipid (soluble) than oxybutynin and crosses the blood–brain barrier to a lesser extent. Tolterodine is non-selective with respect to the muscarinic receptor sub-types but, as shown by data obtained from animals and healthy volunteers in the first clinical trials, showed a greater, more rapid and longer lasting effect on the bladder than on salivary glands *in vivo* [15-17].

Patient tolerability represents a fundamental parameter for the administration of antimuscarinic agents. Given the established role of frequency-dose and patient compliance and its potential effect on tolerability and efficacy, an extended release (ER) formulation was developed for several antimuscarinics. In a large systematic review and meta-analysis [18], all the comparisons among IR (drug intake 2–3 times/day) and ER formulations (drug intake once/day) showed advantages for the latter, either in terms of efficacy or safety.

Few studies investigated the effects of antimuscarinic drugs on male patients with bladder outlet obstruction and OAB/bladder storage symptoms and the results of the use of antimuscarinic agents as monotherapy were conflicting. Starting in 1994, the approach of combination therapy with α-blockers and antimuscarinics has become increasingly popular [19]. Earliest report of Athanasopoulos et al. [20] on the effects of tolterodine 2 mg twice daily combined with tamsulosin 0.4 mg once daily compared with tamsulosin alone in 25 patients showed a better QoL only in the combination therapy group with no acute urinary retention. As a result, there has been a growing interest on the use of antimuscarinics in male LUTS/BPH.

Antimuscarinics have been increasingly used in clinical practice - with caution and regular re-evaluation - in particular for selected patients with moderate to severe LUTS who have predominant bladder storage symptoms and do not have elevated post-void residual urine volumes [21,22]. In the present review we analyzed in detail the mechanism of action of tolterodine ER and its overall safety and efficacy in the treatment of male bladder storage LUTS.

## Methods

A wide Medline search was performed including the combination of following search terms: "LUTS", "BPH", "OAB", "antimuscarinic", "tolterodine", "tolterodine ER". No temporary limits were adopted. IPSS, IPSS storage sub-score and IPSS QoL (International Prostate Symptom Score) were the validated efficacy outcomes. In addition, the numbers of urgency episodes/24 h, urgency incontinence episodes/24 h, incontinence episodes/24 h and pad use were considered. We also evaluated the most common adverse events (AEs) reported for tolterodine ER in selected studies.

## Results

Out of 128 retrieved articles, 109 were excluded for missing or incomplete data, deficiency in methodology (several biases not included), assessment of clinical outcomes without validated instruments. the total flowchart of literature searches is summarized in Figure 1.

## Mechanism of action of tolterodine

### Muscarinic receptors

Five sub-types of muscarinic receptors are presented in the human tissues: even if all these receptors can be found in several tissues, including epithelial cells of the bladder and the salivary glands and nerve cells of the central or peripheral nervous systems, the $M_2$ and $M_3$ are predominantly expressed in detrusor smooth muscle cells [23]. Detrusor contractions are stimulated by the activity of acetylcholine on muscarinic receptors on smooth muscles cells of the bladder.

Tolterodine is a competitive muscarinic receptor antagonist with relative functional selectivity for bladder muscarinic receptors. It is metabolized in microsomes of the human liver by cytochromes P450 (CYP2D6 and CYP3A4) to two primary metabolites: 5-hydroxymethyl tolterodine (5-HMT) (labcode DD 01; PNU-200577) and N-dealkylated tolterodine [23,24]. With the exception of 5-HMT, metabolites of tolterodine are not considered to contribute to the therapeutic effect.

*In vitro* studies in guinea-pig detrusor strips [25] showed a simple competitive blockade of the bladder muscarinic receptors in a concentration-dependent manner after carbachol-induced contractions. Tolterodine was equipotent to oxybutynin and acted as an effective and competitive muscarinic receptor antagonist also in human isolated urinary bladder. Radioligand binding studies in tissue

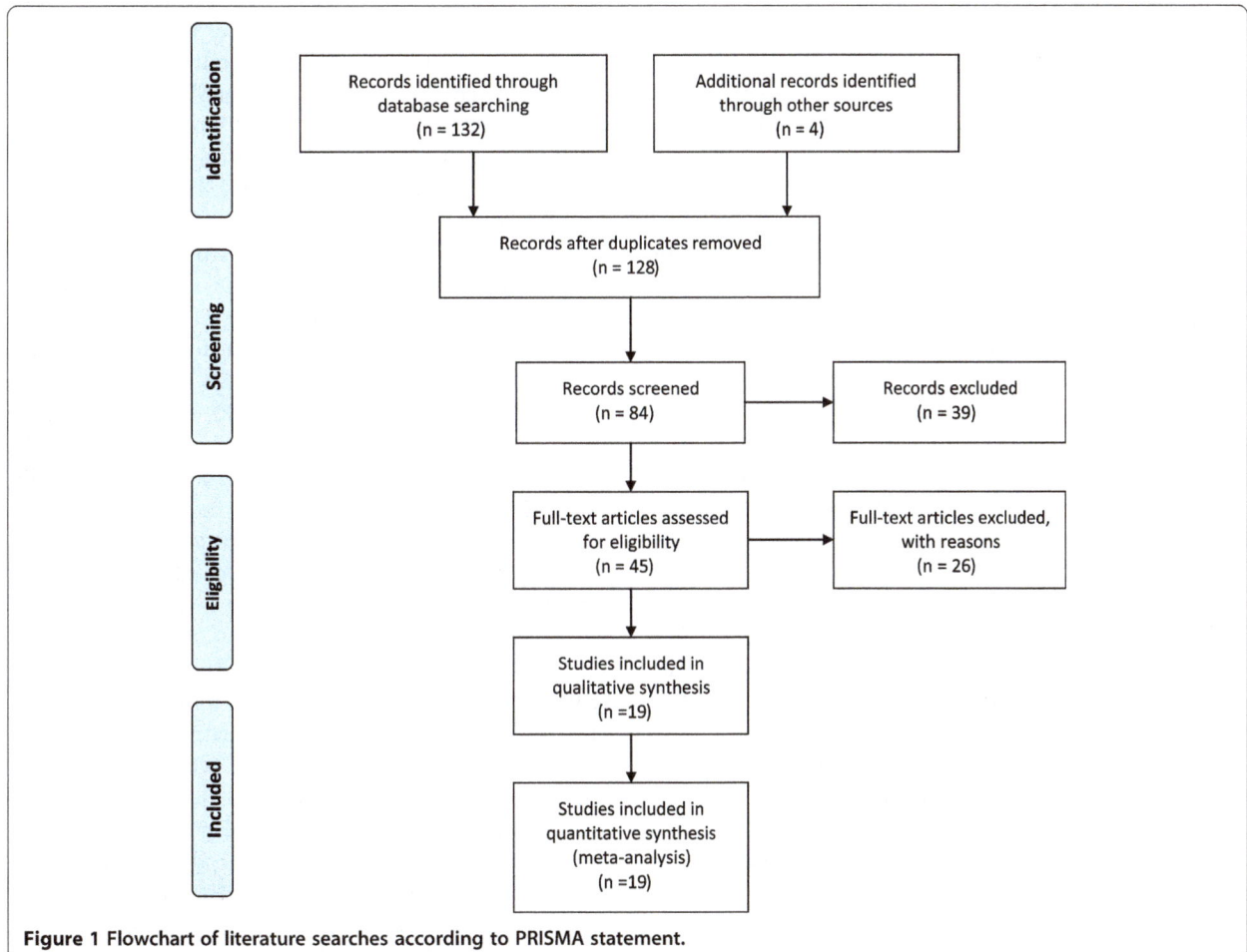

**Figure 1** Flowchart of literature searches according to PRISMA statement.

homogenates showed that the affinities determined and expressed as the dissociation constants ($k_i$), for tolterodine in human bladder were comparable to those in the guinea-pig bladder [25].

### Selectivity profile

The binding affinities determined in the bladder were similar to those in the heart, which can be assumed to contain only muscarinic $M_2$ receptors [25].

Tolterodine and 5-HMT show functional selectivity for the bladder over the salivary glands *in vivo*. In the anaesthetized cats, intravenous injection of tolterodine and 5-HMT resulted in dose-dependent inhibition of acetylcholine-induced urinary bladder contractions and electrically induced salivation. The effect on urinary bladder contractions occurred at significantly lower doses than the effect on salivary secretion, showing favorable tissue selectivity [25-27]. In 2008 Olshansky et al. showed an increase in mean heart rate per 24 hours of ≥5 beats per minute higher with tolterodine than with placebo (p = 0.0114) [28]. Neither oxybutynin nor tolterodine showed clinically significant effects on the heart rate [25,27].

The selectivity profiles in vivo were reflected in the radioligand binding studies. Thus, the affinity profile of tolterodine (cerebral cortex ≥ heart ≈ urinary bladder > parotid gland) differed from those of oxybutynin (cerebral cortex ≈ parotid gland > heart ≈ urinary bladder).

### Pharmacokinetics

The pharmacokinetic properties of tolterodine are influenced by the CYP2D6 polymorphism. The lack or strongly reduced activity of this liver enzyme characterizes poor metabolizers. In these individuals, the active metabolite 5-HMT cannot be formed and the pharmacological effects are mediated exclusively by tolterodine. As shown in a clinical study by Brynne et al. [29], tolterodine was rapidly absorbed in both extensive and poor metabolizer, and the pharmacodynamic effects of tolterodine were not generally influenced by metabolic phenotype. Thus, the same dosage can be used irrespective of CYP2D6 phenotype.

Pharmacokinetic equivalence was demonstrated between IR tolterodine tablets 2 mg twice daily and ER capsule formulation of tolterodine 4 mg once daily ($AUC_{24}$). In addition, tolterodine ER resulted in less serum drug level fluctuation and sustained drug release over 24 hours [27]. This translates into more constant serum concentrations and, in theory, also into better tolerability for patients.

The clearance of tolterodine was considerably lower in patients with liver cirrhosis or impaired renal function [creatinine clearance 10–30 ml/min (0.6 to 1.8 L/h)] compared to healthy volunteers [30].

## Discussion

### Safety and efficacy of tolterodine Er

#### Tolterodine ER vs. Tolterodine IR

Tolterodine intermediate release (IR) was firstly developed and tested in several randomized, double-blind, placebo controlled study which led to drug approval by the FDA in 1998. The efficacy and tolerability of tolterodine IR and oxybutynin IR were found to be comparable [14]. Dry mouth was the only adverse event that occurred significantly more often in patients treated with tolterodine IR (1 mg bid, 30%; 2 mg bid, 48%) in comparison to patients of the placebo group; however, only 3% of the tolterodine IR treated subjects withdrew from treatment because of dry mouth [31].

Regardless of the positive results of the registration trials and confirmation of the excellent efficacy in randomised phase IV studies [32-34], Pfizer laboratories developed an extended release (ER) formulation (approved by the FDA in 2000) to improve patient compliance and to decrease the dry mouth rate which was thought to be dependent from the peak plasma levels of the drug. Tolterodine ER uses a drug delivery system that contains soluble microspheres. The drug is slowly released as the outer layer of the microsphere dissolves, leading to consistent delivery of drug over a 24-hour period [35].

The efficacy and tolerability of tolterodine ER have been evaluated in a multicenter, double-blind, randomized placebo controlled study in 1529 patients with OAB [13,36]. A significant clinical advantage in terms of clinical efficacy and tolerability was associated with tolterodine ER treatment. A 71% mean reduction in urgency incontinence episodes was found in the tolterodine ER group compared to a 60% reduction in the tolterodine IR group (p < 0.05). The incidence of dry mouth was 23% for tolterodine ER versus 30% for tolterodine IR. The overall rate of dry mouth was 23% lower with tolterodine ER than with tolterodine IR. The incidence of other adverse events such as dizziness (ER 2% vs. IR 2%), constipation (ER 7% vs. IR 6%) and somnolence (ER 3% vs. IR 3%) were similar between the treatment groups and comparable with placebo. This pivotal study suggested an improved clinical advantage of tolterodine ER over the IR formulation of the drug in terms of efficacy and tolerability.

### Tolterodine in combination therapies for OAB/LUTS

The theoretical concern about a negative effect on postvoid residual urine or even urinary retention has influenced the use of antimuscarinics for the management of storage LUTS in male patients independent of studies showing no increased risk of urinary tract retention in patients with benign prostatic obstruction. The combined use of antimuscarinics and other drugs currently available for LUTS, including α-blockers, 5α-reductase inhibitors or botulinum toxin A in addition to the introduction of ß3-agonists has recently been investigated to overcome these limitations [37-40].

Few studies have evaluated the clinical efficacy of α-blocker/tolterodine combination therapy [37-39]. The majority are add-on studies, in which tolterodine has been added to an existing $\alpha_1$-blocker therapy. The "Tolterodine and Tamsulosin in Men With LUTS Including OAB: evaluation of Efficacy and Safety" (TIMES) study showed that patients treated with tolterodine/tamsulosin combination therapy, but not with tamsulosin, tolterodine or placebo alone, had a significant treatment benefit as defined by the patient perception questionnaire (80% vs. 71%, 65%, and 62%, respectively) [37,39]. At the end of the study period (12 weeks), only combination therapy significantly improved total IPSS and QoL as well as the IPSS storage sub-score. The TIMES study also identified a subgroup of patients with a PSA value <1.3 ng/ml or prostate volume <29 ml who also significantly profited from tolterodine monotherapy with regard to storage symptom reduction [37,39]. In patients with large prostates (prostate volume >29 cc) only the combination therapy significantly reduced 24-h voiding frequency (2.8 vs. 1.7 with tamsulosin alone, 1.4 with tolterodine alone, or 1.6 with placebo). Adverse events of antimuscarinics (e.g. dry mouth or constipation) occurred in the combination therapy group more often than in patients receiving $\alpha_1$-blocker monotherapy. There was no significant or clinically relevant increase in post-void residual urine or acute urinary retention when the combination treatment arm was compared with mono-therapy of the individual drugs [39].

Another investigational combination therapy with tolterodine ER was with 5α-reductase inhibitors. In particular, Chung et al. demonstrated that in men with persistent OAB symptoms after at least 6 months of treatment with dutasteride the addition of tolterodine ER allowed to significantly reduce frequency and urgency, such as severe OAB episodes and night time voiding (nocturia). Storage LUTS (IPSS storage sub-score) were remarkably reduced from 9.8 to 4.5 (p < 0.001). Regarding tolerability, 7.5% of men experienced dry mouth, but no patient developed urinary retention [40].

The efficacy and safety of tolterodine in combination therapies was reviewed by Athanasopoulos et al. in 2011, concluding that combination therapy was effective and the risk of urinary retention was minimal [41].

Mirabegron, a novel ß3-adrenoceptor agonist, has recently been approved for the treatment of OAB symptoms and is the first of a new class of compounds with a mechanism of action that is different from antimuscarinic agents. Mirabegron represents a new option for the management of OAB, has a comparable efficacy and a better tolerability when compared to tolterodine 4 mg

ER in a large clinical trial dataset in OAB/storage LUTS patients. However, further studies should assess its long term safety and efficacy and the possible role in specific group of patients as male patients with LUTS and benign prostatic obstruction, either alone or in combination with antimuscarinics (e.g. tolterodine ER) [42,43].

## Tolterodine ER vs. other antimuscarinics

Since its introduction in clinical practice, tolterodine has been the active comparator in several studies. The first comparator trial using tolterodine ER was the "Overactive Bladder: Performance of Extended Release Agents" (OPERA) study [44] which compared the efficacy and tolerability of tolterodine ER (4 mg daily) and oxybutynin (10 mg daily). No significant difference was observed in the number of urgency incontinence episodes (tolterodine 20.9% vs. oxybutynin 26.7%) or the total dry rate (tolterodine 16.8% vs. oxybutynin 23%).

Regarding adverse events, the most common side effect in each group was dry mouth, with 29.7% of the patients receiving oxybutynin vs. 22.3% of those receiving tolterodine (p = 0.02). Other adverse events were similar in magnitude and frequency in both groups [18,35]. A recently published study tested the efficacy and tolerability of tolterodine ER versus solifenacin [45]. The STAR-study compared flexible dosing of solifenacin versus tolterodine 4 mg in the primary outcome criteria (change in number of micturitions per 24 hours). Solifenacin flexible dosing proved to be superior to tolterodine ER in reducing the numbers of urgency episodes/24 h (−2.85 vs. −2.42), urgency incontinence episodes/24 h (−1.42 vs. −0-83), incontinence episodes/24 h (−1.60 vs. 1−11), and pad use (−1.72 vs. −1.19). Dry mouth and constipation were significant more common in the solifenacin arm (18.2 vs. 14.5% and 3.0 vs. 1.2%, respectively), although they were mainly of mild to moderate severity [18,45].

In 2008 Chapple et al. compared the antimuscarinic fesoterodine 4 mg or fesoterodine 8 mg once daily to

**Table 1 Comparison of tolterodine ER versus other antimuscarinics as reviewed in the 2012 AHRQ review [49]**

| Experimental drug versus standard drug | No. of studies | Patients | Relative risk (95% CI) |
|---|---|---|---|
| **Efficacy (cure of UI)** | | | |
| Fesoterodine vs tolterodine ER | 2 | 3312 | 1.1 (1.04-1.16) |
| Oxybutynin ER vs tolterodine ER | 3 | 947 | 1.11 (0.94-1.16) |
| Solifenacin vs tolterodine ER | 1 | 1177 | 1.2 (1.08-1.34) |
| **Discontinuation due to adverse events** | | | |
| Solifenacin vs tolterodine ER | 3 | 2755 | 1.28 (0.86-1.91) |
| Fesoterodine vs tolterodine ER | 4 | 4440 | 1.54 (1.21-1.97) |

Efficacy was defined as the achievement of urinary continence.

placebo in a randomized controlled trial and included an active control arm tolterodine ER 4 mg [46]. Fesoterodine 8 mg outperformed tolterodine 4 mg with regard to the median change from baseline in number of UUI episodes (p < 0.05) and volume voided per micturition (p < 0.05), while similar efficacy was shown for fesoterodine 4 mg and tolterodine 4 mg. Fesoterodine 4 mg and tolterodine ER 4 mg had a similar safety profile, while fesoterodine 8 mg was associated with significantly higher rates of dry mouth (p < 0.0001) and dry eyes (p = 0.02) compared to tolterodine 4 mg [18]. In 2013 Ginsberg et al. [47] compared the efficacy of fesoterodine 8 mg vs

tolterodine 4 mg ER for OAB symptoms in terms of patient-reported outcomes in both men and women, supporting the superiority of fesoterodine 8 mg over tolterodine 4 mg ER in improving severe urgency and symptom bother in men.

The EAU Guidelines on Urinary Incontinence recently evaluated and reported data from the Agency for Healthcare Research and Quality (AHRQ) review which included a specific section addressing comparisons of antimuscarinic drugs [48,49] (Table 1). They concluded that there was no evidence that any one antimuscarinic, including tolterodine ER, improved quality of life more

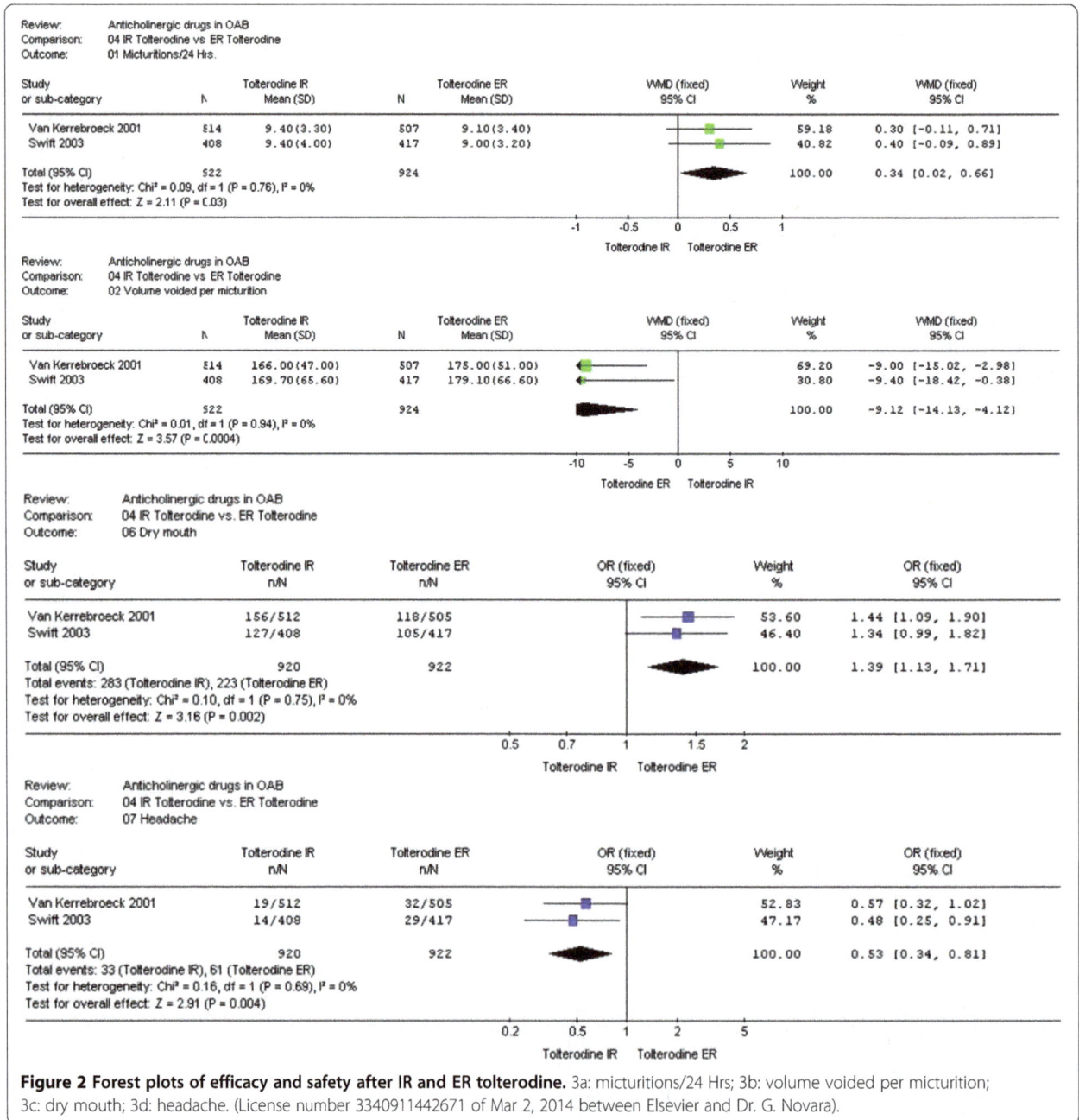

**Figure 2** Forest plots of efficacy and safety after IR and ER tolterodine. 3a: micturitions/24 Hrs; 3b: volume voided per micturition; 3c: dry mouth; 3d: headache. (License number 3340911442671 of Mar 2, 2014 between Elsevier and Dr. G. Novara).

than another agent and there is no consistent evidence for the superiority of one antimuscarinic agent over another for the overall efficacy or discontinuation rate. However, the recently published studies comparing tolterodine with fesoterodine have not been included in this analysis.

A recent network meta-analysis evaluating tolterodine in comparison with other antimuscarinic drugs demonstrated that tolterodine ER was significantly more effective than placebo in reducing micturition/24 h ($-0.76$; $p <0.001$), urinary leakage episodes/24 h ($-0.36$; $p <0.001$), urgency episodes/24 h ($-0.77$; $p <0.001$), and urgency incontinence episodes/24 h ($-0.34$; $p <0.001$) [48]. With regard to adverse events, the same article demonstrated that tolterodine ER was associated with a good adverse event profile resulting in the third most favorable antimuscarinic out of 21 analyzed antimuscarinic drugs, following oxybutynin topical gel 100 mg/g per day and solifenacin 5 mg per day [50] (Figure 2).

## Conclusions

Tolterodine is an effective muscarinic receptor antagonist, with a receptor affinity comparable to oxybutynin in the bladder, and a remarkably lower affinity than oxybutynin in the parotid gland. Immediate-release tablets 2 mg twice daily and extended-release tablets 4 mg once daily have a comparable pharmacokinetic profile.

Tolterodine ER resulted effective in reducing frequency urgency and nocturia and urinary leakage in patients with OAB/storage LUTS. Dry mouth and constipation are the most frequently reported adverse events. The good safety profile, which allow to minimize treatment withdrew, and the adequate effectiveness in the management of storage LUTS, are the strengths of Tolterodine ER.

Further RTCs are needed to identify the best candidates for the treatment with tolterodine ER and to tailor promising combination therapies with other drugs currently available for male LUTS.

### Competing interests

No sources of funding were used to assist in the preparation of this article. Dr Gacci has received Support for travel to meetings for the study, manuscript preparation or other purposes and payment for lectures from GSK, Eli Lilly, MEnarini, Pfizer, Bayer. Dr Novara has been advisory board member or speaker for Astellas, GlaxoSmithKleine, Lilly, Menarini, Nycomed, Pfizer Inc., Pierre Fabre, and Recordati. Dr Oelke has worked on the advisory board for Eli-Lilly and Company, and has received payment for lectures from Eli-Lilly and Company, Pfizer and Bayer. Drs De Nunzio, Tubaro, Schiavina, Brunocilla, Sebastianelli, Salvi, Gravas, Carini and Serni have no competing interest to declare.

### Authors' contributions

Study concept and design: MG. Acquisition of data: AS, MS. Analysis and interpretation of data: MG, GN, CDN, MO. Drafting of the manuscript: MG, CDN, MO, RS, EB. Critical revision of the manuscript for important intellectual content: MC, SG, SS, AT. All authors read and approved the final manuscript.

### Author details

[1]Department of Urology, University of Florence, Careggi Hospital, Viale S. Luca – 50134, Florence, Italy. [2]Department of Surgical, Oncological and Gastroenterological sciences, Urology clinic, University of Padua, Padua, Italy. [3]Department of Urology, Sant'Andrea Hospital, University 'La Sapienza', Rome, Italy. [4]Department of Urology, University of Bologna, Bologna, Italy. [5]Department of Urology, Hannover Medical School, Hannover, Germany. [6]Department of Urology, University Hospital of Larissa, Larissa, Greece.

### References

1. Rosen R, Altwein J, Boyle P, Kirby RS, Lukacs B, Meuleman E, O'Leary MP, Puppo P, Chris R, Giuliano F: **Lower urinary tract symptoms and male sexual dysfunction: the multinational survey of the aging male (MSAM-7).** *Eur Urol* 2003, **44**(6):637–649.
2. Abrams P, Cardozo L, Fall M, Griffiths D, Rosier P, Ulmsten U, Van Kerrebroeck P, Victor A, Wein A, Standardisation Sub-Committee of the International Continence Society: **The standardisation of terminology in lower urinary tract function: report from the standardisation sub-committee of the International Continence Society.** *Urology* 2003, **61**:37–49.
3. Berry SJ, Coffey DS, Walsh PC, Ewing LL: **The development of human benign prostatic hyperplasia with age.** *J Urol* 1984, **132**(3):474–479.
4. Soler R, Andersson KE, Chancellor MB, Chapple CR, de Groat WC, Drake MJ, Gratzke C, Lee R, Cruz F: **Future direction in pharmacotherapy for non-neurogenic male lower urinary tract symptoms.** *Eur Urol* 2013, **64**(4):610–621.
5. Laniado ME, Ockrim JL, Marronaro A, Tubaro A, Carter SS: **Serum prostate-specific antigen to predict the presence of bladder outlet obstruction in men with urinarysymptoms.** *BJ UInt* 2004, **94**:1283–1286.
6. Irwin DE, Milsom I, Hunskaar S, Reilly K, Kopp Z, Herschorn S, Coyne K, Kelleher C, Hampel C, Artibani W, Abrams P: **Population-based survey of urinary incontinence, overactive bladder, and other lower urinary tract symptoms in five countries: Results of the EPIC study.** *Eur Urol* 2006, **50**:1306–1315.
7. Haab F, Castro-Diaz D: **Persistence with antimuscarinic therapy in patients with overactive bladder.** *Int J Clin Pract* 2005, **59**:931–937.
8. Michel MC, Chapple CR: **Basic mechanisms of urgency: roles and benefits of pharmacotherapy.** *World J Urol* 2009, **27**:705–709.
9. Oelke M, Baard J, Wijkstra H, de la Rosette JJ, Jonas U, Höfner K: **Age and bladder outlet obstruction are independently associated with detrusor overactivity in patients with benign prostatic hyperplasia.** *Eur Urol* 2008, **54**:419–426.
10. Gormley EA, Lightner DJ, Burgio KL, Chai TC, Clemens JQ, Culkin DJ, Das AK, Foster HE Jr, Scarpero HM, Tessier CD, Vasavada SP, American Urological Association: Society of Urodynamics, Female Pelvic Medicine & Urogenital Reconstruction. **Diagnosis and treatment of overactive bladder (non-neurogenic) in adults: AUA/SUFU guideline.** *J Urol* 2012, **188**(6 Suppl):2455–2463.
11. De Laet K, De Watcher S, Wyndaele JJ: **Systemic oxybutinin decreases afferent activity of the pelvic nerve of the rat: new insight into the working mechanism of antimuscarinics.** *Neururol Urodyn* 2006, **25**(2):156.
12. Yarker YE, Goa KL, Fitton A: **Oxybutynin: A review of its pharmacodynamics and pharmacokinetic properties, and its therapeutic use in detrusor instability.** *Drugs Aging* 1995, **6**:243–246.
13. Rovner ES, Wein AJ: **Once daily, extended release formulations of antimuscarinics agents in the treatment of overactive bladder: A review.** *Eur Urol* 2002, **41**:6–14.
14. Ulahannan D, Wagg A: **The safety and efficacy of tolterodine extended release in the treatment of overactive bladder in the elderly.** *Clin Interv Aging* 2009, **4**:191–196.
15. Stahl MMS, Ekström B, Sparf B, Mattiasson A, Andersson K-E: **Urodynamic and other effects of tolterodine: a novel antimuscarinic drug for the treatment of detrusor overactivity.** *Neurourol Urodyn* 1995, **14**:647–655.
16. Brynne N, Stahl MMS, Hallén BH, Edlund PO, Palmér L, Höglund P, Gabrielsson J: **Pharmacokinetics and pharmacodynamics of tolterodine in man: a new drug for the treatment of urinary bladder overactivity.** *Int J Clin Pharmacol Therap* 1997, **35**:287–295.

17. Nilvebrant L: Clinical experiences with tolterodine. *Life Sci* 2001, **68**(22–23):2549–2556.

18. Novara G, Galfano A, Secco S, D'Elia C, Cavalleri S, Ficarra V, Artibani W: A systematic review and meta-analysis of randomized controlled trials with antimuscarinic drugs for overactive bladder. *Eur Urol* 2008, **54**:740–763.

19. Chapple CR, Smith D: The pathophysiological changes in the bladder obstructed by benign prostatic hyperplasia. *Br J Urol* 1994, **73**:117–123.

20. Athanasopoulos A, Gyftopoulos K, Giannitsas K, Fisfis J, Perimenis P, Barbalias G: Combination treatment with an alpha-blocker plus an anticholinergic for bladder outlet obstruction: a prospective, randomized, controlled study. *J Urol* 2003, **169**:2253–2256.

21. Oelke M, Bachmann A, Descazeaud A, Emberton M, Gravas S, Michel MC, N'Dow J, Nordling J, de la Rosette JJ: Guidelines on the Management of Male Lower Urinary Tract Symptoms (LUTS) incl. Benign Prostatic Obstruction (BPO). *Eur Urol* 2013, **64**:118–140.

22. McVary KT, Roehrborn CG, Avins AL, Barry MJ, Bruskewitz RC, Donnell RF, Foster HE Jr, Gonzalez CM, Kaplan SA, Penson DF, Ulchaker JC: *AUA Guidelines: Management of BPH, Revision.* ; 2010.

23. Postlind H, Danielson A, Lindgren A, Andersson SH: Tolterodine, a new muscarinic receptor antagonist, is metabolized by cytochromes P450 2D6 and 3A in human liver microsomes. *Drug Metab Dispos* 1998, **26**(4):289–293.

24. Larsson G, Hallén B, Nilvebrant L: Tolterodine in the treatment of overactive bladder: analysis of the pooled phase II efficacy and safety data. *Urology* 1999, **53**(5):990–998.

25. Nilvebrant L, Andersson KE, Gillberg PG, Stahl M, Sparf B: Tolterodine: a new bladder-selective antimuscarinic agent. *Eur J Pharmacol* 1997, **327**(2–3):195–207.

26. Nilvebrant L, Hallén B, Larsson G: Tolterodine: a new bladder selective muscarinic receptor antagonist: preclinical pharmacological and clinical data. *Life Sci* 1997, **60**(13–14):1129–1136.

27. Olsson B, Szamosi J: Multiple Dose Pharmacokinetics of a New Once Daily Extended Release Tolterodine Formulation Versus Immediate Release Tolterodine. *Clinical Pharmacokinetics* 2001, **40**(3):227–235.

28. Olshansky B, Ebinger U, Brum J, Egermark M, Viegas A, Rekeda L: Differential pharmacological effects of antimuscarinic drugs on heart rate: a randomized, placebo-controlled, double-blind, crossover study with tolterodine and darifenacin in healthy participants > or = 50 years. *J Cardiovas Pharmacol Ther* 2008, **13**:241–251.

29. Brynne N, Dalén P, Alván G, Bertilsson L, Gabrielsson J: Influence of CYP2D6 polymorphism on the pharmacokinetics and pharmacodynamic of tolterodine. *Clin Pharmacol Ther* 1998, **63**(5):529–539.

30. Clemett D, Jarvis B: Tolterodine. *Drugs Aging* 2001, **18**(4):277–304.

31. Malone-Lee JG, Walsh JB, Maugourd MF: Tolterodine: a safe and effective treatment for older patients with overactive bladder. *J Am Geriatr Soc* 2001, **49**(6):700–705.

32. Appel RA: Clinical efficacy and safety of tolterodine in the treatment of overactive bladder: a pooled analysisi. *Urology* 1997, **50**(6):90–96.

33. Abrams P, Freeman R, Anderstrom C, Revicki D, Stewart W, Coprey R: Tolterodine, a new antimuscarinic agent: as effective but better tolerated than oxybutinin in patients with overactive bladder. *Br J Urol* 1998, **8**:801–810.

34. Drutz HP, Appel R, Gleason D, Klimberg I, Radomski S: Clinical efficacy and safety of tolterodine comnpared to oxybutynin and placebo in patients with overactive bladder. *Int Urogynecol J* 1999, **10**:283–289.

35. Kanoksky JA, Nitti VW: Tolterodine for treatment of overactive bladder. *Urol Clin N Am* 2006, **33**:447–453.

36. Van Kerrebroeck P, Kreder K, Jonas U, Zinner N, Wein A, Tolterodine Study Group: Tolterodine once-daily: superior effi cacy and tolerability in the treatment of the overactive bladder. *Urology* 2001, **57**(3):414–421.

37. Fullhase C, Chapple C, Cornu JN, De Nunzio C, Gratzke C, Kaplan SA, Marberger M, Montorsi F, Novara G, Oelke M, Porst H, Roehrborn C, Stief C, McVary KT: Systematic Review of Combination Drug Therapy for Non-neurogenic Male Lower Urinary Tract Symptoms. *Eur Urol* 2013, **64**:228–243.

38. Chapple C, Herschorn S, Abrams P, Sun F, Brodsky M, Guan Z: Tolterodine treatment improves storage symptoms suggestive of overactive bladder in men treated with a-blockers. *Eur Urol* 2009, **56**:534–543.

39. Kaplan SA, Roehrborn CG, Rovner ES, Carlsson M, Bavendam T, Guan Z: Tolterodine and tamsulosin for treatment of men with lower urinary tract symptoms and overactive bladder: a randomized controlled trial. *JAMA* 2006, **296**:2319–2328.

40. Chung DE, Te AE, Staskin DR, Kaplan SA: Efficacy and safety of tolterodine extended release and dutasteride in male overactive bladder patients with prostates >30 grams. *Urology* 2010, **75**(5):1144–1148.

41. Athanasopoulosa A, Chapple C, Fowler C, Gratzke C, Kaplan S, Stief C, Tubaro A: The Role of Antimuscarinics in the Management of Men With Symptoms of Overactive Bladder Associated With Concomitant Bladder Outlet Obstruction: An Update. *Eur Urol* 2011, **60**(1):94–105.

42. Nitti V, Auerbach S, Martin N, Calhoun A, Lee M, Herschorn S: Results of a randomized phase III trial of mirabegron in patients with overactive bladder. *J Urol* 2013, **189**:1388–1395.

43. Nitti VW, Khullar V, van Kerrebroeck P, Herschorn S, Cambronero J, Angulo JC, Blauwet MB, Dorrepaal C, Siddiqui E, Martin NE: Mirabegron for the treatment of overactive bladder: a prespecified pooled efficacy analysis and pooled safety analysis of three randomised, double-blind, placebo-controlled, phase III studies. *Int J Clin Pract* 2013, **67**(7):619–632.

44. Diokno AC, Appell RA, Sand PK, Dmochowski RR, Gburek BM, Klimberg IW, Kell SH, OPERA Study Group: Prospective, randomized, double-blind study of the efficacy and tolerability of the extended-release formulations of oxybutynin and tolterodine for overactive bladder: results of the OPERA trial. *Mayo Clin Proc* 2003, **78**:687–695.

45. Chapple CR, Martinez-Garcia R, Selvaggi L, Toozs-Hobson P, Warnack W, Drogendijk T, Wright DM, Bolodeoku J: A comparison of the efficacy and tolerability of solifenacin succinate and extended release tolterodine at treating overactive bladder syndrome: results of the STAR trial. *Eur Urol* 2005, **48**:464–470. overactive bladder syndrome: results of the STAR trial. *Eur Urol* 2005, 48:464–70.

46. Chapple C, Van Kerrebroeck P, Tubaro A, Haag-Molkenteller C, Forst HT, Massow U, Wang J, Brodsky M: Clinical efficacy, safety, and tolerability of once-daily fesoterodine in subjects with overactive bladder. *Eur Urol* 2007, **52**:1204–1212. Corrigendum. Eur Urol 2008, 53:1319.

47. Ginsberg D, Schneider T, Kelleher C, Van Kerrebroeck P, Swift S, Creanga D, Martire DL: Efficacy of fesoterodine compared to extended-release tolterodine in men and women with overactive bladder. *BJU Int* 2013, **112**:373–385.

48. Thüroff JW, Abrams P, Andersson KE, Artibani W, Chapple CR, Drake MJ, Hampel C, Neisius A, Schröder A, Tubaro A: EAU guidelines on urinary incontinence. *Eur Urol* 2011, **59**(3):387–400.

49. Lucas MG, Bedretdinova D, Bosch JLHR, Burkhard F, Cruz F, Nambiar AK, de Ridder DJKM, Tubaro A, Pickard RS: *Guidelines on urinary incontinence.* Arnhem (The Netherlands): European Association of Urology (EAU); 2013:49–65.

50. Buser N, Ivic S, Kessler TM, Kessels AG, Bachmann LM: Efficacy and adverse events of antimuscarinics for treating overactive bladder: network meta-analyses. *Eur Urol* 2012, **62**(6):1040–1060.

# 11

# Prostate volume and biopsy tumor length are significant predictors for classical and redefined insignificant cancer on prostatectomy specimens in Japanese men with favorable pathologic features on biopsy

Masahiro Yashi[1*], Tomoya Mizuno[1], Hideo Yuki[1], Akinori Masuda[1], Tsunehito Kambara[1], Hironori Betsunoh[1], Hideyuki Abe[1], Yoshitatsu Fukabori[1], Osamu Muraishi[2], Koyu Suzuki[3], Yoshimasa Nakazato[4] and Takao Kamai[1]

## Abstract

**Background:** Gleason pattern 3 less often has molecular abnormalities and often behaves indolent. It is controversial whether low grade small foci of prostate cancer (PCa) on biopsy could avoid immediate treatment or not, because substantial cases harbor unfavorable pathologic results on prostatectomy specimens. This study was designed to identify clinical predictors for classical and redefined insignificant cancer on prostatectomy specimens in Japanese men with favorable pathologic features on biopsy.

**Methods:** Retrospective review of 1040 PCa Japanese patients underwent radical prostatectomy between 2006 and 2013. Of those, 170 patients (16.3%) met the inclusion criteria of clinical stage $\leq$ cT2a, Gleason score (GS) $\leq$ 6, up to two positive biopsies, and no more than 50% of cancer involvement in any core. The associations between preoperative data and unfavorable pathologic results of prostatectomy specimens, and oncological outcome were analyzed. The definition of insignificant cancer consisted of pathologic stage $\leq$ pT2, GS $\leq$ 6, and an index tumor volume < 0.5 mL (classical) or 1.3 mL (redefined).

**Results:** Pathologic stage $\geq$ pT3, upgraded GS, index tumor volume $\geq$ 0.5 mL, and $\geq$ 1.3 mL were detected in 25 (14.7%), 77 (45.3%), 83 (48.8%), and 53 patients (31.2%), respectively. Less than half of cases had classical (41.2%) and redefined (47.6%) insignificant cancer. The 5-year recurrence-free survival was 86.8%, and the insignificant cancers essentially did not relapse regardless of the surgical margin status. MRI-estimated prostate volume, tumor length on biopsy, prostate-specific antigen density (PSAD), and findings of magnetic resonance imaging were associated with the presence of classical and redefined insignificant cancer. Large prostate volume and short tumor length on biopsy remained as independent predictors in multivariate analysis.

**Conclusions:** Favorable features of biopsy often are followed by adverse pathologic findings on prostatectomy specimens despite fulfilling the established criteria. The finding that prostate volume is important does not simply mirror many other studies showing PSAD is important, and the clinical criteria for risk assessment before definitive therapy or active surveillance should incorporate these significant factors other than clinical T-staging or PSAD to minimize under-estimation of cancer in Japanese patients with low-risk PCa.

**Keywords:** Predictive factor, Insignificant cancer, Index tumor volume, Prostate volume, Biopsy tumor length

* Correspondence: yashima@dokkyomed.ac.jp
[1]Department of Urology, Dokkyo Medical University, 880 Kitakobayashi, Mibu, Shimotsuga, Tochigi 321-0293, Japan
Full list of author information is available at the end of the article

## Background

The widespread use of prostate-specific antigen (PSA) screening and multiple core biopsy protocol resulted in early detection of prostate cancer (PCa) at a curable stage, and was associated with dramatic decrease in PCa mortality in North America and Europe [1]. The European Randomized Study of Screening for Prostate Cancer (ERSPC) trial showed that PSA-based screening significantly reduced mortality by 21% [2]. The analysis of cancer trends using the national cancer mortality data in Japan also revealed the similar stage migration of PCa. The incidence of localized cancer increased markedly between 2000 and 2003 with an annual percent change of 29.7%, then became stable, while PCa mortality began to decrease in 2004 [3]. The early detection of PCa consequently raises the new issue that the proportion of low-risk cancers for which the definitive therapy will not alter prognosis has been increasing. Potential side effects after definitive therapies for localized cancer worsen the patients' quality of life [4], even with the current advantages of robot-assisted surgery or image-guided radiation therapy.

Gleason pattern 3 less often has molecular abnormalities, so called cancer hallmarks and often behaves indolent compared to Gleason pattern 4 in PCa [5,6]. Although all patients underwent prostatectomy and it was uncertain how therapeutic an effect it had, the 15-year cancer specific mortality rate for pathologic Gleason score (GS) 6 or less was reported as 0.2% [7]. On the other hand, it is controversial whether the low grade and low volume PCa within a few positive biopsy cores could avoid immediate definitive therapy or not, because some cases harbor unfavorable pathologic features at radical prostatectomy specimens with a variety of rates [8]. To predict clinically insignificant cancer in patients with clinical T1c (non-palpable) PCa, Epstein et al. reported a set of criteria [9], and later updated to the contemporary version, including PSA density < 0.15 ng/mL, biopsy Gleason score ≤ 6, the presence of tumor in two or fewer cores, and no more than 50% involvement by tumor in any core [10]. The review of validation studies on Epstein criteria concluded that it had suboptimal accuracy for predicting insignificant cancer from significant heterogeneity in the results of insignificant cancer, GS ≤ 6, and organ-confined status at 37–76%, 54.3–75.9% and 80.0–96.9%, respectively [11]. Currently, active surveillance (AS) has become one of the key treatment options as a strategy for deferring treatment for low-risk PCa in American and European urological associations' guidelines, but the presence of several AS protocols consisting of different clinic-pathologic factors complicate decision making of physicians and patients.

In view of the racial differences, the clinical criteria developed from Western cohort analysis could not be directly applied to Japanese or Asian patients [12]. In addition, the updated definition of index tumor volume threshold to 1.3 mL and total tumor volume threshold to 2.5 mL for insignificant cancer raises reconsideration of the current risk assessment before therapy [13]. To our knowledge, the study using this updated definition has still been insufficient. In this study, we investigated the associations between preoperative clinical data and pathologic results of prostatectomy specimens along with oncological outcome to identify predictors for classical and redefined insignificant cancer in Japanese men who met our expanded inclusion criteria.

## Methods

### Inclusion criteria of patients

The study population consisted of 1040 consecutive patients that underwent radical prostatectomy between January 2006 and December 2013 at 2 Japanese academic institutions. We retrospectively reviewed the records for those pathologic findings of multiple core biopsy and clinical stages. Of those, 170 patients met our inclusion criteria of clinical stage ≤ cT2a [14], GS ≤ 6 without Gleason pattern 4 or 5 as secondary scores, up to two biopsies with cancer, and no more than 50% of cancer involvement in any core; no limitation was set on PSA value and PSA density (PSAD). None of the patients had received hormonal treatments including antiandrogens, luteinizing hormone-releasing hormone analogues, or 5-alpha reductase inhibitors preoperatively.

### Preoperative clinical data including biopsy and radiographic image

Preoperative patient characteristics are provided in Table 1; All prostate volume was measured by magnetic resonance imaging (MRI), which was more accurate than transrectal ultrasound and computed tomography for volume estimation [15], and PSAD was determined as pre-biopsy PSA value divided by MRI-estimated prostate volume. The mean number of biopsy cores per procedure was 13.1 and 19 cases (11.2%) had fewer than 10 cores. Biopsy specimens obtained by transrectal and transperineal approaches were evaluated for GS, number of cores involved with cancer, total length of tissue, and length of cancer measured with subtracting the intervening benign glands. Gleason scoring of the biopsy specimens was done according to the International Society of Urological Pathology (ISUP) Consensus 2005; the second most prevalent pattern to the highest cancer grade observable in the specimen [16]. MRI findings were simply classified according to report by radiologists whether there were typical suspicious lesions for malignancy or not. Seventy patients (41.2%) fulfilled the contemporary Epstein criteria [10], and 103 patients (60.6%) fulfilled the criteria of the Prostate Cancer Research International: Active Surveillance (PRIAS) study [17]. The

## Table 1 Preoperative patient characteristic

|  | Number (%) or Mean value (range) |  |
|---|---|---|
| Number | 170 (100) |  |
| Age (year) |  | 65.5 (40 to 78) |
| PSA (ng/ml) |  | 7.4 (2.8 to 25.9) |
| Prostate volume (cc) |  | 40.2 (13.8 to 87.9) |
| PSA density (ng/ml/cc) |  | 0.208 (0.050 to 1.124) |
| Biospy core (n) |  | 13.1 (6 to 24) |
| Tumor length (mm) |  | 2.1 (0.1 to 7.0) |
| Biopsy approach |  |  |
| Transrectal | 137 (80.6) |  |
| Transperineal | 33 (19.4) |  |
| Positive core |  |  |
| 1 | 120 (70.6) |  |
| 2 | 50 (29.4) |  |
| Biopsy Gleason score |  |  |
| 5 | 7 (4.1) |  |
| 6 | 163 (95.9) |  |
| Clinical T stage(DRE) |  |  |
| cT1c | 154 (90.6) |  |
| cT2a | 16 (9.4) |  |
| MRI findings |  |  |
| Negative | 113 (66.5) |  |
| Positive | 57 (33.5) |  |
| Epstein criteria |  |  |
| Yes | 70 (41.2) |  |
| No | 100 (58.8) |  |
| PRIAS criteria |  |  |
| Yes | 103 (60.6) |  |
| No | 67 (39.4) |  |

*Abbreviations: DRE dicital rectal examination, PRIAS Prostate Cancer Research International: Active Surveillance.*

PRIAS criteria includes clinical stage ≤ T2, PSA ≤10 ng/mL, PSAD <0.2 ng/ml/cc, ≤2 positive cores, and GS ≤ 6.

### Evaluation of prostatectomy specimens

Prostatectomy specimens obtained through 127 open retropubic surgery (74.7%) and 43 through robot-assisted surgery (25.3%) were processed according to the Stanford protocol [18], step sectioned transversely at 5 mm intervals, and mounted as half or quarter sections for microscopic evaluation. Those were evaluated for GS, extraprostatic extension, surgical margin status, seminal vesicle invasion, lymph node involvement when dissection was performed, and tumor volume. Gleason scoring was also done as recommended in the ISUP Consensus 2005 [16]. Prostate cancer volume was calculated from the three-dimensional measurements of the

dominant nodule (index tumor) that correlates with oncological outcome better than total tumor volume [19], using a spherical formula and correcting by shrinkage factor (1.33) due to formalin fixation. Two specialists of urologic pathology from the 2 institutions reported the histopathology of biopsy and prostatectomy specimens, and we retrospectively reviewed the reports.

### Definitions

To avoid confusion of terminology, we describe the following definitions. Classical insignificant cancer was defined by a pathologic stage ≤ pT2, GS ≤ 6, and an index tumor volume < 0.5 mL [8]. Redefined insignificant cancer was characterized as a pathologic stage ≤ pT2, GS ≤ 6, and an updated index tumor volume threshold of 1.3 mL [13]. Both insignificant cancers are results confirmed on prostatectomy specimens. In addition, Epstein criteria and PRIAS criteria are established sets of preoperative factors to predict insignificant cancer [10,17]. Biochemical recurrence was defined as PSA level greater than 0.2 ng/mL with subsequent PSA rising.

### Analyses and statistics

The associations between preoperative clinical data and pathologic characteristics of prostatectomy specimens for targeting the unfavorable pathologic results, and oncological outcome were analyzed. The quantitative data were categorized into two groups by median values, and the qualitative data were compared using a chi-squared test or Fisher's exact test. Recurrence-free survival was estimated using the Kaplan–Meier method and differences were compared with the log-rank test. Logistic regression and Cox proportional hazards regression model were used for multivariate analyses. All statistical analyses were performed with EZR, which is a graphical user interface for R (The R Foundation for Statistical Computing, version 2.13.0). All statistical tests were two-sided, with $p$-value of less than 0.05 considered to be statistically significant.

### Ethics statement

This study was conducted in accordance with the Helsinki Declaration and was approved by the institutional ethical review boards at Dokkyo Medical University Hospital and St. Luke's International Hospital. In addition, each patient signed a consent form with regard to the storage of their information for the purpose of research.

### Results

Tumor characteristics of prostatectomy specimens are provided in Table 2. Pathologic stage ≥ pT3, positive surgical margin (PSM), upgraded GS, index tumor volume ≥ 0.5 mL, and ≥ 1.3 mL were detected in 25 patients (14.7%), 29 patients (17.1%), 77 patients (45.3%), 83 patients (48.8%), and 53 patients (31.2%), respectively. Less

**Table 2 Tumor Characteristic of prostatectomy specimens**

|  | Number (%) or Mean value (range) |
| --- | --- |
| Number | 170 (100) |
| Pathologic T stage |  |
| pT0 | 7 (4.1) |
| pT2 | 138 (80.2) |
| pT3a | 20 (11.8) |
| pT3b | 4 (2.4) |
| pT4 | 1 (0.6) |
| Surgical margin |  |
| Negative | 141 (82.9) |
| Positive | 29 (17.1) |
| Prostatectomy Gleason score |  |
| ≤6 | 86 (50.6) |
| 7 | 71 (41.8) |
| 8 | 6 (3.5) |
| NA | 7 (4.1) |
| Index tumor volume (cc) | 1.42 (0 to 14.62) |
| <0.5 | 87 (51.2) |
| 0.5-1.3 | 30 (17.6) |
| >1.3 | 53 (31.2) |
| Classical insignificant cancer |  |
| Yes | 70 (41.2) |
| No | 100 (58.8) |
| Redefined insignificant cancer |  |
| Yes | 81 (47.6) |
| No | 89 (52.4) |

*Abbreviations: NA* not available due to pT0.

than half of cases had classical (41.2%) and redefined (47.6%) insignificant cancer. Of those with stage ≥ pT3, 23 patients had extraprostatic extension, and 4 patients had seminal vesicle invasion. No lymph node involvement was observed among 158 patients (92.9%) who underwent lymph node dissection that was limited in the obturator areas. In 7 patients, pT0 cancers, namely "vanishing cancer" in prostatectomy specimens were observed. These cases were accounted as insignificant cancers for the following analysis.

Univariate analyses of preoperative factors revealed that the MRI-estimated prostate volume, PSAD, biopsy tumor length, MRI findings, contemporary Epstein criteria, and PRIAS criteria were all or partly associated with unfavorable pathologic results on prostatectomy specimens (Table 3), and all factors were associated with the presence of insignificant cancer of both definitions (Table 4). Meanwhile patient age, PSA value, number of biopsy cores or positive cores, biopsy Gleason score 5 or 6, difference in biopsy approach or institution, and clinical T-stage determined by digital rectal examination did

not hold any associations with unfavorable pathologic results. Multivariate model excluding the established preoperative criteria such as Epstein and PRIAS criteria showed that both large prostate volume (≥35.5 cc) and short tumor length on biopsy (≤2.0 mm) showed independent predictive value for both classical and redefined insignificant cancer. PSAD showed independent value for only redefined insignificant cancer (Table 4). Figure 1 shows the profiles of prostate volume distribution in relation to the unfavorable pathologic features, and the patients with prostate volume larger than 43.3 cc never presented with pathologic stage ≥ pT3, and rarely presented with PSM (only 2 cases).

During a median follow-up of 39.5 months (interquartile range 17.3-58.0), 16 patients developed biochemical recurrence. The estimated 5-year recurrence-free survival and cancer-specific survival were 87.0% and 100%, respectively. PSM was the only independent factor among unfavorable pathologic results. Figure 2 shows the Kaplan–Meier event curves for biochemical recurrence-free survivals. The patients with redefined insignificant cancers essentially did not relapse regardless of the surgical margin status, but 2 cases (2.5%) without PSM relapsed and consequently received salvage radiotherapy.

When statistics were limited in 70 patients who met the contemporary Epstein criteria, the rate of stage ≥ pT3, PSM, upgraded GS, index tumor volume ≥ 1.3 mL, and redefined insignificant cancer reduced to 10.0%, 7.1%, 31.4%, 18.6%, and 64.3%, respectively. In 103 patients who met criteria of the PRIAS study, those rates were 11.7%, 12.6%, 36.9%, 23.3%, and 56.3%, respectively. Furthermore, in 32 patients that were classified as intermediate risk or more because of a PSA value > 10 ng/mL, the rate of redefined insignificant cancer was 43.8%.

## Discussion

Our study demonstrated that prostate volume and biopsy tumor length had independent value for predicting both classical and redefined insignificant cancer, and PSAD showed the independent value for only the redefined insignificant cancer. The different statistics between classical and redefined insignificant cancers in the multivariate analysis might imply that PSAD possibly holds predictive power in larger or aggressive tumors. Substantial overlaps existed in cases with small prostate volume, but large prostate volume firmly had high positive predictive value for tumors of stage ≤ pT2 and negative surgical margins, namely organ-confined cancers. We consider that the finding that prostate volume is important does not simply mirror many other studies showing that PSAD is important. Furthermore, clinical T-staging had little value, and the multiparametric MRI would possibly add some diagnostic value if evaluation was performed in detail.

**Table 3 Preoperative factors associated with unfavorable pathologic results on prostatectomy specimens**

| Factors | pT-stage | | | Surgical margin | | | Gleason score | | | Index tumor volume | | | | | |
|---|---|---|---|---|---|---|---|---|---|---|---|---|---|---|---|
| | ≤pT2 | ≥pT3 | p-value | neg | posi | p-value | ≤6 | ≥7 | p-value | <0.5 mL | ≥0.5 mL | p-value | <1.3 mL | ≥1.3 mL | p-value |
| Prostate volume (cc) | | | | | | | | | | | | | | | |
| ≥35.5 | 81 | 4 | 0.0004 | 79 | 6 | 0.0009 | 61 | 24 | <0.0001 | 60 | 25 | <0.0001 | 71 | 14 | <0.0001 |
| <35.5 | 64 | 21 | | 62 | 23 | | 32 | 53 | | 27 | 58 | | 46 | 39 | |
| PSA density (ng/ml/cc) | | | | | | | | | | | | | | | |
| <0.172 | 78 | 7 | 0.0228 | 78 | 7 | 0.0037 | 58 | 27 | 0.0007 | 56 | 29 | 0.0002 | 69 | 16 | 0.0008 |
| ≥0.172 | 67 | 18 | | 63 | 22 | | 35 | 50 | | 31 | 54 | | 48 | 37 | |
| Tumor length (mm) | | | | | | | | | | | | | | | |
| ≤2.0 | 107 | 11 | 0.0045 | 102 | 16 | 0.0788 | 76 | 42 | 0.0002 | 74 | 44 | <0.0001 | 88 | 30 | 0.0194 |
| >2.0 | 38 | 14 | | 39 | 13 | | 17 | 35 | | 13 | 39 | | 29 | 23 | |
| MRI findings | | | | | | | | | | | | | | | |
| Positive | 99 | 14 | 0.2560 | 99 | 14 | 0.0305 | 69 | 44 | 0.0227 | 68 | 45 | 0.0011 | 83 | 30 | 0.0801 |
| Negative | 46 | 11 | | 42 | 15 | | 24 | 33 | | 19 | 38 | | 34 | 23 | |
| Epstein criteria | | | | | | | | | | | | | | | |
| Yes | 63 | 7 | 0.1880 | 65 | 5 | 0.0038 | 48 | 22 | 0.0029 | 49 | 21 | <0.0001 | 57 | 13 | 0.0040 |
| No | 82 | 18 | | 76 | 24 | | 45 | 55 | | 38 | 63 | | 60 | 40 | |
| PRIAS criteria | | | | | | | | | | | | | | | |
| Yes | 91 | 21 | 0.1870 | 90 | 13 | 0.0633 | 65 | 38 | 0.0075 | 64 | 39 | 0.0005 | 79 | 24 | 0.0070 |
| No | 54 | 13 | | 51 | 16 | | 28 | 39 | | 23 | 44 | | 38 | 39 | |

*Abbreviations: neg negative, posi positive.*

The favorable features on multiple core biopsies consistently harbor unfavorable pathologic results on prostatectomy specimens despite fulfilling the established criteria developed in North America and Europe. Certainly, in our data, patients meeting Epstein and PRIAS criteria harbored clinically significant cancer for one-third and around half of cases, respectively. Oon et al. speculated that the modification to Gleason scoring might be associated with a reduced accuracy of Epstein criteria, because distinct differences were observed in validation studies between pre- and post-2005 [11,18]. In addition, Wolters, et al. presented a recent analysis using a data set from a randomized screening trial that demonstrated that clinically insignificant prostate cancer may include GS 6, pT2 tumors with index tumor volumes of up to 1.3 mL [13] instead of 0.5 mL, which had been used as a threshold for around 20 years [20]. These critical alterations suggest reconsideration of the current methods used for risk assessment before definitive therapy or AS. The established criteria consisting of clinical T-staging by digital rectal examination or PSAD would not be satisfactory for patients in this study, and the clinical criteria should be compiled incorporating the prostate size and biopsy length involved by cancer.

**Table 4 Univariate and multivariate analyses of factors predicting classical and redefined insignificant cancer**

| Factors | Classical insignificant cancer | | | | | | Redefined insignificant cancer | | | | | |
|---|---|---|---|---|---|---|---|---|---|---|---|---|
| | Univariate model | | | Multivariate model | | | Univariate model | | | Multivariate model | | |
| | OR | 95% CI | p-value | OR | 95% CI | p-value | OR | 95% CI | p-value | OR | 95% CI | p-value |
| Prostate volume (≥35.5 vs.<35.5) | 5.87 | 2.97-11.60 | <0.0001 | 4.59 | 2.13-9.90 | 0.0001 | 5.79 | 2.99-11.20 | <0.0001 | 4.31 | 2.07-8.98 | <0.0001 |
| PSA density (<0.172 vs. ≥0.172) | 3.71 | 1.94-7.10 | <0.0001 | 2.12 | 0.99-4.53 | 0.0533 | 3.74 | 1.98-7.06 | <0.0001 | 2.11 | 1.01-4.40 | 0.0460 |
| Tumor length (≤2.0 vs. >2.0) | 5.11 | 2.29-11.40 | <0.0001 | 5.41 | 2.21-13.2 | 0.0001 | 3.57 | 1.75-7.27 | 0.0005 | 3.46 | 1.56-7.69 | 0.0023 |
| MRI findings (neg vs. posi) | 2.43 | 1.22-4.83 | 0.0148 | 2.13 | 0.95-4.75 | 0.0663 | 2.17 | 1.12-4.19 | 0.0210 | 1.84 | 0.86-3.94 | 0.1150 |
| Epstein criteria (yes vs. no) | 3.46 | 1.82-6.58 | 0.0002 | | | | 3.20 | 1.69-6.05 | 0.0003 | | | |
| PRIAS criteria (yes vs. no) | 2.48 | 1.28-4.78 | 0.0068 | | | | 2.47 | 1.30-4.66 | 0.0055 | | | |

*Abbreviations: OR Odds ratio, 95% CI 95% confidence interval, neg negative, posi positive.*

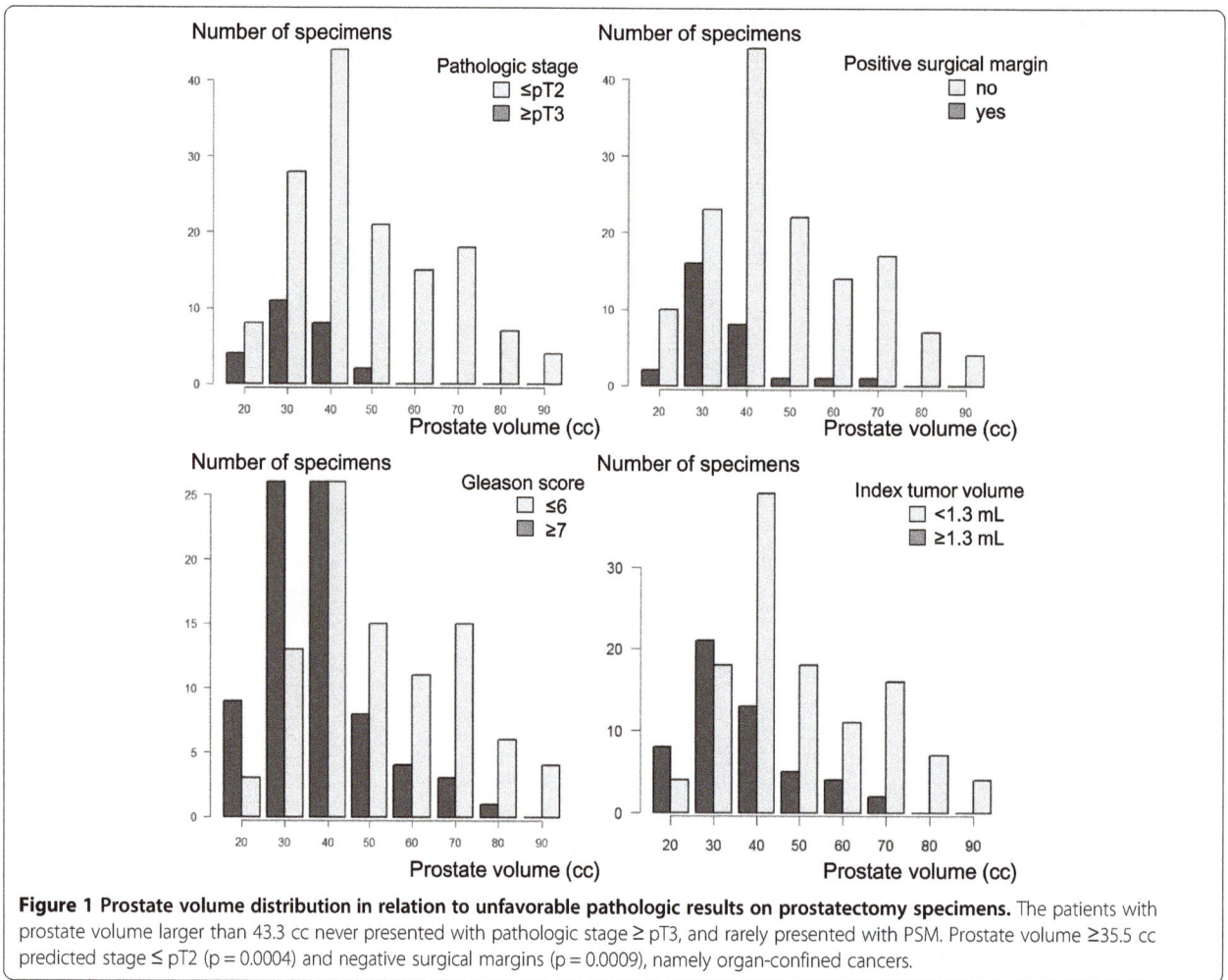

**Figure 1 Prostate volume distribution in relation to unfavorable pathologic results on prostatectomy specimens.** The patients with prostate volume larger than 43.3 cc never presented with pathologic stage ≥ pT3, and rarely presented with PSM. Prostate volume ≥35.5 cc predicted stage ≤ pT2 (p = 0.0004) and negative surgical margins (p = 0.0009), namely organ-confined cancers.

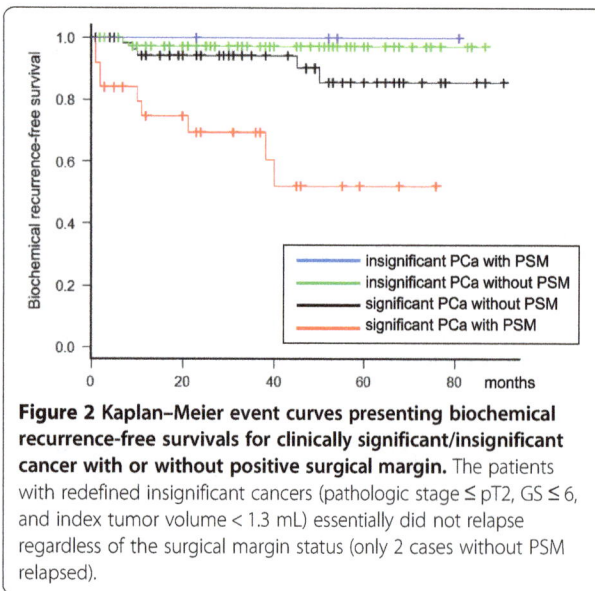

**Figure 2 Kaplan–Meier event curves presenting biochemical recurrence-free survivals for clinically significant/insignificant cancer with or without positive surgical margin.** The patients with redefined insignificant cancers (pathologic stage ≤ pT2, GS ≤ 6, and index tumor volume < 1.3 mL) essentially did not relapse regardless of the surgical margin status (only 2 cases without PSM relapsed).

Prostate volume has been less often mentioned than PSAD or PSA as a predictive factor despite that all of these parameters held independent values [21]. PSAD is a comprehensive parameter considering both serum PSA and prostate size, but the value varies easily based on the fluctuation of PSA. In that sense, prostate volume estimated using MRI is a stable preoperative parameter and the only tumor-unrelated factor in our analysis model. Despite the variations of study design and whether the prostate volume was estimated pre- or postoperatively, small prostate volume is unanimously reported with association between the poor oncological outcomes in several studies. Freedland et al. reported that more high-grade and more advanced cancers were detected in men with smaller prostates along with lower serum testosterone concentrations in a large population ranging from clinical T1 to T3 cancers and suggested that prostate size might be an important prognostic variable that should be evaluated for use pre- and postoperatively [22]. Tilki et al. and Chung et al. reported the associations especially in relation to GS upgrading [21,23]. These trends were also observed even when study populations were limited with GS ≤ 6 by Milonas et al. [24] and with highly selective criteria (T1c, PSA < 10 ng/mL, a single positive biopsy, tumor length < 3 mm, and Gleason score < 7) by Beauval et al. [25]. The prostate volume would be directly affected by age and endocrine factors [26], and the mean prostate size should be significantly different between Japanese and Western populations even after adjusting for differences in age, height, and weight [27]. Although the median prostate volume was obviously different between 35.5 cc in our study and more than 40 to 50 cc in the Western study, our study confirmed that prostate volume retained its predictive ability for both classical and redefined insignificant cancer in Japanese men.

The percentage and length of cancer involvement in biopsy core are also significant predictors, and have already been incorporated in the major prediction models before developing AS protocols [28]. Russo et al. reported that inclusion of the percentage of cancer involvement contributed to reducing the misclassification in patients eligible for AS according to the PRIAS criteria, which does not reference any cancer involvement in the core [29]. Antonelli et al. used the updated definition of total tumor volume and determined its optimal cutoff to be 20% for the diagnosis of insignificant cancer using the receiver operating characteristic curve [30]. Freedland et al. reported the same threshold of 20% for predicting PSA recurrence after prostatectomy [31]. We agree with their strict threshold despite the fact that our data were analyzed in terms of tumor length but not in the percentage of tumor involvement, and we consider the threshold of 50%, which is used in the many AS protocols, to be too relaxed to avoid under-estimation of cancer. However, a more stringent threshold, namely minute or microfocal cancer defined by ≤ 5% or ≤ 1 mm in a single core, is not a guarantee of insignificant cancer [8].

The current established clinical criteria can-not eliminate the risk of over- and under- estimation of cancer. A stringent selection criteria excludes a considerable number of patients who are willing to be managed by AS, even those having potentially insignificant cancer, and therefore, well-balanced criteria between sensitivity and specificity are required for patients. The implication of increasing the index tumor volume threshold to 1.3 mL is that we should miss small-volume cancer and set the AS protocols to be more expanded. In the recent report of head-to-head comparison of contemporary AS protocols, Iremashvili et al. revealed that the PRIAS and University of Miami criteria demonstrated the best balance between sensitivity and specificity for insignificant prostate cancer among the existing AS protocols, and the contemporary Epstein criteria demonstrated high specificity but low sensitivity for all end points [32].

Nevertheless, clinically significant cancer might not always progress, and some cases might remain indolent for a substantial duration of time. A validation of AS protocol should not be a surrogate endpoint, such as the analysis of the pathologic results of prostatectomy specimens, but should be a long-term outcome of a prospective cohort. According to the review of AS in the large prospective series, approximately one-third of patients were treated after a median surveillance of about 2.5 years because of histologic reclassification on biopsy or a PSA doubling time of less than 3 years, while some cases were treated with no evidence of progression [33]. The short- to mid-term estimated treatment-free survivals were reported as 62 to 72% at 5 years and at 43 to 62% at 10 years [34,35]. These data characterize AS as a strategy for deferring treatment and justify it as an optimal choice for patients with low-risk PCa that can accept the confirmatory biopsy within 1 to 2 years and the slight increased risk of late metastasis.

To develop a model to discriminate clinically indolent from aggressive disease efficiently, advances in biochemical markers replacing PSA or PSA derivatives such as prostate cancer antigen 3 or transmembrane protease serine 2 will be required in addition to the existing factors [36]. In addition, a more detailed analysis of multiparametric MRI, including number of lesions, lesion suspicion, and lesion density (calculated as total lesion volume/prostate volume) [37], and image-guided targeted biopsy should play a positive role [38]. The current study has some limitations; there is no control population outside of Japan other than the published literature. It is a retrospective study based on a relatively small Japanese population, and the pathologic examination was performed at 2 institutions. The median follow-up time was also relatively short to determine oncological outcomes. Thus, the results may not apply to the Western population. Nonetheless, it is valuable to give insight into ethnic differences, and these data provide useful information that could help predict insignificant cancer in Japanese or Asian patients with favorable features on needle biopsy. The findings of this study should be validated in a larger, independent dataset.

## Conclusions

The favorable features of biopsy often are followed by adverse pathologic findings on prostatectomy specimens despite fulfilling the established criteria. Large prostate volume and short tumor length on biopsy remained as independent predictors for classical and redefined insignificant prostate cancer in Japanese patients with favorable pathologic features on needle biopsy. The clinical criteria for risk assessment before definitive therapy or AS should incorporate these factors to minimize under-estimation of cancer in Japanese patients with low-risk PCa.

## Competing interests
The authors declare that they have no competing interests.

## Authors' contributions
MY, TM and OM initiated this study, participated in its design and coordination, carried out the study, performed the statistical analysis. MY, TM drafted the manuscript. HY, AM, TK, HB, HA, YF, KS, YN and TK carried out the study. All authors read and approved the final manuscript.

## Acknowledgement
The authors are special thanks to Toshihisa Iwabuchi, Chief Director of Urology at Yamato Hospital, Tokyo, Japan, for his practical advice in conducting this study, and assistance in statistical work.

## Author details
[1]Department of Urology, Dokkyo Medical University, 880 Kitakobayashi, Mibu, Shimotsuga, Tochigi 321-0293, Japan. [2]Department of Urology, St. Luke's International Hospital, Tokyo, Japan. [3]Department of Pathology, St. Luke's International Hospital, Tokyo, Japan. [4]Department of Pathology, Dokkyo Medical University, Tochigi, Japan.

## References
1. Jemal A, Siegel R, Xu J, Ward E: **Cancer statistics, 2010.** *CA Cancer J Clin* 2010, **60:**277–300.
2. Schröder FH, Hugosson J, Roobol MJ, Tammela TL, Ciatto S, Nelen V, Kwiatkowski M, Lujan M, Lilja H, Zappa M, Denis LJ, Recker F, Páez A, Määttänen L, Bangma CH, Aus G, Carlsson S, Villers A, Rebillard X, van der Kwast T, Kujala PM, Blijenberg BG, Stenman UH, Huber A, Taari K, Hakama M, Moss SM, de Koning HJ, Auvinen A, ERSPC Investigators: **Prostate-cancer mortality at 11 years of follow-up.** *N Engl J Med* 2012, **366:**981–990.
3. Katanoda K, Matsuda T, Matsuda A, Shibata A, Nishino Y, Fujita M, Soda M, Ioka A, Sobue T, Nishimoto H: **An updated report of the trends in cancer incidence and mortality in Japan.** *Jpn J Clin Oncol* 2013, **43:**492–507.
4. Johansson E, Steineck G, Holmberg L, Johansson JE, Nyberg T, Ruutu M, Bill-Axelson A, SPCG-4 Investigators: **Long-term quality-of-life outcomes after radical prostatectomy or watchful waiting: the Scandinavian Prostate Cancer Group-4 randomised trial.** *Lancet Oncol* 2011, **12:**891–899.
5. Ahmed HU, Arya M, Freeman A, Emberton M: **Do low-grade and low-volume prostate cancers bear the hallmarks of malignancy?** *Lancet Oncol* 2012, **13:**e509–e517.
6. Hanahan D, Weinberg RA: **Hallmarks of cancer: the next generation.** *Cell* 2011, **144:**646–674.
7. Eggener SE, Scardino PT, Walsh PC, Han M, Partin AW, Trock BJ, Feng Z, Wood DP, Eastham JA, Yossepowitch O, Rabah DM, Kattan MW, Yu C, Klein EA, Stephenson AJ: **Predicting 15-year prostate cancer specific mortality after radical prostatectomy.** *J Urol* 2011, **185:**869–875.
8. Ploussard G, Epstein JI, Montironi R, Carroll PR, Wirth M, Grimm MO, Bjartell AS, Montorsi F, Freedland SJ, Erbersdobler A, van der Kwast TH: **The contemporary concept of significant versus insignificant prostate cancer.** *Eur Urol* 2011, **60:**291–303.
9. Epstein JI, Walsh PC, Carmichael M, Brendler CB: **Pathologic and clinical findings to predict tumor extent of nonpalpable (stage T1c) prostate cancer.** *JAMA* 1994, **271:**368–374.
10. Bastian PJ, Mangold LA, Epstein JI, Partin AW: **Characteristics of insignificant clinical T1c prostate tumors. A contemporary analysis.** *Cancer* 2004, **101:**2001–2005.
11. Oon SF, Watson RW, O'Leary JJ, Fitzpatrick JM: **Epstein criteria for insignificant prostate cancer.** *BJU Int* 2011, **108:**518–525.
12. Lee SE, Kim DS, Lee WK, Park HZ, Lee CJ, Doo SH, Jeong SJ, Yoon CY, Byun SS, Choe G, Hwang SI, Lee HJ, Hong SK: **Application of the Epstein criteria for prediction of clinically insignificant prostate cancer in Korean men.** *BJU Int* 2010, **105:**1526–1530.
13. Wolters T, Roobol MJ, van Leeuwen PJ, van den Bergh RC, Hoedemaeker RF, van Leenders GJ, Schröder FH, van der Kwast TH: **A critical analysis of the tumor volume threshold for clinically insignificant prostate cancer using a data set of a randomized screening trial.** *J Urol* 2011, **185:**121–125.
14. Reese AC, Landis P, Han M, Epstein JI, Carter HB: **Expanded criteria to identify men eligible for active surveillance of low risk prostate cancer at johns hopkins: a preliminary analysis.** *J Urol* 2013, **190:**2033–2038.
15. Karademir I, Shen D, Peng Y, Liao S, Jiang Y, Yousuf A, Karczmar G, Sammet S, Wang S, Medved M, Antic T, Eggener S, Oto A: **Prostate volumes derived from MRI and volume-adjusted serum prostate-specific antigen: correlation with Gleason score of prostate cancer.** *AJR Am J Roentgenol* 2013, **201:**1041–1048.
16. Egevad LL; ISUP Grading Committee, Epstein JI, Allsbrook WC Jr, Amin MB: **The 2005 International Society of Urological Pathology (ISUP) Consensus Conference on Gleason Grading of Prostatic Carcinoma.** *Am J Surg Pathol* 2005, **29:**1228–1242.
17. Bul M, Zhu X, Valdagni R, Pickles T, Kakehi Y, Rannikko A, Bjartell A, van der Schoot DK, Cornel EB, Conti GN, Boevé ER, Staerman F, Vis-Maters JJ, Vergunst H, Jaspars JJ, Strölin P, van Muilekom E, Schröder FH, Bangma CH, Roobol MJ: **Active surveillance for low-risk prostate cancer worldwide: the PRIAS study.** *Eur Urol* 2013, **63:**597–603.
18. McNeal JE, Redwine EA, Freiha FS, Stamey TA: **Zonal distribution of prostatic adenocarcinoma. Correlation with histologic pattern and direction of spread.** *Am J Surg Pathol* 1988, **12:**897–906.
19. Billis A, Meirelles LR, Freitas LL, Polidoro AS, Fernandes HA, Padilha MM, Magna LA, Ferreira U: **Prostate total tumor extent versus index tumor extent–which is predictive of biochemical recurrence following radical prostatectomy?** *J Urol* 2013, **189:**99–104.
20. Stamey TA, Freiha FS, McNeal JE, Redwine EA, Whittemore AS, Schmid HP: **Localized prostate cancer. Relationship of tumor volume to clinical significance for treatment of prostate cancer.** *Cancer* 1993, **71**(Suppl):933–938.
21. Tilki D, Schlenker B, John M, Buchner A, Stanislaus P, Gratzke C, Karl A, Tan GY, Ergün S, Tewari AK, Stief CG, Seitz M, Reich O: **Clinical and pathologic predictors of Gleason sum upgrading in patients after radical prostatectomy: results from a single institution series.** *Urol Oncol* 2011, **29:**508–514.
22. Freedland SJ, Isaacs WB, Platz EA, Terris MK, Aronson WJ, Amling CL, Presti JC Jr, Kane CJ: **Prostate size and risk of high-grade, advanced prostate cancer and biochemical progression after radical prostatectomy: a search database study.** *J Clin Oncol* 2005, **23:**7546–7554.
23. Chung MS, Lee SH, Lee DH, Chung BH: **Is small prostate volume a predictor of Gleason score upgrading after radical prostatectomy?** *Yonsei Med J* 2013, **54:**902–906.
24. Milonas D, Grybas A, Auskalnis S, Gudinaviciene I, Baltrimavicius R, Kincius M, Jievaltas M: **Factors predicting Gleason score 6 upgrading after radical prostatectomy.** *Cent Eur J Urol* 2011, **64:**205–208.
25. Beauval JB, Ploussard G, Soulié M, Pfister C, Van Agt S, Vincendeau S, Larue S, Rigaud J, Gaschignard N, Rouprêt M, Drouin S, Peyromaure M, Long JA, Iborra F, Vallancien G, Rozet F, Salomon L, Members of Committee of Cancerology of the French Association of Urology (CCAFU): **Pathologic findings in radical prostatectomy specimens from patients eligible for active surveillance with highly selective criteria: a multicenter study.** *Urology* 2012, **80:**656–660.
26. Partin AW, Oesterling JE, Epstein JI, Horton R, Walsh PC: **Influence of age and endocrine factors on the volume of benign prostatic hyperplasia.** *J Urol* 1991, **145:**405–409.
27. Masumori N, Tsukamoto T, Kumamoto Y, Miyake H, Rhodes T, Girman CJ, Guess HA, Jacobsen SJ, Lieber MM: **Japanese men have smaller prostate volumes but comparable urinary flow rates relative to American men: results of community based studies in 2 countries.** *J Urol* 1996, **155:**1324–1327.
28. Steyerberg EW, Roobol MJ, Kattan MW, van der Kwast TH, de Koning HJ, Schröder FH: **Prediction of indolent prostate cancer: validation and updating of a prognostic nomogram.** *J Urol* 2007, **177:**107–112.
29. Russo GI, Cimino S, Castelli T, Favilla V, Urzì D, Veroux M, Madonia M, Morgia G: **Percentage of cancer involvement in positive cores can predict unfavorable disease in men with low-risk prostate cancer but eligible for the prostate cancer international: Active surveillance criteria.** *Urol Oncol* 2014, **32:**291–296.
30. Antonelli A, Vismara Fugini A, Tardanico R, Giovanessi L, Zambolin T, Simeone C: **The percentage of core involved by cancer is the best predictor of insignificant prostate cancer, according to an updated definition (tumor volume up to 2.5 cm3): analysis of a cohort of 210 consecutive patients with low-risk disease.** *Urology* 2014, **83:**28–32.

31. Freedland SJ, Aronson WJ, Csathy GS, Kane CJ, Amling CL, Presti JC Jr, Dorey F, Terris MK, SEARCH Database Study Group: **Comparison of percentage of total prostate needle biopsy tissue with cancer to percentage of cores with cancer for predicting PSA recurrence after radical prostatectomy: results from the SEARCH database.** *Urology* 2003, **61**:742–747.

32. Iremashvili V, Pelaez L, Manoharan M, Jorda M, Rosenberg DL, Soloway MS: **Pathologic prostate cancer characteristics in patients eligible for active surveillance: a head-to-head comparison of contemporary protocols.** *Eur Urol* 2012, **62**:462–468.

33. Dall'Era MA, Albertsen PC, Bangma C, Carroll PR, Carter HB, Cooperberg MR, Freedland SJ, Klotz LH, Parker C, Soloway MS: **Active surveillance for prostate cancer: a systematic review of the literature.** *Eur Urol* 2012, **62**:976–983.

34. Klotz L, Zhang L, Lam A, Nam R, Mamedov A, Loblaw A: **Clinical results of long-term follow-up of a large, active surveillance cohort with localized prostate cancer.** *J Clin Oncol* 2010, **28**:126–131.

35. van den Bergh RC, Roemeling S, Roobol MJ, Aus G, Hugosson J, Rannikko AS, Tammela TL, Bangma CH, Schröder FH: **Outcomes of men with screen-detected prostate cancer eligible for active surveillance who were managed expectantly.** *Eur Urol* 2009, **55**:1–8.

36. Dijkstra S, Birker IL, Smit FP, Leyten GH, de Reijke TM, van Oort IM, Mulders PF, Jannink SA, Schalken JA: **Prostate Cancer Biomarker Profiles in Urinary Sediments and Exosomes.** *J Urol* 2014, **191**:1132–1138.

37. Stamatakis L, Siddiqui MM, Nix JW, Logan J, Rais-Bahrami S, Walton-Diaz A, Hoang AN, Vourganti S, Truong H, Shuch B, Parnes HL, Turkbey B, Choyke PL, Wood BJ, Simon RM, Pinto PA: **Accuracy of multiparametric magnetic resonance imaging in confirming eligibility for active surveillance for men with prostate cancer.** *Cancer* 2013, **119**:3359–3366.

38. Haffner J, Lemaitre L, Puech P, Haber GP, Leroy X, Jones JS, Villers A: **Role of magnetic resonance imaging before initial biopsy: comparison of magnetic resonance imaging-targeted and systematic biopsy for significant prostate cancer detection.** *BJU Int* 2011, **108**(8 Pt 2):E171–E178.

# 12

# Flexible ureteroscopy training for surgeons using isolated porcine kidneys in vitro

Dongliang Hu, Tongzu Liu* and Xinghuan Wang

## Abstract

**Background:** To evaluate the feasibility of flexible ureteroscopy training by using isolated porcine kidneys and ureters in vitro.

**Methods:** Twenty young urologists were randomly divided into four groups. Overall performance was assessed based on a global rating scale, pass/fail rating, total time to complete task, learning curve, incidence of trauma, and perforations. The effect of training was determined by comparing their performance in baseline with that in the post-test.

**Results:** After the training, average operation time significantly decreased from $18 \pm 3.4$ min to $11 \pm 1.2$ min ($P < 0.05$). The urologists exhibited a relatively stable performance level after the sixth operation. Significant differences were observed between pre-test and post-test with respect to the global rating scale and the pass/fail rating ($P < 0.05$). However, the incidence of mucosal trauma and perforations did not change significantly ($P = 0.26$ and 0.35, respectively).

**Conclusions:** The isolated porcine kidneys are convenient and intuitive models for young urologists to practice flexible ureteroscopy on.

**Keywords:** Ureteroscopes, Training, Porcine kidney, Teaching

## Background

Minimally invasive technologies, including flexible ureteroscopy, on kidney stones have developed rapidly. Flexible ureteroscopy is characterized by a relatively high safety and less injuries. It is widely used in urological diagnoses and treatments [1]; the indications are summarized in Table 1. The disadvantages of flexible ureteroscopy include high price, high repair cost, and low reusability, thereby limiting its application in clinical practice [2, 3]. Young urologists need a long learning curve, but they are given less operation opportunity. Thus, simulated training or actual practice is particularly crucial to them [4].

Unlike laparoscopic technique, flexible ureteroscopy is characterized by a relatively narrow field and a small operating channel. Flexible ureteroscopy training focuses on finding and locating renal calyces instead of on operating skills. To enable young urologists to understand and master flexible ureteroscopy intuitively within a short period, we trained 20 young urologists by using porcine kidneys in vitro. All operations were performed via modular flexible ureteroscopy. We report our experience in this paper.

## Methods

### Experimental preparation

Four pairs of fresh porcine kidneys (including the ureter) were purchased from a slaughterhouse on the day of the experiment. To achieve smooth insertion of the ureteroscope access sheath, all specimens were soaked in warm water before training to thaw or avoid stiffness. The modular semi-disposable PolyScope system has a deflexion angle of 225 ° and a working channel diameter of 3.6 F [5, 6]. The rigid ureteroscope and guidewire were prepared to deal with a few difficult operations.

Researchers often choose residents or medical students as training subjects. To avoid wasting time on training students with basic skills, we trained 20 urologists who have 5 years to 8 years of experience and who are qualified attending physicians because flexible ureteroscopy typically requires rigid ureteroscopy and cystoscopy skills. All the participants had assisted in flexible ureteroscopy surgeries, but none had performed the operation as lead surgeon.

* Correspondence: 513199176@qq.com
Department of Urology, Zhongnan Hospital of Wuhan University, Wuhan, China

**Table 1** The indications for flexible ureteroscopy

| | Indications |
|---|---|
| Flexible Ureteroscopy | holmium: YAG laser lithotripsy for treatment |
| | diagnostic ureteroscopy |
| | patients with hematuria but CT and fluorescence in situ hybridization (FISH) negative result |
| | solitary kidney |
| | hard to percutaneous nephroscope lithotripsy |
| | kidney stone less than 2 cm in diameter |
| | etc. |

The participants have not yet performed this operation independently.

The study was approved by the Ethical Committee of Zhongnan Hospital of Wuhan University and carried out in compliance with the Helsinki declaration. Participants signed an informed consent prior to enrolment in the study.

## Surgical methods
### Brief steps
The isolated porcine kidneys and ureters were placed and fixed on the net bar of the operating platform (Fig. 1). The ureteroscope access sheath was inserted into the ureteral orifice to establish a working channel for washing. The modular semi-disposable flexible ureteroscope was ready, and the focal distance was adjusted in vitro.

### Pre-test preparation
A total of 20 young urologists were randomly divided into 4 groups. They attended a didactic teaching session given by a tutor, who provided a review of genitourinary anatomy, instruments, endoscopic techniques, and related knowledge. A supervised hands-on practice session

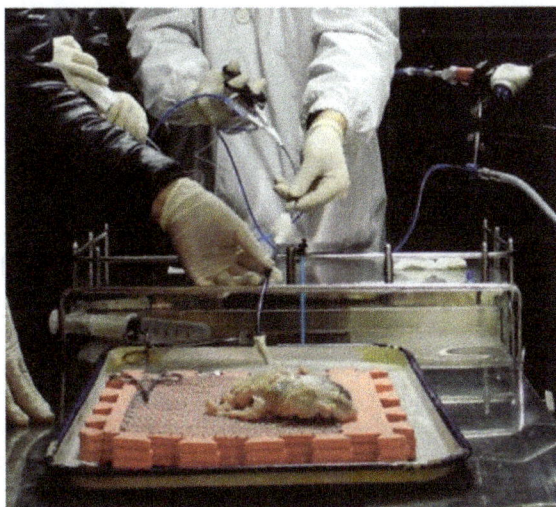

**Fig. 1** Isolated porcine kidney and ureter

was conducted. The urologists were allowed to practice repeatedly with the instruments to familiarize themselves with the task. During this session, the tutor provided instructive feedback.

### Main assessments
A pre-test was administered to all the urologists to assess their baseline endoscopic ability before the study, and then, a post-test was given after the training intervention. The urologists were evaluated during the procedure by an experienced tutor by using a global rating scale that assesses performance parameters (see Additional file 1) [7]. Other data included total time to complete the task, incidence of mucosal trauma from the endoscope or instruments, and the number of perforations. An evaluation (pass/fail rating) was also conducted after the training program (see Additional file 1). In this program, operation time was defined as the time elapsed between access sheath insertion and task completion.

### Training contents
The urologists were instructed to insert the ureteroscope access sheath and finish the required task. To compare operation time easily and uniformly, the tutor assigned the same training content to all participants in each operation: looking for the foreign body placed randomly in the kidneys and telling the specific renal calix. The tutor explained the key differences between flexible and rigid ureteroscopies, such as hand–eye coordination during examination, cooperation points in moving the ureteroscope, and handling strength in transforming the visual field. To save time, other skills that are identical or similar to rigid ureteroscopy were not emphasized during training. All the urologists observed the left and right kidneys separately (i.e., from easy to complicated) step by step. We trained a total of four operations, and thus, each participant was provided with eight operating opportunities. In the training, the tutor reviewed their shortcomings and time-consuming points after each operation. As a result, the urologists can improve their skills in the next operation based on their own understanding, thus indicating the efficiency of training.

To make the training impressive, intuitive, and clear, we enhanced light-source intensity and observed its shadow through a renal capsule. In this manner, the urologists can expediently achieve real-time positioning, and the training results can be verified after surgery through renal parenchyma incision.

### Statistical analyses
All results were expressed as mean ± SE. The data was analyzed for statistical significance by using $t$-test, chi-square, and Mann–Whitney $U$ test (SPSS 15.0 software). The differences were considered significant at $P < 0.05$.

## Results

All the urologists finished the training contents according to the assignment. Five urologists from each group individually practiced the procedure by using four pairs of left and right isolated porcine kidneys; thus, a total of eight operation times for each urologist were recorded.

After the training, the average operation time significantly decreased from the initial $18 \pm 3.4$ min to $11 \pm 1.2$ min ($P < 0.05$). Significant differences were found between the pre-test and post-test with respect to the global rating scale and the pass/fail rating ($P < 0.05$, Table 2). However, the difference between the incidence of mucosal trauma and the number of perforations from the pre-test to post-test was insignificant ($P = 0.26$ and $0.35$, respectively; Table 2). Based on the learning curve (Fig. 2), we found that the urologists achieved a relatively stable performance level after the sixth operation.

## Discussion

Compared with laparoscopic training, reports on flexible ureteroscopy training are relatively rare. Urologists have been trained by using validated simulators or computer-based models [8, 9] without true anatomical experience and simulation environment [10]. Animal surgery has also been performed by using pigs under general endotracheal anesthesia [11]. By using pigs as models, the following factors should be considered before training. A double J tube must be placed on the pigs 2 weeks to 4 weeks before surgery to insert the ureteroscope access sheath that will be used as a working channel during surgery. This process is complex and time consuming with disregard to anesthesia or operating procedures. The key point of flexible ureteroscopy training is to observe the different renal calyces, particularly the lower ones, and thus, a live/intact pig or an enclosed abdomen is unnecessary. By contrast, carbon dioxide pneumoperitoneum is needed in laparoscopic training to perform the operation in a closed space. We conducted trainings by using pigs in the early stages, and found that inserting an ureteroscope access sheath and performing the subsequent operations are difficult because experimental pigs are relatively young. Unlike adult pigs, the urethra and ureter of young pigs are considerably thinner, and thus, the trainees cannot finish the training program easily.

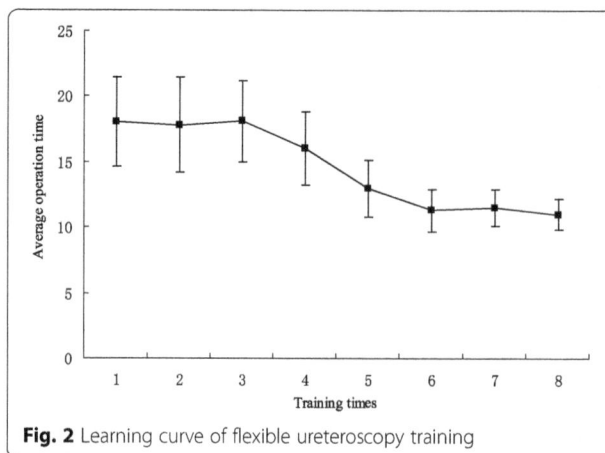

**Fig. 2** Learning curve of flexible ureteroscopy training

**Table 2** Testing performance

| Variable | Pre-test | Post-test | P value |
|---|---|---|---|
| Global rating scale | $19.3 \pm 0.8$ | $28.7 \pm 1.1$ | <0.05 |
| Pass rating | 6/20 | 19/20 | <0.05 |
| Time to complete task (min) | $18 \pm 3.4$ | $11 \pm 1.2$ | <0.05 |
| Mucosal trauma (No.) | $0.8 \pm 0.5$ | $0.6 \pm 0.3$ | 0.26 |
| Number of perforations | $0.23 \pm 0.2$ | $0.19 \pm 0.1$ | 0.35 |

Based on these situations, we used isolated porcine kidneys as training objects. Compared with a live/intact pig, the main advantages and characteristics of isolated porcine kidneys are summarized as follows. (1) Omission of the preoperative preparation, thereby increasing training and learning time. (2) As training objects, isolated kidneys are cheaper and easier to obtain than experimental pigs, thereby reducing training cost. (3) Changes in the visual field caused by different handling manipulations can be shown intuitively and clearly. The specific advantage of a modular flexible ureteroscope is its lens, which can only bend in one direction. However, the ureteroscope body and handle can be moved forward and backward and rotated 360°. In addition, the visual field of flexible ureteroscopy is different from that of rigid ureteroscopy, which has a linear scan imaging characteristic because unconscious shaking and handle grip strength change the direction of the lens and the visual range. All these differences emphasize the difficulty of flexible ureteroscopy training. To enable the urologists to master a sense of position as soon as possible, we enhanced the brightness of light to allow it to penetrate the surface of the kidney. Under such condition, verifying whether target renal calyces are reached accurately is convenient, and positioning differences between rigid and flexible ureteroscopy can then be compared visually. However, these experiences could not be accumulated in an experimental pig during endoscopic operation. (4) Side injury and complications of flexible ureteroscopy can be summarized intuitively. At the start of the preliminary training, the urologists inserted a flexible ureteroscope directly without placing an access sheath because of the relatively low temperature and stiff ureter. As a result, renal subcapsular edema and swelling occurred during water irrigation several minutes later. Afterward, the sheath could be inserted smoothly when the isolated kidneys and ureters have been soaked in warm water for a certain period of time. This process cautions the young urologists to learn from the training and avoid side injury during actual clinical work because we could not find any kidney and perirenal tissue damage in vivo. (5) Various training programs are easy to increase. At the end of the training, we placed small stones or mung beans in the renal pelvis through the access sheath to simulate a realistic experience. The foreign bodies were washed with water randomly into one of the renal calyx, and then the trainees were instructed to find the foreign bodies accurately by using a flexible ureteroscope. After several trainings, the urologists gradually accumulated operating experience.

After the training, the ability of the urologists was significantly improved. The global rating scale and the pass/fail rating verified their advancement. In addition, with the improvement in proficiency, the time to finish the task was decreased gradually and a relatively stable level was achieved after several operations. Thus, for urologists with endourological experiences, mastering this technique is possible, primarily through animal training, as long as they mastered the differences and features of the two types of ureteroscopes, particularly eye–hand–ureteroscope coordination. In the subsequent study, we decided to train the 20 urologists during actual operations with patients to verify their performance. Moreover, the differences in side injuries, such as trauma and perforation, between the pre-test and the post-test were insignificantly different. We thought that these complications could be easily experienced by junior residents. Our subjects had endourological experience on rigid ureteroscopy and cystoscopy. Thus, with regard to flexible ureteroscopy training, the main differences are the visual field and the manipulation habit rather than the basic skills required in rigid ureteroscopy. Surgical errors/injuries are unrelated to technical skills, but to other skills, such as communication, teamwork, supervision, and decision making [12]. Different medical environments may also affect the occurrence of injuries.

## Conclusions

To flexible ureteroscopy, young urologists need a long learning curve, but they are given less operation opportunity. The isolated porcine kidneys are convenient and intuitive models for young urologists to practice flexible ureteroscopy on.

**Competing interests**
The authors declare that they have no competing interests.

**Authors' contributions**
DH participated in the design of the study, performed the statistical analysis, reviewed the literature and drafted the manuscript. TL participated in the design and coordination of the study, performed the tests and collected the data. XW conceived of the study, and participated in its design and coordination. All authors read and approved the final manuscript.

**Acknowledgements**
This study was supported by the grants from the National Natural Science Foundation of China (No. 81200579).

**References**

1. Dasgupta P, Cynk MS, Buhitude MF, Tiptaft RC, Glass JM. Flexible ureterorenoscopy: prospective analysis of the Guy's experience. Ann R Coll Surg Engl. 2004;86:367–70.
2. Knudsen B, Miyaoka R, Shah K, Holden T, Turk TM, Pedro RN, et al. Durability of the next generation flexible flberoptic ureteroscopes: a randomized prospective multi-institutional clinical trial. Urology. 2010;75:534–8.
3. Carey RI, Gomez CS, Maurici G, Lynne CM, Leveillee RJ, Bird VG. Frequency of ureteroscope damage seen at a tertiary care center. J Urol. 2006;176:607–10.
4. Wignall GR, Denstedt JD, Preminger GM, Cadeddu JA, Pearle MS, Sweet RM, et al. Surgical simulation: a urological perspective. J Urol. 2008;179:1690–9.
5. Bader MJ, Gratzke C, Wahher S, Schlenker B, Tilki D, Hocaoglu Y, et al. The polyseope: a modular design, semidisposable flexible ureterorenoscope system. J Endourol. 2010;24:1061–6.
6. Bansal H, Swain S, Sharma GK, Mathanya M, Trivedi S, Dwivedi US, et al. Polyscope: a new era in flexible ureterorenoscopy. J Endourol. 2011;25:317–21.
7. Matsumoto ED, Hamstra S, Radomski S, Cusimano M. A novel approach to endourological training: training at the Surgical Skills Center. J Urol. 2001;166:1261–6.
8. Knoll T, Trojan L, Haecker A, Alken P, Michel MS. Validation of computer-based training in ureterorenoscopy. BJU Int. 2005;95:1276–9.
9. Michel MS, Knoll T, Köhrmann KU, Alken P. The URO Mentor: development and evaluation of a new computer-based interactive training system for virtual life-like simulation of diagnostic and therapeutic endourological procedures. BJU Int. 2002;89:174–7.
10. Brehmer M, Tolley DA. Validation of a bench model for endoscopic surgery in the upper urinary tract. Eur Urol. 2002;42:175–9.
11. Desai MM, Aron M, Gill IS, Pascal-Haber G, Ukimura O, Kaouk JH, et al. Flexible robotic retrograde renoscopy: description of novel robotic device and preliminary laboratory experience. Urology. 2008;72:42–6.
12. Gawande AA, Zinner MJ, Studdert DM, Brennan TA. Analysis of errors reported by surgeons at three teaching hospitals. Surgery. 2003;133:614–21.

# 13

# A rare case of unilateral adrenal hyperplasia accompanied by hypokalaemic periodic paralysis caused by a novel dominant mutation in *CACNA1S*: features and prognosis after adrenalectomy

Bo Yang[1], Yuan Yang[2], Wenling Tu[2], Ying Shen[2] and Qiang Dong[1*]

## Abstract

**Background:** Acute hypokalaemic paralysis is characterised by acute flaccid muscle weakness and has a complex aetiological spectrum. Herein we report, for the first time, a case of unilateral adrenal hyperplasia accompanied by hypokalaemic periodic paralysis type I resulting from a novel dominant mutation in *CACNA1S*. We present the clinical features and prognosis after adrenalectomy in this case.

**Case presentation:** A 43-year-old Han Chinese male presented with severe hypokalaemic paralysis that remitted after taking oral potassium. The patient had suffered from periodic attacks of hypokalaemic paralysis for more than 20 years. A computed tomography (CT) scan of the abdomen showed a nodular mass on the left adrenal gland, although laboratory examination revealed the patient had not developed primary aldosteronism. The patient underwent a left adrenalectomy 4 days after admission, and the pathological examination further confirmed a 1.1 cm benign nodule at the periphery of the adrenal gland. Three months after the adrenalectomy, a paralytic attack recurred and the patient asked for assistance from the Department of Medical Genetics. His family history showed that two uncles, one brother, and a nephew also had a history of periodic paralysis, although their symptoms were milder. The patient's *CACNA1S* and *SCN4A* genes were sequenced, and a novel missense mutation, c.1582C > T (p.Arg528Cys), in *CACNA1S* was detected. Detection of the mutation in five adult male family members, including three with periodic paralysis and two with no history of the disease, indicated that this mutation caused hypokalaemic periodic paralysis type I in his family. Follow-up 2 years after adrenalectomy showed that the serum potassium concentration was increased between paralyses and the number and severity of paralytic attacks were significantly decreased.

**Conclusion:** We identified a novel dominant mutation, c.1582C > T (p.Arg528Cys), in *CACNA1S* that causes hypokalaemic periodic paralysis. The therapeutic effect of adrenalectomy indicated that unilateral adrenal hyperplasia might make paralytic attacks more serious and more frequent by decreasing serum potassium. This finding suggests that the surgical removal of hyperplastic tissues might relieve the symptoms of patients with severe hypokalaemic paralysis caused by other incurable diseases, even if the adrenal lesion does not cause primary aldosteronism.

**Keywords:** Unilateral adrenal hyperplasia, Hypokalaemic periodic paralysis, *CACNA1S*, Adrenalectomy

* Correspondence: dqiang418@163.com
[1]Department of Urology, West China Hospital, Sichuan University, Chengdu 610041, China
Full list of author information is available at the end of the article

## Background

Adrenal hyperplasia (AH) is a common endocrine disease, and unilateral adrenal hyperplasia (UAH) is a common cause of primary aldosteronism (PA) [1,2]. Muscular paralysis and decreased serum potassium are two of the initial symptoms in some patients with PA-causing UAH, which can be corrected by adrenalectomy [3,4]. However, it is unclear whether adrenalectomy in patients with non-PA-causing UAH increases serum potassium, which would indicate that this surgery could relieve symptoms caused by hypokalaemia resulting from other incurable diseases.

Hypokalaemic periodic paralysis (HOKPP), including HOKPP1 (OMIM #170400) and HOKPP2 (OMIM #613345), is a rare autosomal dominant inherited disease characterised by episodic muscle weakness with significant hypokalaemia (< 0.9 to 3.0 mmol/L) during attacks [5,6]. HOKPP1 and HOKPP2 are caused by mutations in CAC-NA1S (calcium channel, voltage-dependent, L type, alpha 1S subunit) (OMIM #114208) and SCN4A (sodium channel, voltage-gated, type IV, alpha subunit) (OMIM #603967), respectively [7,8]. The frequency of HOKPP attacks varies from daily to yearly, and the attacks typically last from 3–4 hours up to a day or longer [9]. The frequency of attacks varies significantly among members of families with HOKPP, and the cause for this variation remains unknown.

In this case, we report the clinical features, diagnosis, and prognosis after adrenalectomy in a patient with non-PA-causing UAH and HOKPP and discuss the potential of this surgery to relieve the symptoms of hypokalaemic periodic paralysis.

## Case presentation

A 43-year-old male presented to the outpatient Department of Urology of West China Hospital in March 2012 with severe paralytic attacks characterised by palpitations and muscle weakness starting in the right thigh and spreading to all limbs. A significant reduction in the serum potassium concentration (1.89 mmol/L, reference value 3.5–5.0 mmol/L) was found during laboratory examination, and an ECG indicated severe potassium deficiency. Symptoms remitted after taking oral potassium (50 ml of 10% potassium chloride was administered immediately followed by an additional 50 ml over 24 h for a total dose of 10 g). After the paralytic attack, a CT scan of the abdomen was performed, which revealed left UAH characterised by a nodular mass on the left adrenal gland. Laboratory examination showed a slight elevation in norepinephrine (602 ng/L, reference value, 272–559 ng/L) and a reduction in adrenaline (< 25 ng/L, reference value 54–122 ng/L) in the serum. Other data, including the serum concentrations of potassium (3.71 mmol/L), aldosterone (11.41 ng/dL, reference value 9.8–27.5 ng/dl), cortisol (7.3 μg/dL, reference value 7.2–18.2 μg/dL), renin (2.22 ng/mL, reference value

0.56–2.79 ng/ml), calcium (2.27 mmol/L, reference value 2.1–2.7 mmol/L), creatine kinase (58 IU/L, reference value 19–226 IU/L), lactate dehydrogenase (167 IU/L, reference value 110–220 IU/L), alanine aminotransferase (19 IU/L, reference value <55 IU/L), aspartate transaminase (15 IU/L, reference value <46 IU/L), creatinine (74.5 μmol/L, reference value 53–140 μmol/L), blood urea nitrogen (7.69 mmol/L, reference value 3.30–8.22 mmol/L), thyroid-stimulating hormone (6.3 mU/L, reference value 2–10 mU/L), total-triiodothyronine (2.14 nmol/L, reference value 1.8–2.9 nmol/L), and total thyroxine (87 nmol/L, reference value 65156 nmol/L), were normal. The patient did not have hypertension (117/83 mm Hg).

Patient history showed that the paralytic attacks were usually triggered by physical labour or stress and were periodic. Attack frequency varied from weekly during the summer to bimonthly in the winter; each attack lasted 4–6 hours. This attack was the most severe of the attacks he had experienced during the past decade. Although these paralytic attacks were associated with hypokalaemia, the aetiology had not been previously established, and the patient had not received any treatment, including potassium supplement, between attacks. Two years before this attack, serum potassium had been measured several times between attacks; the results of three of these tests were available and were 3.74, 3.69 and 3.63 mmol/L.

Because of the presence of severe hypokalaemic periodic paralysis, the patient underwent a left adrenalectomy after admission. Examination of the adrenal gland revealed a 1.1-cm benign nodule at the periphery of the gland with multiple cortical nodular hyperplasias. The patient did not have any complications during the perioperative period and laboratory results were normal (serum potassium .87 mmol/L, serum sodium 143.9 mmol/L, norepinephrine 452 ng/L, adrenaline 60 ng/L, aldosterone 12.24 ng/dL, cortisol 8.1 μg/dL, renin 2.13 ng/mL, creatine kinase 60 IU/L, lactate dehydrogenase 168 IU/L, alanine aminotransferase 20 IU/L, aspartate transaminase 16 IU/L, creatinine 81.3 μmol/L, blood urea nitrogen 8.01 mmol/L). He was discharged 4 days after surgery. During the next 3 months, while recovering at home, no paralytic attacks occurred. The patient then returned to work, and the acute paralytic crises soon recurred. A colour Doppler ultrasound examination did not show any abnormality of the right adrenal gland. The patient then asked for help from the Department of Medical Genetics. His serum potassium was monitored three times with a frequency of once per month with results of 4.12, 3.97, and 4.27 mmol/L, respectively. As shown in Figure 1, in addition to the patient (II₂), four other adult male family members, including two uncles (I₅ and I₆), one brother (II₃), and one nephew (III₁), also had a history of paralytic attacks, although their attacks were milder and less

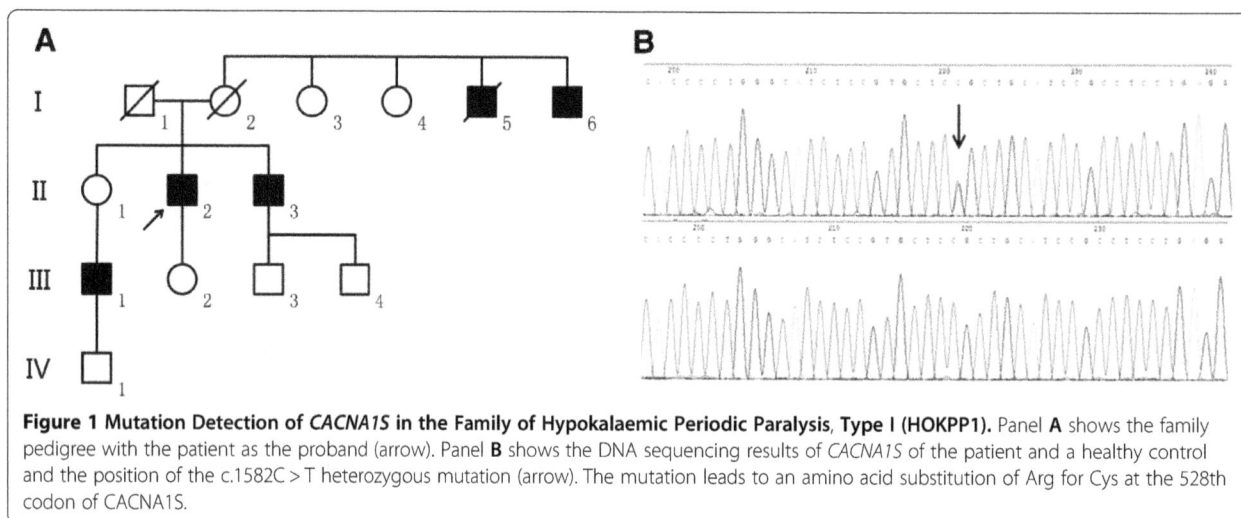

**Figure 1 Mutation Detection of CACNA1S in the Family of Hypokalaemic Periodic Paralysis, Type I (HOKPP1).** Panel **A** shows the family pedigree with the patient as the proband (arrow). Panel **B** shows the DNA sequencing results of CACNA1S of the patient and a healthy control and the position of the c.1582C > T heterozygous mutation (arrow). The mutation leads to an amino acid substitution of Arg for Cys at the 528th codon of CACNA1S.

frequent (yearly to decadal). These members refused examination to determine the presence or absence of UAH.

Because of the positive family history of periodic paralysis with potential autosomal dominant inheritance, the diagnosis of HOKPP was considered, and genetic testing of the CACNA1S and SCN4A genes was performed using Sanger sequencing of all exons and their splice sites. Consequently, the patient was identified as a heterozygote carrying a novel missense mutation, c.1582C > T, in CACNA1S (p.Arg528Cys) (Figure 1). In his family, the mutation was also detected in three other adult males with periodic paralysis ($I_6$, $II_3$, and $III_1$) and in two asymptomatic females ($II_1$ and $III_2$). This mutation was absent in two male family members who did not have a history of symptoms ($III_3$ and $III_4$). Furthermore, the targeted Sanger sequencing did not detect the mutation in 130 adult male controls.

During the following 2 years, the patient maintained the same diet as before surgery. He did not receive any potassium supplement treatment and suffered 12 paralytic attacks. However, there were considerably fewer attacks (monthly in the summer and no attacks in the winter), and the attacks were shorter in duration (2–3 hours) than the attacks before adrenalectomy.

## Discussion

Periodic paralysis caused by hypokalaemia possesses significant aetiological heterogeneity. A recent study [10] concluded that 42.9% of patients had a secondary cause, including renal tubular acidosis, Gitelman syndrome, thyrotoxicosis, alcoholism, hypothyroidism, Liddle's syndrome, gastroenteritis, and primary hyperaldosteronism. In the other cases of primary periodic paralysis, 48.2% were sporadic and 8.9% had a positive family history [10]. Some of the cases with a positive family history might be attributed

to mutations in a single gene, such as CACNA1S or SCN4A.

CACNA1S and SCN4A encode the human skeletal muscle α1-subunit of a dihydropyridine-sensitive calcium channel and the α-subunit of a sodium channel, respectively [7,8]. Previous studies have linked mutations in these genes to HOKPP. The mutant CACNA1S and SCN4A have a partial loss of function, leading to reduced calcium or sodium current density, which is followed by membrane depolarisation. Membrane depolarisation is coupled with the inflow of potassium into skeletal muscle cells, causing paroxysmal hypokalaemia and periodic paralysis [11,12]. In the present case, genetic testing revealed a missense mutation in CACNA1S, resulting in p.Arg528Cys. This mutation had not been reported previously. A genotype-phenotype correlation was identified in the patient's family by the cosegregation of the mutation with all of the affected adult male members and a higher penetrance in males. In all of the seven HOKPP1–causing mutations that have been reported, two different mutations involve the 528th codon of CACNA1S, including p.Arg528His and p.Arg528Gly [5,13]. The arginine residue encoded by the wild-type 528th codon is highly conserved among different species from C. elegans to humans, and it is located in the critical voltage sensor region of the transmembrane segment of the calcium channel [13]. The above evidence combined with the absence of the mutation in the matched male controls strongly suggests that the Arg528Cys substitution is a novel dominant HOKPP1-causing mutation accounting for the onset of hypokalaemic periodic paralysis in this patient's family.

The patient also had UAH identified by a CT scan and pathological examination. UAH possesses a pathogenic mechanism distinct from HOKPP; however, the clinical manifestations of the two diseases are similar when UAH causes PA followed by hypokalaemia and muscular paralysis [14]. UAH was previously considered a rare sub-type of PA [15], whereas recent studies suggest that the contribution of UAH to PA might have been underestimated because high-resolution multi-slice CT and other new screening tests have shown more patients with PA to have UAH [2]. This finding is encouraging because PA caused by UAH has been confirmed to be surgically correctable by adrenalectomy with excellent long-term results [3]. In the present case, the patient did not display PA, but his clinical manifestation was the most severe of his family members with periodic paralysis based on attack frequency and duration. In addition, there was no remission although he was over 43 years old, which could not be completely explained by HOKPP1 alone. After adrenalectomy, the symptoms of the patient were significantly relieved, including increased serum potassium concentrations ($t$ test, $\alpha = 0.05$: $P = 0.009$) between crises and decreased paralytic attack frequency and duration. This observation suggests a close association between the decreased serum potassium caused by UAH and the severity of HOKPP and supports the hypothesis that adrenalectomy may be an effective treatment for relieving the symptoms of patients with both UAH and severe hypokalaemic paralysis resulting from some incurable genetic diseases such as HOKPP and Gitelman syndrome [10,16].

## Conclusions

In this first reported case of unilateral adrenal hyperplasia in concurrence with hypokalaemic periodic paralysis, we identified a novel dominant mutation, p.Arg528Cys, of *CACNA1S* causing HOPPK, which is the third known pathogenic mutation involving the 528th code of *CACNA1S*. These results emphasise the importance of CACNA1S Arg528 in maintaining calcium channel function. The prognosis after adrenalectomy suggests that the presence of UAH might increase the severity of hypokalaemic paralysis caused by other diseases. Operative treatment may be a rational choice for relieving the symptoms of hypokalaemic paralysis by increasing serum potassium, even if the UAH does not cause primary aldosteronism or clinical hypokalaemia.

## Consent

This study was approved by the Ethics Committee of Clinical Trials and Biomedical Research, West China Hospital, Sichuan University. Written informed consent for reporting results of genetic testing was obtained from the patient and his seven family members. A copy of the written consent is available for review by the Editor of this journal.

**Competing interests**
The authors declare that they have no competing interests.

**Authors' contributions**
QD and BY cared for the patient. WT and YS performed the genetic testing. YY was responsible for genetic counselling. BY wrote the manuscript. All of the authors discussed the content of the manuscript and approved the final version of the manuscript.

**Acknowledgements**
This work was supported by Science and Technology Support Project of Sichuan province (Grant No.2012SZ0025).

**Author details**
[1]Department of Urology, West China Hospital, Sichuan University, Chengdu 610041, China. [2]Department of Medical Genetics, West China Hospital, Sichuan University, Chengdu 610041, China.

**References**
1. Jiang SB, Guo XD, Wang HB, Gong RZ, Xiong H, Wang Z, Zhang HY, Jin XB: A retrospective study of laparoscopic unilateral adrenalectomy for primary hyperaldosteronism caused by unilateral adrenal hyperplasia. *Int Urol Nephrol* 2014, **46:**1283–1288.
2. Sigurjonsdottir HA, Gronowitz M, Andersson O, Eggertsen R, Herlitz H, Sakinis A, Wangberg B, Johannsson G: Unilateral adrenal hyperplasia is a usual cause of primary hyperaldosteronism. Results from a Swedish screening study. *BMC Endocr Disord* 2012, **12:**17.
3. Iacobone M, Citton M, Viel G, Boetto R, Bonadio I, Tropea S, Mantero F, Rossi GP, Fassina A, Nitti D, Favia G: Unilateral adrenal hyperplasia: a novel cause of surgically correctable primary hyperaldosteronism. *Surgery* 2012, **152:**1248–1255.
4. Huang YY, Hsu BR, Tsai JS: Paralytic myopathy-a leading clinical presentation for primary aldosteronism in Taiwan. *J Clin Endocrinol Metab* 1996, **81:**4038–4041.
5. Elbaz A, Vale-Santos J, Jurkat-Rott K, Lapie P, Ophoff RA, Bady B, Links TP, Piussan C, Vila A, Monnier N, Padberg GW, Abe K, Feingold N, Guimaraes J, Wintzen AR, van der Hoeven JH, Saudubray JM, Grunfeld JP, Lenoir G, Nivet H, Echenne B, Frants RR, Fardeau M, Lehmann-Horn F, Fontaine B: Hypokalemic periodic paralysis and the dihydropyridine receptor (CACNL1A3): genotype/phenotype correlations for two predominant mutations and evidence for the absence of a founder *effect in 16 caucasian families. Am J Hum Genet* 1995, **56:**374–380.
6. Sternberg D, Maisonobe T, Jurkat-Rott K, Nicole S, Launay E, Chauveau D, Tabti N, Lehmann-Horn F, Hainque B, Fontaine B: Hypokalaemic periodic paralysis type 2 caused by mutations at codon 672 in the muscle sodium channel gene SCN4A. *Brain* 2001, **124:**1091–1099.
7. Fontaine B, Vale-Santos J, Jurkat-Rott K, Reboul J, Plassart E, Rime CS, Elbaz A, Heine R, Guimarães J, Weissenbach J, Baumann N, Fardeau M, Lehmann-Horn F: Mapping of the hypokalaemic periodic paralysis (HypoPP) locus to chromosome 1q31-32 in three European families. *Nat Genet* 1994, **6:**267–272.
8. Bulman DE, Scoggan KA, van Oene MD, Nicolle MW, Hahn AF, Tollar LL, Ebers GC: A novel sodium channel mutation in a family with hypokalemic periodic paralysis. *Neurology* 1999, **53:**1932–1936.
9. Weiner ID, Wingo CS: Hypokalemia-consequences, causes, and correction. *J Am Soc Nephrol* 1997, **8:**1179–1188.
10. Kayal AK, Goswami M, Das M, Jain R: Clinical and biochemical spectrum of hypokalemic paralysis in North: East India. *Ann Indian Acad Neurol* 2013, **16:**211–217.
11. Morrill JA, Cannon SC: Effects of mutations causing hypokalaemic periodic paralysis on the skeletal muscle L-type Ca2+ channel expressed in Xenopus laevis oocytes. *J Physiol* 1999, **520:**321–336.
12. Jurkat-Rott K, Mitrovic N, Hang C, Kouzmekine A, Iaizzo P, Herzog J, Lerche H, Nicole S, Vale-Santos J, Chauveau D, Fontaine B, Lehmann-Horn F: Voltage-sensor sodium channel mutations cause hypokalemic periodic paralysis type 2 by enhanced inactivation and reduced current. *Proc Natl Acad Sci U S A* 2000, **97:**9549–9554.
13. Wang Q, Liu M, Xu C, Tang Z, Liao Y, Du R, Li W, Wu X, Wang X, Liu P, Zhang X, Zhu J, Ren X, Ke T, Wang Q, Yang J: Novel CACNA1S mutation causes autosomal dominant hypokalemic periodic paralysis in a Chinese family. *J Mol Med (Berl)* 2005, **83:**203–208.

14. Kotsaftis P, Savopoulos C, Agapakis D, Ntaios G, Tzioufa V, Papadopoulos V, Fahantidis E, Hatzitolios A: **Hypokalemia induced myopathy as first manifestation of primary hyperaldosteronism - an elderly patient with unilateral adrenal hyperplasia: a case report.** *Cases J* 2009, **2:**6813.

15. Amar L, Plouin PF, Steichen O: **Aldosterone-producing adenoma and other surgically correctable forms of primary aldosteronism.** *Orphanet J Rare Dis* 2010, **5:**9.

16. Ng HY, Lin SH, Hsu CY, Tsai YZ, Chen HC, Lee CT: **Hypokalemic paralysis due to Gitelman syndrome: a family study.** *Neurology* 2006, **67:**1080–1082.

# 14

# Could Hyaluronic acid (HA) reduce Bacillus Calmette-Guérin (BCG) local side effects?

Luca Topazio[1], Roberto Miano[2], Valentina Maurelli[1], Gabriele Gaziev[1], Mauro Gacci[3], Valerio Iacovelli[1] and Enrico Finazzi-Agrò[2,4*]

**Abstract**

**Background:** Bacillus Calmette-Guérin (BCG) is considered the most effective treatment to reduce recurrence and progression of non-muscle invasive bladder cancer (NMIBC) but can induce local side effects leading to treatment discontinuation or interruption. Aim of this exploratory study is to investigate if the sequential administration of Hyaluronic acid (HA) may reduce local side effects of BCG.

**Methods:** 30 consecutive subjects undergoing BCG intravesical administration for high risk NMIBC were randomized to receive BCG only (Group A) or BCG and HA (Group B). A 1 to 10 Visual Analog Scale (VAS) for bladder pain, International Prostate Symptom Score (IPSS) and number of micturitions per day were evaluated in the two groups before and after six weekly BCG instillations. Patients were also evaluated at 3 and 6 months by means of cystostopy and urine cytology.

**Results:** One out of 30 (3,3%) patients in group A dropped out from the protocol, for local side effects. Mean VAS for pain was significantly lower in group B after BCG treatment (4.2 vs. 5.8, p = 0.04). Post vs. pre treatment differences in VAS for pain, IPSS and number of daily micturitions were all significantly lower in group B. Three patients in group A and 4 in group B presented with recurrent pathology at 6 month follow up.

**Conclusions:** These preliminary data suggest a possible role of HA in reducing BCG local side effects and could be used to design larger randomized controlled trials, assessing safety and efficacy of sequential BCG and HA administration.

**Keywords:** BCG, Hyaluronic acid, Non-muscle invasive bladder cancer, Non bacterial cystitis

## Background

Bacillus Calmette–Guérin (BCG) is considered the most effective treatment to increase disease-free interval and reduce progression of non-muscle invasive bladder cancer (NMIBC) [1]. Although considered safe, BCG can produce both local and systemic side effects leading to treatment discontinuation or interruption. The most common local side-effects of BCG intravesical instillations include cystitis, characterized by irritative voiding symptoms and hematuria, which occur in approximately 75% of all patients. More rarely, serious local adverse events as a result of BCG infection, such as symptomatic granulomatous prostatitis and epididymo-orchitis, might occur and require permanent discontinuation of BCG treatment. Systemic side-effects include flu-like symptoms, such as general malaise and fever, occuring in approximately 40% of patients. A high persistent fever might be related to BCG infection or sepsis. Local and systemic side-effects might lead to discontinue intravesical BCG treatment in approximately 20% of patients [2]. Up to 54% of the

* Correspondence: efinazzi@tin.it
[2]Department of Experimental Medicine and Surgery, Tor Vergata University, Rome, Italy
[4]Unit for Functional Urology, Department of Urology, Policlinico Tor Vergata, Rome, Italy
Full list of author information is available at the end of the article

patients undergoing intravesical therapy with chemotherapeutic agents to treat superficial bladder tumours can be affected by nonbacterial cystitis [3].

Several solutions have been proposed to reduce the occurrence of side effects from BCG with the aim to limit BCG discontinuation and the concomitant discomfort during endovesical treatment. Some Authors have proposed to avoid BCG administration in case of TUR within previous 2 weeks, traumatic catheterization, macroscopic hematuria, urethral stenosis, active tuberculosis, prior Bacillus Calmette–Guérin sepsis, immuno-suppression or urinary tract infection [4]. Other procedures include the prophylactic administration of isoniazid [5] or ofloxacin [6,7] or usually involve BCG dose reductions [8]. In common practice antimicrobials, anticholinergics, anaesthetics and analgesics are often used to relieve patients' symptoms.

Glycosaminoglycan (GAG) substitution therapy is an emerging treatment of Bladder Pain Syndrome/Interstitial Cystitis (BPS/IC) and response rates between 30% and 80% have been described with intravesical administration of various GAGs (hyaluronic acid, pentosan polysulfate, heparin, chondroitin sulfate, and dimethyl sulfoxide) [9,10]. Few papers report the results of GAG substitution therapy in the treatment of radiation and chemical cystitis [9,10]. To our knowledge, to date, only two papers have described GAG use in the treatment of BCG local side effects; this papers show very good results, with significant reduction of lower urinary tract symptoms after intravesical administration of HA [11,12].

Aim of the present randomized pilot study was to evaluate if the sequential administration of HA and BCG could be safe in prevention of early recurrence and progression of bladder tumor, and safe in reduction of local side-effects in patients with high risk NMIBC.

## Methods

This is a prospective randomized pilot study approved by our institutional review board (Policlinico Tor Vergata Ethics Committee, resolution n° 69–2011). Patients with a diagnosis of a intermediate/high risk NMIBC, according to the European Organization for Research and Treatment of Cancer (EORTC) score [13] after transurethral resection of bladder tumor (TURBT) were eligible for this study.

Inclusion criteria were:

1. Hystologically proven non-muscle invasive bladder cancer;
2. Indication to intravesical instillation of BCG according to EAU guidelines;
3. Age > 18 years;
4. Willingness, to participate to the study;
5. Written informed consent.

Exclusion criteria were:

1. Previous or ongoing BCG or different intravesical instillations;
2. Urinary tract infections (UTI) or other known pathologies of the lower urinary tract;
3. Indication for a radical cystectomy;
4. Severe systemic disorders, including neurological pathologies, kidney, liver or heart failure;
5. Contraindications to BCG use.

Patients enrolled in the study started the intravesical therapies within 4 weeks from the TURBT and were randomized in two groups. We a priori decided to stop this pilot study after reaching the number of 15 patients in each group. Group A was sent to receive BCG (Immucist®81 mg, Sanofi-Aventis Group) alone and Group B to receive BCG (see previous reference) and HA 40 mg (Cystistat, Mylan, Pittsburgh, PA, U.S.A.). BCG strain used in our study was Connaught $3,4 \pm 3 \times 10(8)$ CFU, 81 mg (Immucist®) in 50 cc of saline. BCG was administered by means of a 2 ways 14 Ch Foley catheter latex and left inside the bladder for 60 minutes. After 60 minutes BCG was evacuated, the bladder washed with saline and the catheter removed. HA was administered intravesically after every BCG evacuation in Group B. After HA administration and catheter removal, patients were instructed to maintain HA in the bladder as long as possible, for at least 2 hours after administration. In Group A normal saline was administered, so that all patients were blinded to the administration of HA. Both groups received an induction course of 6 weekly instillations of BCG.

A 1 to 10 Visual Analog Scale (VAS) for bladder pain was considered the primary outcome measure of the study and was evaluated in both groups before and after the treatment. International Prostate Symptom Score (IPSS) and number of micturitions per day were also evaluated in both groups before starting and at the end of the induction cycle of BCG instillations.

Patients were evaluated at three and six months by means of cystoscopy and urine cytology for oncologic follow-up. The number of patients with bladder tumor recurrence was recorded in both groups at 6 month follow-up.

Data are presented as mean ± standard deviation (SD). The statistical analysis was conducted with a t Student Test using a software Stata 12.0, and considering as significant a *p value* ≤0.05.

Our manuscript adheres to CONSORT guidelines. CONSORT checklist is shown in Additional file 1.

## Results and discussion

30 subjects were enrolled in the study between January and December 2011. Mean age was 67 (range 54–81): 23

(76%) were male while 7 (24%) female. All Patients had BCa with intermediate/high risk of progression according to the European Organization for Research and Treatment of Cancer (EORTC) score. Fifteen patients (12 male and 3 female) were randomly assigned to Group A and 15 patients (11 male and 4 female) to Group B. Clinical and pathologic features of patients are shown in Table 1.

Only one out of 30 (3,3%) patients in Group A dropped out from the protocol, for local side effects (urgency, frequency and burning micturition), while all Patients in Group B completed the induction cycle with intravesical BCG. The results are shown in Table 2.

Mean pre-treatment VAS was comparable in the two groups (4.46 (2;10) for Group A and 4.86 (2;8) for Group B, $p = 0.56$). After treatments mean VAS was significantly lower in group B (4.2 (2;7) vs. 5.53 (4;7) in Group A, $p = 0.04$). VAS post treatment was increased in Group A and reduced in Group B: difference in post vs pre-treatment VAS was significantly lower in Group B ($-0.66$ ($-4$;1) vs. 1.06 ($-4$;3) in Group A, $p = 0.0001$).

Mean pre-treatment IPSS was comparable in both groups (13.93 (8;24) in Group A and 14.73 (9;22) in Group B, $p = 0.6$). After treatment, mean IPSS was slightly lower in group B (15.26 (11;21) vs. 17.46 (13;21) in Group A, even if the difference was not statistically significant $p = 0.1$). IPSS increase post treatment was significantly lower in Group B than in Group A (0.53 ($-3$;2) vs. 3.53 ($-3$;10) in Group A, $p = 0.02$).

Mean pre-treatment number of daily micturitions was comparable in the two groups (10.26 (7;15) for Group A and 10.8 (7;16) for Group B, $p = 0.53$). After treatment, we failed to find a significant difference in number of daily micturitions between the two groups (11.26 (9;13) in Group A and 10.73 (7;14) in Group B, $p = 0.44$). On the other hand, there was no increase in number of daily micturitions in Group B and a slight increase in Group A: this difference was significant ($-0.066$ ($-2$;1) for Group B and 1 ($-2$;5) for Group A, $p = 0.04$).

At 6 month follow-up 3/15 (21%) pts of Group A (including the patient who dropped out from the induction

## Table 1 Clinical and pathologic features of pts

|  | Tot | Group A (BCG) | Group B (BCG + HA) |
|---|---|---|---|
| **Gender** | | | |
| M | 23 (76%) | 12 (80%) | 11 (73%) |
| F | 7 (24%) | 3 (20%) | 4 (27%) |
| **Age** | | | |
| Mean | 67 | 66 | 68 |
| Range | 54-81 | 54-75 | 60-81 |
| **N° of tumors** | | | |
| Single | 9 (30%) | 5 (33%) | 4 (27%) |
| Multiple | 21 (70%) | 10 (67%) | 11 (53%) |
| **Tumor diameter** | | | |
| Mean | 1,5 cm | 1,5 cm | 1,5 cm |
| Range | 5 cm – 50 cm | 5 cm – 40 cm | 5 cm – 50 cm |
| **pT** | | | |
| Ta | 17 (56%) | 9 (60%) | 8 (53%) |
| T1 | 13 (44%) | 6 (40%) | 7 (47%) |
| CIS | 8 (27%) | 3 (20%) | 5 (33%) |
| **WHO grade 1973** | | | |
| G1 | 8 (27%) | 4 (27%) | 4 (27%) |
| G2 | 10 (33%) | 6 (40%) | 4 (27%) |
| G3 | 12 (40%) | 5 (33%) | 7 (46%) |
| **EORTC recurrence score** | | | |
| ≤ 9 intermediate | 10 (33%) | 6 (40%) | 4 (27%) |
| 10-17 high | 20 (67%) | 9 (60%) | 11 (73%) |
| **EORTC progressive score** | | | |
| ≤6 intermediate | 11 (36%) | 6 (40%) | 5 (33%) |
| 7-23 high | 19 (64%) | 9 (60%) | 10 (67%) |

**Table 2 Results of VAS, IPSS and bladder diaries at baseline and at the end of BCG induction cycle**

| Mean (SD) | Group A Pre | Group B Pre | p | Group A Post | Group B Post | p | Group A | Group B | p |
|---|---|---|---|---|---|---|---|---|---|
| | | | | | | | Difference | | |
| VAS (1–10) | 4.5 (±2) | 4.9 (±1.8) | .56 | 5.8 (±1) | 4.2 (±1.6) | .04 | 1.5 (±0.7) | −0.7 (±1.6) | .0001 |
| IPSS | 13.9 (±4.4) | 14.7 (±4.0) | .60 | 17.5 (±2.6) | 15.3 (±4) | .10 | 3 (±3.5) | 0.53 (±1.6) | .02 |
| n° daily micturitions | 10.3 (±2.2) | 10.8 (±2.4) | .53 | 11.5 (±1.3) | 10 .9 (±2.1) | .44 | 1.23 (±1.7) | 0.13 (±1) | .04 |

BCG cycle for severe LUTS) and 4/15 (26.7%) pts in Group B had a recurrence of BCa. None of them had BCa progression to muscle-invasive disease.

Several trials in the last two decades have investigated BCG efficacy in reducing the risk of recurrence and progression in intermediate/high risk BCa showing that BCG after TUR is superior to TUR alone or TUR and conventional chemotherapy [14,15]. Two meta-analyses have demonstrated that BCG therapy prevents, or at least delays, the risk of tumour progression [16,17].

Despite of its great efficacy, BCG therapy has potential local and systemic side effects that may either lead to treatment cessation in up to 30% of patients or lead to a delay or reduction in the number of instillations in 55–83% of patients [18].

The risk of increased toxicity during maintenance has been questioned. According to the results of a European Organization for Research and Treatment of Cancer (EORTC) phase 3 trial [18], local side effects of BCG do not increase during maintenance and systemic side effects are more frequent during the first 6 mo of treatment. However, a significant proportion of patients (84% [19], 67.3% [18]), 86% [20] in the three most representative series) failed to complete the 3-yr maintenance course for various reasons.

Several options have been proposed to decrease the occurrence of BCG side effects including the prophylactic administration of isoniazid or ofloxacin, modifications to the BCG treatment schedule and dose reductions. The concomitant administration of isoniazid, has not been found to decrease the incidence of BCG related side-effects [5]. In contrast, ofloxacin reduced the incidence of moderate to severe BCG related adverse events when given prophylactically in a randomized double blind trial in 115 patients [6,7]. However, further studies are required to confirm these initial findings and to ensure that there is no impairment of treatment efficacy. Martinez-Pineiro et al. investigated the BCG side effects rate using a reduced dose of BCG. They found significantly less toxicity on the reduced dose but recommended the use of a full dose in the treatment of high-risk patients [8]. In a second study in high-risk patients with T1G3 tumors and/or carcinoma in situ (CIS) they concluded that one-third dose was indeed as effective as full dose, but was associated with significantly less toxicity [21]. The final results of an EORTC-GU Cancers

Group Randomized Study of Maintenance Bacillus Calmette-Guerin in Intermediate- and High-risk Ta, T1 Papillary Carcinoma of the Urinary Bladder showed no significant differences in toxicity between 1/3 dose and full dose (FD) BCG. 1/3 dose with 1 yr of maintenance was considered suboptimal compared with the standard FD during 3 yr [22].

Despite of this great number of papers on BCG toxicity in literature, only two papers investigated the possible use of HA for treatment of BCG induced cystitis [11,12] showing interesting results.

GAGs have been used extensively in BPS/IC with response rates between 30% and 80% described with intravesical administration of various substances such as HA, PPS, heparin; chondroitin sulfate, and DMSO [23,24]. The efficacy of HA is based on several mechanisms that aim on the urothelial function disorder present in BPS/IC: on one side, HA reinforces the urine-tissue barrier by integration in the GAG layer on the luminal surface and the base of urothelial cells; on the other side, unique anti-inflammatory mechanisms have been identified, like inhibition of leukocyte migration, adherence of immune complexes, and binding to specific receptors (I-CAM 1, CD 44) involved in the inflammatory process [25-27].

Moreover studies on rat models have shown that HA can inhibit bladder mast cell activation as well as the inflammatory mediator release of urinary histamine, rat mast cell protease-I and IL-6 [28] thus reducing their pro-inflammatory activity.

Because of GAGs documented anti-inflammatory and protective activity on the urothelium we considered the possible use of these devices on the treatment of BCG induced cystitis, even if one can argue that reducing BCG side-effects can even impair BCG efficacy.

A correlation between BCG side-effects and treatment efficacy has been reported by various authors, suggesting that local side-effects have a significantly longer time to first recurrence. However, patients with a better outcome remain on treatment for a longer period of time and receive more BCG, thus increasing their risk of developing side-effects. Neither local nor systemic BCG toxicity before 6 months was found to be a prognostic factor for subsequent recurrence. Thus, it is not possible to confirm that BCG toxicity is actually responsible for an improved outcome and a causal effect cannot be inferred from the data [29].

Our preliminary results show a possible role of HA in reducing BCG side-effects during the induction cycle when their frequency is higher than in the maintenance period [18]. As described in the Results and discussion section, VAS for bladder pain was significantly lower, at the end of the induction cycle, in Group B (patients treated with HA). It is important to underline that baseline VAS was relatively high because obtained in patients who recently underwent a TURBT. Interestingly, patients in Group B showed a reduction, whilst those in Group A presented an increase of VAS for pain. Indeed we failed to show between groups a statistically significant difference in IPSS and number of daily micturitions; nevertheless, the use of HA seems to have reduced the appearance of lower urinary tract symptoms in Group B, with an increase of IPSS of only 0.53 points vs. a significantly higher increase in group A (3.53). The same could be said about number of daily micturitions that remained almost unchanged in Group B whilst was increased after treatment in Group A. These results could indicate a protective function of HA on the urothelium of the bladder against the irritative activity of BCG.

One can argue that even ofloxacin when given prophylactically before each BCG administration [6,7] can achieve good results with a lower cost for the Health Care System. Actually the use of Ofloxacin has significantly decreased the incidence of class 2 or higher AEs, but has not improved class 1 AEs [6] while HA in our paper has demonstrated to significantly reduce class 1 AEs. Moreover it should be discussed if the prophylactic use of Ofloxacin for 9 weeks could increase bacterial resistance.

These very preliminary data seem to support a possible role of HA in reducing BCG local side effects. Nevertheless, our study has some limitations:

1. We have only a short follow up time;
2. It is a pilot study, with no power calculation;
3. Does not provide data on maintenance treatment;
4. Does not provide data on possible long term interactions of HA with BCG efficacy;
5. It remains to be seen whether the administration of HA after BCG is worth the benefit and increased costs.

The only outcome measures evaluated (VAS, IPSS, daily micturitions) may have not detected important efficacy end points, such as quality of life and relief of painful micturition.

For all these reasons, no definitive conclusions should be drawn. Nevertheless the data coming from this study should be used to design a randomized controlled study aimed to verify this hypothesis.

## Conclusions

This pilot study provides, for the first time to our knowledge, evidence of a possible reduction of BCG local adverse events by using a sequential administration of HA. Larger randomized controlled study, designed on the basis of this pilot study are needed to assess how clinically significant the association of HA to BCG could be. In other words, further studies will have to investigate if this association is worthy, having proven (statistically and clinically) significant reduction of local adverse events of BCG, possibly causing a reduction of the number of patients who have to suspend or discontinue the treatment with BCG, with a consequent reduction of its efficacy. Furthermore, a possible interaction of HA with BCG efficacy must be excluded before this association could become part of a standard care. In conclusion, this pilot study is only the first step, but further research is needed to investigate the exact potentialities and role of HA administered in patients treated by means of BCG for NMIBC.

### Abbreviations
HA: Hyaluronic acid; BCG: Bacillus Calmette-Guérin; NMIBC: Non-muscle invasive bladder cancer; VAS: Visual analog scale; IPSS: International Prostate Symptom Score; GAG: Glycosaminoglycan; BPS/IC: Bladder pain syndrome/interstitial cystitis; EORTC: European Organization for Research and Treatment of Cancer; TUR: Trans-urethral resection; BCa: Bladder cancer.

### Competing interests
Enrico Finazzi-Agrò is consultant for Mylan Inc. Luca Topazio, Roberto Miano, Valentina Maurelli, Gabriele Gaziev, Valerio Iacovelli and Mauro Gacci declare that they have no conflict of interest.

### Authors' contributions
LT has been involved in drafting the manuscript. VI and GG have made substantial contributions to acquisition and analysis of data. VM has made substantial contributions to conception and design of the study. EFA, MG and RM have made substantial contributions to conception and design and interpretation of data; they have been involved in revising the manuscript critically for important intellectual content. All authors read and approved the final manuscript.

### Funding
Departmental; Cystistat supplied by Mylan, Pittsburgh, PA, U.S.A.

### Author details
[1]School of Specialization in Urology, Tor Vergata University, Rome, Italy. [2]Department of Experimental Medicine and Surgery, Tor Vergata University, Rome, Italy. [3]Department of Urology, University of Florence, Florence, Italy. [4]Unit for Functional Urology, Department of Urology, Policlinico Tor Vergata, Rome, Italy.

### References
1.  Gontero P, Bohle A, Malmstrom PU, O'Donnell MA, Oderda M, Sylvester R, Witjes F: **The role of bacillus Calmette-Guérin in the treatment of non-muscle-invasive bladder cancer.** *Eur Urol* 2010, **57**(3):410–429. doi:10.1016/j.eururo.2009.11.023. Epub 2009 Nov 13.
2.  Lamm DL, van der Meijden PM, Morales A, Brosman SA, Catalona WJ, Herr HW, Soloway MS, Steg A, Debruyne FM: **Incidence and treatment**

of complications of bacillus Calmette-Guerin intravesical therapy in superficial bladder cancer. *J Urol* 1992, **147**(3):596–600.

3. Drake MJ, Nixon PM, Crew JP: **Drug-induced bladder and urinary disorders. Incidence, prevention and management.** *Drug Saf* 1998, **19**(1):45–55.

4. Witjes JA, Palou J, Soloway M, Lamm D, Brausi M, Spermon JR, Persad R, Buckley R, Akaza H, Colombel M, Böhle A: **Clinical practice recommendations for the prevention and management of intravesical therapy-associated adverse events.** *Eur Urol Suppl* 2008, **7**(10):667–674.

5. Vegt PD, van der Meijden AP, Sylvester R, Brausi M, Höltl W, de Balincourt C: **Does isoniazid reduce side effects of intravesical bacillus Calmette-Guerin therapy in superficial bladder cancer? Interim results of European Organization for Research and Treatment of Cancer Protocol 30911.** *J Urol* 1997, **157**(4):1246–1249.

6. Colombel M, Saint F, Chopin D, Malavaud B, Nicolas L, Rischmann P: **The effect of ofloxacin on bacillus Calmette-Guérin induced toxicity in patients with superficial bladder cancer: results of a randomized, prospective, double blind, placebo controlled, multicenter study.** *J Urol* 2006, **176**:935.

7. O'Donnell M: **Does ofloxacin protect against BCG related toxic effects in patients with bladder cancer?** *Nat Clin Pract Urol* 2007, **4**:304.

8. Martínez-Piñeiro JA, Flores N, Isorna S, Solsona E, Sebastián JL, Pertusa C, Rioja LA, Martínez-Piñeiro L, Vela R, Camacho JE, Nogueira JL, Pereira I, Resel L, Muntañola P, Galvis F, Chesa N, De Torres JA, Carballido J, Bernuy C, Arribas S, Madero R, for CUETO (Club Urológico Español de Tratamiento Oncológico): **Long-term follow-up of a randomized prospective trial comparing a standard 81 mg dose of intravesical bacille Calmette-Guérin with a reduced dose of 27 mg in superficial bladder cancer.** *BJU Int* 2002, **89**(7):671–680.

9. Iacovelli V, Topazio L, Gaziev G, Bove P, Vespasiani G, Finazzi Agrò E: **Intravesical glycosaminoglycans in the management of chronic cystitis.** *Minerva Urol Nefrol* 2013, **65**(4):249–262.

10. Madersbacher H, van Ophoven A, van Kerrebroeck PE: **GAG layer replenishment therapy for chronic forms of cystitis with intravesical glycosaminoglycans–a review.** *Neurourol Urodyn* 2013, **32**(1):9–18. doi:10.1002/nau.22256. Epub 2012 Jul 10.

11. Sommariva ML, Sandri SD, Guerrer CS: **Treatment of acute iatrogenic cystitis secondary to bladder chemo-immuno-instillation or pelvic radiotherapy.** *Urologia* 2010, **77**:187.

12. Fowler S, Daukeh M, Thompson A: **Intravesical sodium hyaluronate (Cystistat®) as a treatment for chronic BCG Cystitis: a discussion of two successful cases.** [http://www.bjui.org/ContentFullItem.aspx?id=638]

13. Sylvester RJ, van der Meijden AP, Oosterlinck W, Witjes JA, Bouffioux C, Denis L, Newling DW, Kurth K: **Predicting recurrence and progression in individual patients with stage Ta T1 bladder cancer using EORTC risk tables: a combined analysis of 2596 patients from seven EORTC trials.** *Eur Urol* 2006, **49**(3):466–4755. discussion 475–7. Epub 2006 Jan 17.

14. Shelley MD, Kynaston H, Court J, Wilt TJ, Coles B, Burgon K, Mason MD: **A systematic review of intravesical bacillus Calmette-Guérin plus transurethral resection vs transurethral resection alone in Ta and T1 bladder cancer.** *BJU Int* 2001, **88**(3):209–216.

15. Han RF, Pan JG: **Can intravesical bacillus Calmette-Guérin reduce recurrence in patients with superficial bladder cancer? A meta-analysis of randomized trials.** *Urology* 2006, **67**(6):1216.

16. Böhle A, Bock PR: **Intravesical bacillus Calmette-Guerin versus mitomycin C in superficial bladder cancer: formal meta-analysis of comparative studies on tumour progression.** *Urology* 2004, **63**(4):682.

17. Sylvester RJ, van der Meijden AP, Lamm DL: **Intravesical bacillus Calmette-Guerin reduces the risk of progression in patients with superficial bladder cancer: a meta-analysis of the published results of randomized clinical trials.** *J Urol* 2002, **168**(5):1964.

18. Van der Meijden APM, Sylvester RJ, Oosterlinck W, Hoeltl W, Bono AV, EORTC Genito-Urinary Tract Cancer Group: **Maintenance bacillus Calmette-Guerin for TaT1 bladder tumors is not associated with increased toxicity: results from a European Organisation for Research and Treatment of Cancer Genito-Urinary Group phase III trial.** *Eur Urol* 2003, **44**:429.

19. Lamm DL, Blumenstein BA, Crissman JD, Montie JE, Gottesman JE, Lowe BA, Sarosdy MF, Bohl RD, Grossman HB, Beck TM, Leimert JT, Crawford ED: **Maintenance bacillus Calmette-Guerin immunotherapy for recurrent TA, T1 and carcinoma in situ transitional cell carcinoma of the bladder: a randomized Southwest Oncology Group Study.** *J Urol* 2000, **163**(4):1124–1129.

20. Saint F, Irani J, Patard JJ, Salomon L, Hoznek A, Zammattio S, Debois H, Abbou CC, Chopin DK: **Tolerability of bacille Calmette-Guérin maintenance therapy for superficial bladder cancer.** *Urology* 2001, **57**(5):883–888.

21. Martínez-Piñeiro JA, Martínez-Piñeiro L, Solsona E, Rodríguez RH, Gómez JM, Martín MG, Molina JR, Collado AG, Flores N, Isorna S, Pertusa C, Rabadán M, Astobieta A, Camacho JE, Arribas S, Madero R, Club Urológico Español de Tratamiento Oncológico (CUETO): **Has a 3-fold decreased dose of bacillus Calmette-Guerin the same efficacy against recurrences and progression of T1G3 and Tis bladder tumors than the standard dose? Results of a prospective randomized trial.** *J Urol* 2005, **174**(4 Pt 1):1242–1247.

22. Oddens J, Brausi M, Sylvester R, Bono A, van de Beek C, van Andel G, Gontero P, Hoeltl W, Turkeri L, Marreaud S, Collette S, Oosterlinck W: **Final results of an EORTC-GU cancers group randomized study of maintenance bacillus Calmette-Guérin in intermediate- and high-risk Ta, T1 papillary carcinoma of the urinary bladder: one-third dose versus full dose and 1 year versus 3 years of maintenance.** *Eur Urol* 2013, **63**(3):462–472. doi: 10.1016/j.eururo.2012.10.039. Epub 2012 Nov 2.

23. Toft BR, Nordling J: **Recent developments of intravesical therapy of painful bladder syndrome/interstitial cystitis: a review.** *Curr Opin Urol* 2006, **16**:268.

24. Nickel JC, Egerdie B, Downey J, Singh R, Skehan A, Carr L, Irvine-Bird K: **A real-life multicentre clinical practice study to evaluate the efficacy and safety of intravesical chondroitin sulphate for the treatment of interstitial cystitis.** *BJU Int* 2009, **103**(1):56–60. doi:10.1111/j.1464-410X.2008.08028.x. Epub 2008 Sep 3.

25. Hurst RE: **Structure, function, and pathology of proteoglycans and glycosaminoglycans in the urinary tract.** *World J Urol* 1994, **12**:3.

26. Leppilahti M, Hellström P, Tammela TLJ: **Effect of diagnostic hydrodistension and four intravesical Hyaluronan Instillations on bladder ICAM-1 intensity and association of ICAM-1 intensity with clinical response in patients with interstitial cystitis.** *Urology* 2002, **60**:46.

27. Schulz A, Vestweber AM, Dressler D: **Anti-inflammatory action of a hyaluronic acid-chondroitin sulphate preparation in an in vitro bladder model.** *Akt Urol* 2009, **40**(2):109.

28. Boucher WS, Letourneau R, Huang M, Kempuraj D, Green M, Sant GR, Theoharides TC: **Intravesical sodium hyaluronate inhibits the rat urinary mast cell mediator increase triggered by acute immobilization stress.** *J Urol* 2002, **167**(1):380–384.

29. Sylvester RJ, van der Meijden APM, Oosterlinck W, Hoeltl W, Bono AV, EORTC Genito-Urinary Tract Cancer Group: **The side effects of bacillus Calmette-Guérin in the treatment of TaT1 bladder cancer do not predict its efficacy: results from a European Organization for Research and Treatment of Cancer Genito-Urinary Group phase III trial.** *Eur Urol* 2003, **44**:423.

# 15

# Evaluation of the learning curve for thulium laser enucleation of the prostate with the aid of a simulator tool but without tutoring: comparison of two surgeons with different levels of endoscopic experience

Giovanni Saredi[1], Giacomo Maria Pirola[2*], Andrea Pacchetti[1], Jon Alexander Lovisolo[3], Giacomo Borroni[4], Federico Sembenini[5] and Alberto Mario Marconi[1]

**Abstract**

**Background:** The aim of this study was to determine the learning curve for thulium laser enucleation of the prostate (ThuLEP) for two surgeons with different levels of urological endoscopic experience.

**Methods:** From June 2012 to August 2013, ThuLEP was performed on 100 patients in our institution. We present the results of a prospective evaluation during which we analyzed data related to the learning curves for two surgeons of different levels of experience.

**Results:** The prostatic adenoma volumes ranged from 30 to 130 mL (average 61.2 mL). Surgeons A and B performed 48 and 52 operations, respectively. Six months after surgery, all patients were evaluated with the International Prostate Symptom Score questionnaire, uroflowmetry, and prostate-specific antigen test. Introduced in 2010, ThuLEP consists of blunt enucleation of the prostatic apex and lobes using the sheath of the resectoscope. This maneuver allows clearer visualization of the enucleation plane and precise identification of the prostatic capsule. These conditions permit total resection of the prostatic adenoma and coagulation of small penetrating vessels, thereby reducing the laser emission time. Most of the complications in this series were encountered during morcellation, which in some cases was performed under poor vision because of venous bleeding due to surgical perforation of the capsule during enucleation.

**Conclusions:** Based on this analysis, we concluded that it is feasible for laser-naive urologists with endoscopic experience to learn to perform ThuLEP without tutoring. Those statements still require further validation in larger multicentric study cohort by several surgeon. The main novelty during the learning process was the use of a simulator that faithfully reproduced all of the surgical steps in prostates of various shapes and volumes.

**Keywords:** Benign prostatic hyperplasia, Endourology, Laser surgery, Prostate disease, Simulator

* Correspondence: gmo.pirola@gmail.com
[2]Department of Urology, University of Modena e Reggio Emilia, viale Borri, 57, 21100 Varese, Modena, Italy
Full list of author information is available at the end of the article

## Background

Since 1998, holmium laser enucleation of the prostate (HoLEP) has been increasingly used as an alternative to the classic transurethral endoscopic resection of the prostate (TURP) and open prostatectomy [1]. HoLEP is currently considered to be at least equivalent to, or better than, TURP [2]. It shortens the catheterization time and the overall hospital stay. Its functional outcomes are reported to have the same long-term record as open prostatectomy. It has thus been proposed as an endourological procedure that could replace open prostatectomy [3].

Thulium laser, which was introduced in 2005, was found to offer all the advantages of HoLEP for treating bladder outlet obstruction (BOO). The difference between the holmium and thulium beams lies in the latter's continuous wave mode [4] and tissue penetration of 0.1–0.2 mm compared with the 0.3- to 0.4-mm penetration of holmium [5]. Thulium-YAG laser has been applied during various procedures, such as prostate vaporization (ThuVAP), vaporesection (ThuVARP), vapoenucleation (ThuVEP), and more recently thulium laser enucleation of the prostate (ThuLEP) [6].

ThuLEP was introduced as a minimally invasive, size-independent treatment for BOO using an approach comparable to that for HoLEP [4, 7]. When compared with a holmium laser, thulium seems to deliver improved vaporization ability, ensuring smooth tissue incisions. Because this plane is now more easily distinguishable with ThuLEP, the surgeon is able to remove the adenoma accurately at the level of the surgical capsule. Virtually any prostate size can be removed transurethrally using this technique [8].

For HoLEP, it has been shown that at least 50 cases must be undertaken to achieve a safe learning curve [9]. To date, there are no such data for ThuLEP. Hence, in 2012, two laser-naive surgeons with consolidated experience in traditional urological endoscopy embarked on a pathway to perform this innovative technique after visiting several centers where urological laser surgery was regularly performed.

The aim of this study was to compare retrospectively the learning curves of these two surgeons. Each was an experienced urological surgeon: one had more than 25 years of experience in endoscopic urological surgery (surgeon A), and the other had about 15 years of practice (surgeon B). Both surgeons practiced the steps involved in ThuLEP on a dedicated simulator before performing the procedure on humans but had no formal tutoring.

## Methods

Between June 2012 and August 2013, a total of 100 patients underwent ThuLEP at our institution. Two laser-naive surgeons (A and B) who had long-term experience in traditional urological endoscopy performed all of the ThuLEP procedures.

A novelty in this case series was the availability of a new tool (CyberSim; Quanta System, Solbiate Olona VA, Italy). This simulation instrument clearly reproduces the various steps of the operation [10, 11]. The simulator is able to reproduce prostatic adenomas of different volumes and shapes, different lengths of the prostatic urethra, and particularly different median lobe morphologies. After each simulated procedure, the system gives a report on the resection rate (with preoperative and postoperative views) and shows the areas of residual adenoma. It also reports errors, such as surgical capsule perforation, and the presence of striated sphincter lesions. To test various modalities of coagulation, it is possible to induce "bleeding" during the procedure. Each of the two surgeons was offered the possibility of practicing for a 2-week period.

Prior to surgery all patients underwent clinical evaluation including assessment of the International Prostate Symptom Score (IPSS) questionnaire, uroflowmetry, post-void residual urine evaluation, and transrectal ultrasonography (TRUS). Patients with prostatic adenoma volumes of 30–150 mL were considered candidates for ThuLEP, whereas those with adenomas <30 mL underwent ThuVAP (150 W). Those with adenomas >150 mL were treated by open simple prostatectomy. Patients with cardiovascular disease (assuming that the patient was under care with anti-platelet drugs) were not excluded, except for one case in which the patient was receiving doubled anti-platelet therapy. Additionally, patients on oral anticoagulant therapy were shifted to low-molecular-weight heparin.

We obtained institutional review board approval for this study. Written informed consent was always obtained from the patient before surgery.

Exclusion criteria were a low IPSS score (<7 points), urodynamic evidence of neurogenic acontractile bladder detrusor, and/or a history of prostate surgery. We recorded the total surgical time, total laser emission time, total delivered laser energy (joules), laser fiber caliber, days of postoperative catheterization with and without continuous saline bladder irrigation, and the length of postoperative hospital stay.

Spinal anesthesia was mainly used. All operations were performed with the same laser machine (Cyber TM 150; Quanta System, Solbiate Olona VA, Italy) using two different end-firing fibers (calibers of 600 and 800 μm, depending on the prostate volume and the surgeon's preference). A mechanical tissue morcellator (Piranha; Wolf, Knittlingen, Germany) was used in all but five cases, in which a different device (DRILLCUT; Karl Storz, Tuttlingen, Germany) was used. Continuous bladder irrigation was employed for the first 12 h postoperatively in all cases. Indwelling catheters were removed on the first postoperative day if hematuria was not present. The Clavien–Dindo classification was used to assess early and late surgical complications. All patients were followed for at least 6 months postoperatively, at which time functional and subjective outcomes were recorded using the same tests that were applied as preoperative baseline studies (IPSS questionnaire, uroflowmetry, prostate-specific antigen [PSA] test) as well as urinalysis, urine culture, and echography to evaluate the post-void residual volume. Intraoperative data and data regarding clinical outcome were compared between surgeons A and B. Multivariate analysis was used to compare laser emission time (min) and prostatic adenoma volume (mL). We did not consider the total surgical time as it was influenced by variables not directly related to the intervention itself (e.g., instrument changes, technical delays, initial cystoscopy). We also created another variable linked to experience in an attempt to determine if it influenced the laser emission time. We verified our data with the Student's $t$-test and the Shapiro-Wilk test.

A "stepwise" multiple regression analysis was performed on data from 90 of the participants. Patients who underwent multiple procedures simultaneously—ureterorenoscopy (two cases) and bladder calculus lithotripsy (eight cases)—were excluded. The Ethics Committee of the Faculty of Medicine, University of Insubria, Varese e Como, Italy, approved this study.

### Surgical technique

We employed the classic technique [4] with the Quanta System Cyber TM 150. First, the ureteral orifices were identified, and a coagulation marker (60 W) was placed approximately 1 cm away from each orifice. Then, after identifying the edge of the external urethral sphincter, two mucosal incisions were made (as wide as possible) at the level of the distal third of the verumontanum toward the 12 o'clock position using a thulium laser set at 60 W. Subsequently, the prostatic median lobe was removed starting from a bilateral bladder neck incision that followed the lateral edges of the prostatic median lobe and extended to the verumontanum, where an inverted-U incision was made close to it. The resectoscope was gradually moved under the enucleation edge of the median lobe, and blunt dissection towards 12 o'clock was performed with laser emission of 110 W. In the absence of a median lobe, we performed incisions at 5 and 7 o'clock, creating an artificial median lobe, or a deep incision on the bladder neck at 6 o'clock that extended to the verumontanum, with subsequent lateral shifting of prostatic lobes (110 W).

We next made an anterior incision that extended from 12 o'clock on the bladder neck to the verumontanum. After identifying the "white plane" of the capsule, we mobilized the anterolateral aspect of the adenoma with a bilateral semicircular motion of the resectoscope towards 2 and 10 o'clock, respectively.

The lateral lobes were enucleated separately, beginning with the left lobe. After deepening the apical incision from 6 o'clock to 2 o'clock, the apical edge of the lateral lobes was bluntly exposed by moving the resectoscope and pushing the lobes in the 2 o'clock direction. After identifying the capsular plane (a white plane with small vessels running in parallel fashion), the perforating vessels were coagulated. The entire lateral lobe was then bluntly and progressively released towards the bladder neck. The released lobe was then dissected, joining the anterior and lateral incision at the 2 o'clock position. After complete mobilization of the apex, we completed the blunt disconnection towards the 12 o'clock position. The same procedure was completed on the opposite side. The prostate fragments were pushed into the bladder by continuous irrigation and were totally morcellated at the end of the enucleation.

### Results

The average patient age was 68.8 years (range 52–85 years, median 69 years) (Table 1). The prostatic adenoma volume ranged from 30 to 130 mL (mean 61.2 mL). For surgeon B, the maximum adenoma volume was 105 mL. Surgeon A performed 48 operations, and surgeon B performed 52. Surgical durations were similar: 34–160 min (median 92 min) for surgeon A and 40–127 min (median 86 min) for surgeon B. Laser emission time ranged from 16.0 to 58.4 min (median 28 min) for surgeon A and from 19.0 to 37.1 min (median 24 min) for surgeon B. The total amount of energy delivered was 84,820–386,920 joules (J) (median 165,650 J) for surgeon A and 87,540–358,327 J (median 163,445 J) for surgeon B. Surgeon A used 600 μm of laser fiber in 18 patients (37.5 %) and 800 μm in 30 patients (62.5 %). Surgeon B used the same fibers in 11 patients (21.1 %) and 41 patients (78.9 %), respectively.

Surgeon A performed a consensual endolithotripsy of bladder calculi in three patients, and surgeon B did the same in five patients. Surgeon B performed two consensual ureterorenoscopies—one in a patient with urolithiasis and the other in a second patient who was suspected to have a ureteral neoplasm.

Intraoperative complications occurred in two patients treated by surgeon A: a bladder perforation managed with intraoperative monopolar coagulation, prolonged bladder catheterization (5 days) [Clavien–Dindo (C–D) grade 1], and a case of intraoperative bleeding that required a second procedure to complete the morcellation the following day (C–D grade 3b). Surgeon B experienced one case of bladder perforation during morcellation that was identified and managed conservatively (C–D grade 1).

**Table 1** Perioperative data (Varese, 2014)

| | Surgeon A | Surgeon B |
|---|---|---|
| Cases (n) | 48 | 52 |
| Median age (yrs, range) | 71 (50–86) | 68 (51–84) |
| Median Adenoma volume (TRUS, ml, range) | 61 (30–130) | 60 (30–105) |
| Median PSA (ng/dl, range) | 6.32 (1.2–37.1) | 5.98 (0.7–23.6) |
| I-PSS moderate/high | 24/ 17 (7 n.v.) | 25/ 17 (10 n.v.) |
| Median Surgical time (min, range) | 92 (34–160) | 86 (40–127) |
| Median Laser emission time (min, range) | 28 (16–58,44) | 24 (19–37,16) |
| Median Total energy delivered (J, range) | 165,650 (84,820–386,920) | 163,445 (87,540–358,327) |
| 600 μm fiber use (no. cases) | 18 | 11 |
| 800 μm fiber use (no. cases) | 30 | 41 |
| Intraoperative complications | •1 Bladder perforation | •1 Bladder perforation |
| | •1 Intraoperative bleeding, with necessity to delay morcellation | |
| Contemporary procedures | •3 bladder ELT | •2 URS |
| | | •5 bladder ELT |
| Reoperations | •1 Morcellation on first postoperative day | •1 Hemostatic TUR (first postoperative day) |
| | •1 TURP for chronic retention (6 months later) | •1 Morcellation of a residual fragment (1 month later) |
| | | •1 Urethrotomy for bulbar urethral stenosis (9 months later) |

Reoperations were necessary in four other cases. One patient required TURP for chronic retention 6 months later (surgeon A); one required hemostatic TURP for massive postoperative bleeding 24 h after surgery (surgeon B); there was one case of incomplete morcellation that caused urinary retention and required a second look 1 month later (C–D grade 3b) (surgeon B); and there was one case of urethral stenosis 9 months after ThuLEP (surgeon B).

Patients were discharged after urinating spontaneously on the same day on which the bladder catheter was removed. This occurred on the first postoperative day in 75.0 % ($n = 36$) of patients operated on by surgeon A and in 67.3 % ($n = 35$) of patients operated on by surgeon B. The bladder catheter was removed on the second postoperative day in 13 patients (6 for surgeon A, 7 for surgeon B) and on the third postoperative day in 11 patients (5 for surgeon A, 6 for surgeon B). Five patients retained the bladder catheter for more than 3 days: two for 4 days (hematuria, surgeon B) (C–D grade 2), one for 5 days (bladder perforation, surgeon A) (C–D grade 1), and two for a week because of urinary retention after catheter removal in one case (surgeon B) (C–D grade 1) and a renal injury that occurred during ureteroscopy performed in a patient with a solitary kidney (surgeon B) (C–D grade 1).

The 2-month follow-up consisted of clinical evaluation and administration of the IPSS questionnaire. At the 6-month follow-up, we undertook a new clinical evaluation,

PSA testing, and uroflowmetry with a sonographic post-void residual determination. Resolution of the symptoms was reflected in a low postoperative IPSS evaluation (<4 points, with a clear patient statement of improved quality of life) and by ecographic assessment of the absence of post-void residual urine, with normal urinary outflow. These data are summarized in Table 2.

We evaluated our data using a statistical multivariate analysis, noting the laser emission time and prostatic adenoma volume for each surgeon and comparing them. There was a positive linear correlation between these two variables, with a correlation index of 0.856. This model explains the 73 % ($R^2$ adjusted = 72.74 %) variability in laser emission time relative to the prostatic adenoma volume. At each 1-mL increment in the prostatic adenoma volume, the laser emission time increased by 0.3232 min. These data were confirmed by the Student's $t$-test and the Shapiro–Wilk test. All regression coefficients were statistically significant, as shown in Fig. 1.

In the second part of our statistical analysis, we sought a possible relation of the laser emission time (normalized by prostate size) with the amount of urological endoscopic experience. Analyzing the effect of experience (calculated as the number of total operations by an operator) on the laser emission time normalized by prostate size, the linear regression showed that this variable is not statistically significant. The laser emission time did not change significantly during this 100-patient series.

Evaluation of the learning curve for thulium laser enucleation of the prostate with the aid of a simulator tool...

95

**Table 2** Postoperative and follow-up data (Varese, 2014)

|  | Surgeon A | Surgeon B |
| --- | --- | --- |
| Bladder catheter removal on 1 st postoperative day | 36 patients | 35 patients |
| Bladder catheter removal on 2 nd postoperative day | 6 patients | 7 patients |
| Bladder catheter removal on 3 rd postoperative day | 5 patients | 6 patients |
| Bladder catheter removal after 3 rd postoperative day | 1 patient<br>Bladder perforation | 4 patients<br>2 cases hematuria<br>1 Respiratory illness<br>1 post URS ARI in patient with solitary kidney |
| 2 months- IPSS symptoms resolution | 40 cases (83.3 %) | 47 cases (90.38 %) |
| Median 6 months- PSA (ng/dl) | 0.83 (0.20–3.56) | 0.91 (0.27–3.75) |
| 6 months- Qmax, ml/s (median) | 24.8 (17–31) | 24.4 (18–30) |
| 6 months- PVR, ml (Eco) | 5.8 (0–22) | 7.2 (0–30) |

## Discussion

As there is still a lack of studies regarding the learning curve for applying thulium laser surgery to BOO, we tried to compare our data to those obtained using other techniques, such as ThuVEP [12, 13] and HoLEP [8]. HoLEP has been proven to be an effective, minimally invasive, size-independent procedure for the surgical treatment of benign prostatic hyperplasia (BPH). Its prolonged learning curve (requiring specific tutoring for 30–50 cases), however, has prevented this technique from being widely adopted [14].

In 2009, Bach et al. [15] introduced Tm:YAG laser prostatectomy, which initially involved both enucleation of the prostatic lobes and vaporization (Tm-YAG vapoenucleation of the prostate, or ThuVEP). Herrmann et al. [4] introduced the ThuLEP technique in 2010, which involves blunt enucleation of the prostatic apex and lobes using the sheath of the resectoscope. This technique permits easier enucleation because of better visualization and thus the ability to identify precisely the prostatic capsule. This condition, in turn, permits total resection of adenomatous tissue and coagulation of small penetrating vessels. The incidence of postoperative edema and potential complications (e.g., urinary retention, hematuria) is thus reduced [16]. We have refined our technique with the aid of a simulator (Cybersim), which

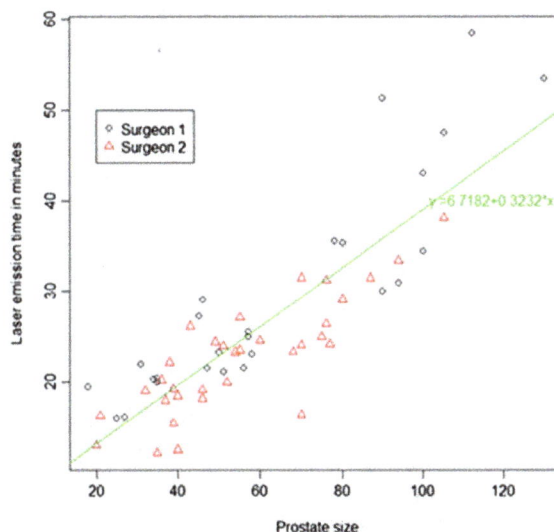

**Fig. 1** Our Statystical regression model in a scatter plot, showing a linear relation between prostatic adenoma volume (ml) and laser emission time (min). It's visually clear the absence of statistical differences between the two Surgeons. Varese, 2014

allowed us to practice with "prostatic adenomas" of different sizes and shapes and to focus on the various steps of the operation.

ThuLEP appears to be safe and effective regardless of prostate size, with outcomes comparable to those achieved in case series using HoLEP and ThuVEP [5, 14]. However, there is still a lack of studies concerning the learning curve for mastering the ThuLEP technique. We presented herein the results we obtained for the first 100 consecutive patients who underwent ThuLEP at our institution. The procedures were performed by two surgeons who were laser naive but had 25 years (surgeon A) and 15 years (surgeon B) of experience with traditional urological endoscopy.

Patients with adenoma volumes of 30–50 mL were considered for ThuLEP. Those with adenomas <30 mL were treated by ThuVEP, and those with adenomas >150 mL underwent simple open prostatectomy. As we do not believe that there is an upper size limit for the procedure, our current practice is to employ ThuLEP in all patients with an enlarged prostate.

Our results have shown a low incidence of complications with ThuLEP, comparable to that for HoLEP [14] and ThuVEP [12] and fewer than are seen with classic endoscopic procedures for BPH treatment [16]. The excellent hemostatic properties of thulium laser provides safety for the surgeon, who can avoid important complications even without any tutoring. In this consecutive case series, we faced all types of prostatic adenoma from the beginning, and among the first 100 cases we handled adenoma volumes up to 130 mL. We believe that this demonstrates the safety and efficacy of the method we employed. Our follow-up data confirm complete removal of the adenomatous tissue according to the PSA values, uroflowmetry, sonographic evaluation, and "symptomatic" IPSS score resolution.

Symptomatic evaluation using the IPSS questionnaire 2 months after surgery revealed that 13 patients reported persistence of nocturia at least three times per night. All other respondents reported complete resolution of their symptoms. No patients complained about voiding—only about irritative symptoms (nocturia, pollakiuria). Among those with irritative symptoms, most had had adenomas with volumes of <40 mL, so the symptoms were probably due to the large amount of laser energy delivered. The same evaluation at 6 months showed that only four patents still had those symptoms.

The postoperative outcomes of this study appear comparable to those of other case series in the literature. As all surgical complications were verified within the first 60 cases, we might say that it was sufficient experience to perform the operation well and safely after about 30 cases. All complications were managed successfully, and of the five patients who required reoperation (two for surgeon A, three for surgeon B) only three could be viewed as complications caused by inexperience. Most of the complications in our series were observed during morcellation, and the biggest problem we had was related to poor vision as a result of venous bleeding caused by perforation of the prostatic capsule during enucleation. Obviously, the prior endourological experience of the two operators was beneficial for their rapid learning of the technique. The absence of noticeable differences in the perioperative data and urodynamic results for the patients treated by the two surgeons shows that this technique is feasible even without direct tutoring.

Our results are comparable to those published by high-volume centers, where the technique was performed by various surgeons [12]. Our study has shown that a learning curve of about 30 cases is sufficient for performing this technique without difficulty. This number of cases clearly provides less experience than is needed for HoLEP, which requires 30–50 cases [9].

Our statistical analysis showed a linear correlation between the laser emission time and the prostatic adenoma volume. We did not find any statistically significant influence on the laser emission times by each of the two surgeons' experience from the beginning to the end of the study period, which could be interpreted to mean that more cases are needed to show this parameter. Furthermore, a possible bias of this work is the fact that we considered the learning curves of only two surgeons, both with a previous consolidated endoscopic urology experience, without being able to demonstrate clear difference between them. Larger multicentric cohort studies of patients operated by several surgeons with different endoscopic experience are still required to provide further validity to Our statements.

**Conclusion**

The aim of this study was to evaluate the learning curve for ThuLEP required by two surgeons with different levels of urological endoscopic experience. The learning process began with visits to some centers with experience in HoLEP and ThuLEP. It continued with practicing the ThuLEP procedure with a new simulator (Cybersim). Surgical complications were mostly due to morcellation—not to the enucleation itself—and were easily managed. The results of the study are similar to those from other case studies in the literature for laser treatment of BPH. Our data suggest that the number of cases necessary for an endoscopically experienced urological surgeon to learn ThuLEP is lower than that for HoLEP and that tutoring for this technique is not mandatory. The main novelty in our experience is the long-term use of a new simulator tool that precisely reproduces all the step of this procedure. To the best of our knowledge, simulation of ThuLEP has not been previously described. We found that practicing the procedure in 30 cases is sufficient for a single operator to complete the learning curve. In this 100-patient series, there was no significant reduction in laser emission time from the first cases to the last with the same size adenomas for the two surgeons. The only parameter that showed a linear influence on enucleation time was the adenoma volume. Further validity to those statements will be provided by larger multicentric cohort studies considering the outcomes of several surgeons with different urologic endoscopy experience.

## Abbreviations

ThuLEP: Thulium laser enucleation of the prostate; IPSS: International Prostate Symptoms Score; TRUS: Transrectal ultrasonography; PSA: Prostate-specific antigen; HoLEP: Holmium laser enucleation of the prostate; TURP: Transurethral endoscopic resection of the prostate; BOO: Bladder outlet obstruction; ThuVAP: Thulium prostate vaporization; ThuVARP: Thulium vaporesection of the prostate; ThuVEP: Thulium vapoenucleation of the prostate; PVR: Post-void residual volume.

## Competing interests

The authors declare that they have no conflict of interest.

## Authors' contributions

GS created the conception and design of the study and analyzed and interpreted the data. GMP drafted the manuscript and worked on most of the data presented. AP and GB aided in data collection and interpretation. JAL revised the manuscript, especially improving the Discussion section. FS statistically analyzed the data. AMM supervised the overall work. All authors read and approved the final manuscript.

## Acknowledgments

We thank the engineer Filippo Fagnani, who provided technical support for the thulium laser settings on behalf of Quanta System DNA Laser Technology throughout the study.

## Author details

[1]Department of Urology, Ospedale di Circolo e Fondazione Macchi, Varese, Italy. [2]Department of Urology, University of Modena e Reggio Emilia, viale Borri, 57, 21100 Varese, Modena, Italy. [3]Department of Urology, Ospedale di Circolo di Busto Arsizio, Saronno, Italy. [4]Department of Surgery, Ospedale di Circolo e Fondazione Macchi, Varese, Italy. [5]Department of Statistics, Bicocca University, Milan, Italy.

## References

1. Gilling PJ, Fraundorfer MR. Holmium laser prostatectomy: a technique in evolution. Curr Opin Urol. 1998;8(1):11–5.
2. Ahyai SA, Gilling P, Kaplan SA, et al. Meta-analysis of functional outcomes and complications following transurethral procedures for lower urinary tract symptoms resulting from benign prostatic enlargement. Eur Urol. 2010;58(3):384–97.
3. Kuntz RM, Lehrich K, Ahyai SA. Holmium laser enucleation of the prostate versus open prostatectomy for prostates greater than 100 grams: 5-year follow-up results of a randomised clinical trial. Eur Urol. 2008;53(1):160–6.
4. Fried NM, Murray KE. High-power thulium fiber laser ablation of urinary tissues at 1.94 microm. J Endourol. 2005;19(1):25–31.
5. Gravas S, Bachmann A, Reich O, Roehrborn CG, Gilling PJ, De La Rosette J. Critical review of lasers in benign prostatic hyperplasia (BPH). BJU Int. 2011;107(7):1030–43.
6. Zarrabi A, Gross AJ. The evolution of lasers in urology. Ther Adv Urol. 2011;3(2):81–9.
7. Herrmann TR, Bach T, Imkamp F, et al. Thulium laser enucleation of the prostate (ThuLEP): transurethral anatomical prostatectomy with laser support. Introduction of a novel technique for the treatment of benign prostatic obstruction. World J Urol. 2010;28(1):45–51.
8. Maheshwari PN, Joshi N, Maheshwari RP. Best laser prostatectomy in the year 2013. Indian J Urol. 2013;29(3):236–43.
9. El-Hakim A, Elhilali MM. Holmium laser enucleation of the prostate can be taught: the first learning experience. BJU Int. 2002;90(9):863–9.
10. Brewin J, Ahmed K, Challacombe B. An update and review of simulation in urological training. Int J Surg. 2014;12(2):103–8.
11. Khan R, Aydin A, Khan MS, Dasgupta P, Ahmed K. Simulation-based training for prostate surgery. BJU Int. 2014
12. Gross AJ, Netsch C, Knipper S, Hölzel J, Bach T. Complications and early postoperative outcome in 1080 patients after thulium vapoenucleation of the prostate: results at a single institution. Eur Urol. 2013;63(5):859–67.
13. Netsch C, Bach T, Herrmann TR, Neubauer O, Gross AJ. Evaluation of the learning curve for Thulium VapoEnucleation of the prostate (ThuVEP) using a mentor-based approach. World J Urol. 2013;31(5):1231–8.
14. Zhang F, Shao Q, Herrmann TR, Tian Y, Zhang Y. Thulium laser versus holmium laser transurethral enucleation of the prostate: 18-month follow-up data of a single center. Urology. 2012;79(4):869–74.
15. Bach T, Wendt-Nordahl G, Michel MS, Herrmann TR, Gross AJ. Feasibility and efficacy of Thulium:YAG laser enucleation (VapoEnucleation) of the prostate. World J Urol. 2009;27(4):541–5.
16. Tang K, Xu Z, Xia D, et al. Early outcomes of thulium laser versus transurethral resection of the prostate for managing benign prostatic hyperplasia: a systematic review and meta-analysis of comparative studies. J Endourol. 2014;28(1):65–72.

# 16

# Prediction of clinical manifestations of transurethral resection syndrome by preoperative ultrasonographic estimation of prostate weight

Atsushi Fujiwara[1], Junko Nakahira[1*], Toshiyuki Sawai[1], Teruo Inamoto[2] and Toshiaki Minami[1]

## Abstract

**Background:** This study aimed to investigate the relationship between preoperative estimated prostate weight on ultrasonography and clinical manifestations of transurethral resection (TUR) syndrome.

**Methods:** The records of patients who underwent TUR of the prostate under regional anesthesia over a 6-year period were retrospectively reviewed. TUR syndrome is usually defined as a serum sodium level of < 125 mmol/l combined with clinical cardiovascular or neurological manifestations. This study focused on the clinical manifestations only, and recorded specific central nervous system and cardiovascular abnormalities according to the checklist proposed by Hahn. Patients with and without clinical manifestations of TUR syndrome were compared to determine the factors associated with TUR syndrome. Receiver operating characteristic curve analysis was used to determine the optimal cutoff value of estimated prostate weight for the prediction of clinical manifestations of TUR syndrome.

**Results:** This study included 167 patients, of which 42 developed clinical manifestations of TUR syndrome. There were significant differences in preoperative estimated prostate weight, operation time, resected prostate weight, intravenous fluid infusion volume, blood transfusion volume, and drainage of the suprapubic irrigation fluid between patients with and without clinical manifestations of TUR syndrome. The preoperative estimated prostate weight was correlated with the resected prostate weight (Spearman's correlation coefficient, 0.749). Receiver operator characteristic curve analysis showed that the optimal cutoff value of estimated prostate weight for the prediction of clinical manifestations of TUR syndrome was 75 g (sensitivity, 0.70; specificity, 0.69; area under the curve, 0.73).

**Conclusions:** Preoperative estimation of prostate weight by ultrasonography can predict the development of clinical manifestations of TUR syndrome. Particular care should be taken when the estimated prostate weight is > 75 g.

**Keywords:** TUR syndrome, Hyponatremia, Transurethral resection of prostate

## Background

Benign prostatic hyperplasia (BPH) is common in elderly men. The risk of BPH increases with age, approaching 50% by the age of 60 years and 90% by the age of 85 years [1]. Numerous therapeutic options are available for BPH, including pharmacological treatment, minimally invasive surgery, and open prostatectomy. Preoperative ultrasonography is often performed to confirm the diagnosis of BPH and to measure the shape, volume, and structure of the prostate.

Transurethral resection of the prostate (TURP) is a standard surgical treatment for BPH. Non-conductive irrigation fluid is used during TURP to maintain good visibility of the operating field during resection of the prostate with monopolar cutting diathermy. The non-conductive irrigation fluid contains no electrolytes, and absorption of this hypotonic solution into the bloodstream can cause fluid overload and dilutional hyponatremia, resulting in adverse cardiovascular and central nervous system effects. Transurethral resection (TUR) syndrome is usually defined as a serum sodium level of < 125 mmol/l combined with clinical cardiovascular or neurological manifestations [2,3]. However, the clinical manifestations can also occur with a serum sodium

* Correspondence: ane052@poh.osaka-med.ac.jp
[1]Department of Anesthesiology, Osaka Medical College, 2-7 Daigaku-machi, Takatsuki, Osaka 569-8686, Japan
Full list of author information is available at the end of the article

level of > 125 mmol/l. Because of the multifactorial pathophysiology of TUR syndrome, few studies have used a clear and consistent definition of this condition. This study used the severity score for TUR syndrome proposed by Hahn, which is based on a checklist of central nervous system and cardiovascular abnormalities (Table 1) [4].

The theoretical risk factors for TUR syndrome include patent prostatic sinuses, high irrigation pressure, prolonged operation time, and use of hypotonic irrigation fluid [5]. It was reported that 77% of patients undergoing TURP had significant pre-existing medical conditions, and that resection time > 90 min, estimated prostate weight > 45 g, acute urinary retention, age > 80 years, and African descent were associated with increased morbidity [2,5]. This study aimed to determine the risk factors for development of the clinical manifestations of TUR syndrome, and to investigate whether these clinical manifestations could be predicted by preoperative estimation of prostate weight by ultrasonography.

## Methods

After obtaining approval from the Ethical Committee of Osaka Medical College (reference number: 898), patients at our institution were informed of this retrospective observational study on a bulletin board. We retrospectively reviewed the records of patients who underwent TURP under combined spinal and epidural anesthesia from April 2006 to March 2011. Spinal anesthesia was administered at L2/3, L3/4, or L4/5, and the epidural space was catheterized at L1/2 or L2/3. Intrathecal bupivacaine

hydrochloride (hyperbaric, 0.5%, 2.0–3.0 ml) was administered to achieve a T10 sensory level. Patients who underwent surgery under general anesthesia because spinal anesthesia failed were excluded from the study. If the sensory level was lower than T10, or the duration of surgery was > 90 min, 0.375% ropivacaine hydrochloride (3.0–5.0 ml) was administered via the epidural catheter. Postoperative analgesia was provided by continuous epidural infusion of 0.2% ropivacaine at 2–5 ml/h. All surgical procedures were performed using an electronic resectoscope with a monopolar view, by surgeons with the same qualifications and clinical experience. D-sorbitol 3% was used as the non-conductive irrigation fluid, with the bags positioned 90 cm above the operating table. Hemodynamic monitoring included non-invasive measurement of systolic and diastolic blood pressure every 2 min and continuous monitoring of the heart rate, electrocardiogram, and pulse oximetry. Patients with bleeding disorders, renal insufficiency, and contraindications to spinal anesthesia were excluded. All patients received intravenous infusion of lactated Ringer's solution before spinal anesthesia.

Clinical manifestations of TUR syndrome were scored using the checklist proposed by Hahn, which recorded central nervous system abnormalities (such as nausea, vomiting, restlessness, and coma) and intra- or postoperative cardiovascular abnormalities (Table 1) [4]. At least one neurological and one cardiovascular abnormality were required for patients to be included in the TUR syndrome group. For cardiovascular abnormalities, such as hypertension (systolic blood pressure > 30% above the baseline),

**Table 1 Severity score checklist**

| | Severity score | | |
|---|---|---|---|
| | 1 | 2 | 3 |
| Circulatory | | | |
| Chest pain | Duration < 5 min | Duration > 5 min | Repeated attacks |
| Bradycardia | HR decrease 10–20 bpm | HR decrease > 20 bpm | Repeated decreases |
| Hypertension | SAP up 10–20 mmHg | SAP up > 30 mmHg | Score (2) for 15 min |
| Hypotension | SAP down 30–50 mmHg | SAP down > 50 mmHg | Repeated drops > 50 mmHg |
| Poor urine output | Diuretics needed | Repeated use | Diuretics ineffective |
| Neurological | | | |
| Blurred vision | Duration < 10 min | Duration > 10 min | Transient blindness |
| Nausea | Duration < 5 min | Duration 5–120 min | Intense or > 120 min |
| Vomiting | Single instance | Repeatedly, < 60 min | Repeatedly, > 60 min |
| Uneasiness | Slight | Moderate | Intense |
| Confusion | Duration < 5 min | Duration 5–60 min | Duration > 60 min |
| Tiredness | Patient says so | Objectively exhausted | Exhausted for > 120 min |
| Consciousness | Mildly depressed | Somnolent < 60 min | Needs ventilator |
| Headache | Mild | Severe < 60 min | Severe > 60 min |

A checklist used to define and score the clinical manifestations of TUR syndrome [2].
HR, heart rate; SAP, systolic arterial pressure.

hypotension (systolic blood pressure < 80 mmHg), bradycardia, and arrhythmia, immediate treatment was administered to avoid further deterioration. For systolic blood pressure < 80 mmHg, 4 mg ephedrine hydrochloride was administered intravenously. The medical and nursing staff closely monitored patients during and after the procedure to detect and treat complications, and to evaluate the severity of clinical manifestations of TUR syndrome. All anesthetic charts included detailed records of patient status. Manifestations of TUR syndrome were differentiated from manifestations of a vasovagal reflex caused by filling of the bladder or by the epidural and spinal anesthesia.

Patients were divided into groups with and without clinical manifestations of TUR syndrome, and potential risk factors were compared between the two groups. Patient characteristics, dose of regional anesthetic, duration of surgery, resected prostate weight, intravenous infusion volume, blood transfusion volume, and whether the irrigation fluid was continuously drained through a suprapubic pigtail drainage catheter (C. R. Bard, Karlsruhe, Germany; Figure 1) [6] were recorded. Potential manifestations of TUR syndrome were treated to prevent further complications. Blood sampling was performed at the discretion of the anesthesiologist and surgeon. The anesthesiologist determined whether clinical abnormalities were caused by TUR syndrome or by the anesthesia or sedation.

The prostate size was estimated preoperatively by transrectal longitudinal ultrasonography with a real-time linear scanner and 5.0-MHz transducer (Hitachi Aloka Medical Ltd, Tokyo, Japan). The maximal length (A) and maximal width (B) of the prostate were measured. Assuming that the prostate is ellipsoid in shape in patients with BPH, the volume (V) was calculated according to the formula $V = \pi AB^2 / 6$. The prostate weight was assumed to be approximately equal to V as the specific gravity of prostatic tissue in patients with BPH is 1.05–1.06 $g/cm^3$ [7]. The hand-rolling method was used to measure the resected prostate weight after TURP [8].

The Mann–Whitney U test and unpaired t-test were used to compare potential risk factors for TUR syndrome, including age, prostate weight, and operating time [9], between patients with and without clinical manifestations of TUR syndrome. Spearman's rank correlation coefficient was used to evaluate the relationship between the preoperative estimated prostate weight and the resected prostate weight. Receiver operator characteristic curve analysis was performed to determine the predictive value and optimal cutoff point of preoperative estimated prostate weight for prediction of the development of clinical manifestations of TUR syndrome. A $p$ value of < 0.05 was considered statistically significant. All analyses were performed using GraphPad Prism version 5.0 for Mac (GraphPad Software, San Diego, CA, USA).

**Results**

A total of 167 patients were included in this study, of which 42 developed clinical manifestations of TUR syndrome (24.2%; 95% confidence interval, 18.5%–31.8%). The majority of initial cardiovascular abnormalities were either hypertension with reflex bradycardia, or sudden hypotension. There were no significant differences in preoperative characteristics between patients with and without clinical manifestations of TUR syndrome, except for the preoperative estimated prostate weight (Table 2). There were significant differences in the duration of surgery, resected prostate weight, intravenous infusion volume, blood transfusion volume, and continuous drainage of irrigation fluid via suprapubic cystostomy between patients with and without clinical manifestations of TUR syndrome (Table 3). The postoperative serum sodium level and hemoglobin concentration were significantly lower in patients with than without clinical manifestations of TUR syndrome. All patients who developed clinical manifestations of TUR syndrome had a severity score of ≥ 2 according to Hahn's checklist at the end of surgery (Table 1). Patients with a score of ≥ 3 required additional intravenous anesthetic agents such as propofol or midazolam. One patient developed severe hyponatremia and required tracheal intubation to manage his cardiovascular and neurological abnormalities. One patient without clinical manifestations of TUR syndrome developed postoperative esophageal hemorrhage from ruptured esophageal varices, which was judged to be unrelated to the TURP procedure. One patient without intraoperative manifestations of TUR syndrome developed postoperative

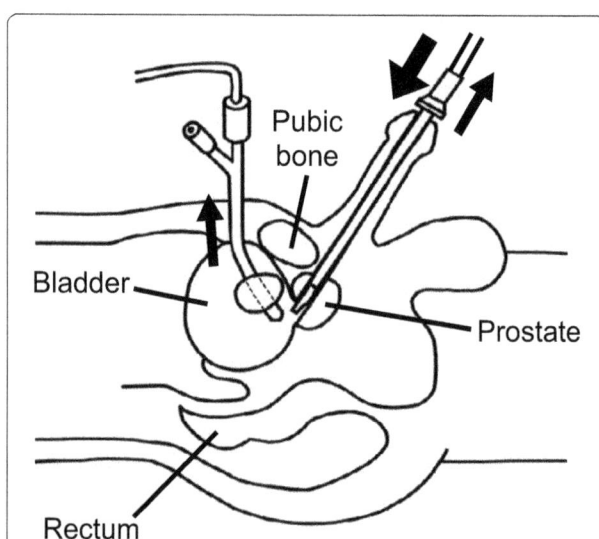

**Figure 1 Continuous drainage of irrigation fluid.** Irrigation fluid drains from the bladder via the resectoscope and the drainage catheter inserted through a suprapubic cystostomy. This image was reproduced from reference [6].

## Table 2 Patient characteristics

|  | Symptomatic (n = 42) | Asymptomatic (n = 125) | p value |
|---|---|---|---|
| Age, years | 72 ± 8 | 70 ± 7 | 0.202 |
| Height, cm | 164.6 ± 6.1 | 164.6 ± 5.8 | 0.989 |
| Body weight, kg | 63.2 ± 10.6 | 63.0 ± 9.2 | 0.925 |
| Diabetes mellitus | 2 (4.8%) | 9 (7.2%) | 0.732 |
| Hypertension | 3 (7.1) | 9 (7.2%) | 1.000 |
| Arrhythmia | 0 (0.0%) | 1 (0.8%) | 1.000 |
| Preoperative blood data |  |  |  |
| Creatinine, mg/dl | 0.9 ± 0.2 | 0.9 ± 0.2 | 0.718 |
| BUN, mg/dl | 15.7 ± 5.9 | 15.2 ± 4.0 | 0.912 |
| Sodium, mmol/l | 140.5 ± 2.2 | 140.5 ± 2.4 | 0.942 |
| Hemoglobin, g/dl | 13.6 ± 1.6 | 14.1 ± 1.5 | 0.321 |
| Hematocrit,% | 39.5 ± 4.5 | 40.7 ± 4.9 | 0.218 |
| Estimated prostate weight, g | 99.0 ± 45.6 | 64.6 ± 26.4 | < 0.001 |

Data are expressed as mean ± SD or number (%). Symptomatic = the presence of central nervous system abnormalities such as nausea, vomiting, restlessness, pain, confusion, and coma together with intra- or postoperative cardiovascular abnormalities; BUN = blood urea nitrogen.

## Table 3 Intraoperative and postoperative data

| Parameter | Symptomatic (n = 42) | Asymptomatic (n = 125) | p value |
|---|---|---|---|
| Continuous drainage of irrigation fluid | 23 (54.8%) | 17 (13.6%) | < 0.001 |
| Intrathecal 0.5% bupivacaine, ml | 2.4 ± 0.4 | 2.5 ± 0.5 | 0.869 |
| Resected prostate weight, g | 52.3 ± 29.7 | 29.8 ± 18.7 | < 0.001 |
| Operation time, min | 101 ± 34 | 71 ± 26 | < 0.001 |
| Operation time > 90 min | 25 (59.5%) | 32 (25.6%) | < 0.001 |
| Total infusion volume, ml | 903 ± 598 | 578 ± 284 | 0.002 |
| Symptoms | 42 (100.0%) | - | NA |
| Restlessness | 24 (57.1%) | - | NA |
| Vomiting | 14 (33.3%) | - | NA |
| Nausea | 22 (52.3%) | - | NA |
| Pain | 17 (40.5%) | - | NA |
| Confusion | 11 (26.2%) | - | NA |
| Blood transfusion | 26 (61.9%) | 24 (19.2%) | < 0.001 |
| Diuretics | 6 (14.3%) | 1 (0.8%) | 0.003 |
| Saline infusion | 0 (0.0%) | 1 (0.8%) | 0.001 |
| Postoperative blood data |  |  |  |
| Creatinine, mg/dl | 0.9 ± 0.3 | 0.9 ± 0.2 | 0.943 |
| BUN, mg/dl | 12.4 ± 5.0 | 12.8 ± 4.1 | 0.441 |
| Sodium, mmol/l | 133.4 ± 7.9 | 138.0 ± 3.8 | < 0.001 |
| Hemoglobin, g/dl | 11.0 ± 1.8 | 12.8 ± 1.6 | < 0.001 |
| Hematocrit,% | 32.0 ± 5.6 | 37.4 ± 4.6 | < 0.001 |

Data are expressed as mean ± SD or number (%). Symptomatic = the presence of central nervous system abnormalities such as nausea, vomiting, restlessness, pain, confusion, and coma together with circulatory intra- or postoperative cardiovascular abnormalities; BUN = blood urea nitrogen.

nausea and vomiting. All blood transfusions were autologous, except in one of the patients who developed clinical manifestations of TUR syndrome who received an allogeneic transfusion.

The preoperative estimated prostate weight was correlated with the resected prostate weight (Spearman's correlation coefficient, 0.749; Figure 2). Receiver operator characteristic curve analysis showed that the optimal cutoff value of estimated prostate weight for the prediction of clinical manifestations of TUR syndrome was 75 g (sensitivity, 0.70; specificity, 0.69; area under the curve, 0.73; Figure 3).

## Discussion

The incidence of TUR syndrome was higher in our cohort than in previous studies, which reported rates from 0.5% to 10.5% [2,3,7]. This can be explained by the varying definitions of TUR syndrome used. Many previous studies defined TUR syndrome as a serum sodium level of ≤125 mmol/l after TURP with two additional abnormalities such as nausea, vomiting, bradycardia, hypotension, chest pain, mental confusion, anxiety, paresthesia, or visual impairment [3]. The proportion of patients in our study that met this definition based on the sodium level was 13.2%. This study focused on the clinical manifestations of TUR syndrome, regardless of the serum sodium level. The clinical manifestations included central nervous system abnormalities such as nausea, vomiting, restlessness, and coma, and intra- and postoperative cardiovascular abnormalities, according to the checklist proposed by Hahn [4]. Some of our patients with neurological and cardiovascular manifestations of

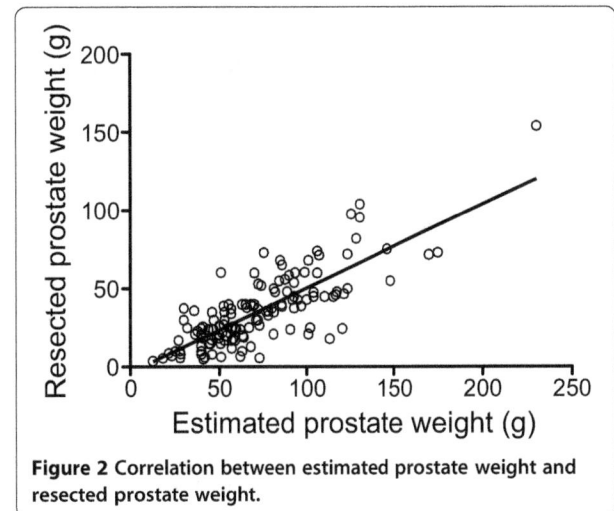

**Figure 2** Correlation between estimated prostate weight and resected prostate weight.

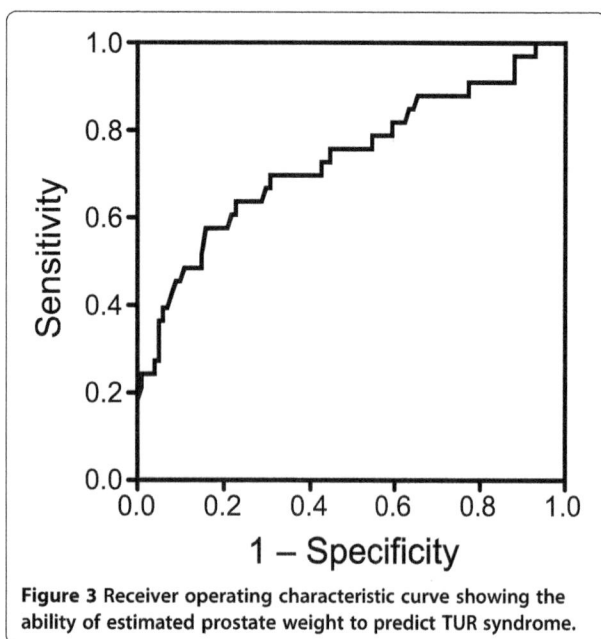

**Figure 3** Receiver operating characteristic curve showing the ability of estimated prostate weight to predict TUR syndrome.

TUR syndrome did not have a serum sodium level of < 125 mmol/l. Patients with a severity score of 1 were treated to avoid further deterioration, regardless of the serum sodium level.

Our results show an optimal cutoff value for estimated prostate weight of 75 g to predict the development of clinical manifestations of TUR syndrome, which is heavier than previously suggested weights. Previous studies reported that the most significant risk factors for TUR syndrome were an operation time of > 90 min, a heavier prostate weight such as > 45 g, acute urinary retention, and age > 80 years [2]. These factors increase the risk of TUR syndrome because of the larger quantity of irrigation fluid absorbed. Technical advances and resection speeds of 0.5–0.9 g/min have not resulted in a significant reduction in the incidence of TUR syndrome [10]. This study was conducted in our specialized college hospital that is associated with satellite hospitals, and the patients who undergo TURP at our hospital tend to have relatively large prostate glands, resulting in longer operation times and a higher incidence of TUR syndrome. Some centers may perform open prostatectomy in patients with large prostate glands, but TURP is the standard procedure for such cases in Japan.

This is the first study to investigate the relationship between prostate weight and the development of clinical manifestations of TUR, regardless of serum sodium levels. Preoperative ultrasonography is commonly used to diagnose BPH and to estimate prostate weight. In this study, there was a strong correlation between the preoperative estimated prostate weight on ultrasonography and the resected prostate weight, indicating that preoperative

estimation of prostate weight by ultrasonography may be useful for predicting the risk of TUR syndrome. The optimal cutoff value of estimated prostate weight to predict the development of clinical manifestations of TUR syndrome was 75 g. However, there is also a risk of TUR syndrome when resecting prostates of lower weights. Akata et al. reported that changes in the serum sodium level during TURP correlated with incision of the capsular veins and prostatic sinuses, but not with operation time [11]. It is important to carefully monitor patients for the development of TUR syndrome, especially patients with larger prostates, and we recommend measurement of the serum sodium level during and after surgery.

In this study, continuous drainage of irrigation fluid through a suprapubic cystostomy was found to be a risk factor for TUR syndrome. Our previous study also found this to be an important risk factor for TUR syndrome in older patients [12]. Such continuous drainage of irrigation fluid facilitates the removal of debris, blood, and clots from the operating field. Blood clots and debris may obstruct the drainage catheter, thereby raising the fluid pressure and increasing the volume absorbed [13]. Drainage catheters with small diameters may be less effective than catheters with larger diameters. A number of patients in this study were noted to have abdominal swelling caused by leakage of irrigation fluid through the drainage site into the extraperitoneal space and abdominal cavity. When this occurs, extracellular electrolytes diffuse into the accumulated irrigation fluid [14], resulting in dilutional hyponatremia and increasing the risk of TUR syndrome. The hyponatremia is most pronounced at 2–4 h after surgery, but may go undetected until the next day [15].

Patients with a preoperative prostate weight of > 75 g should receive additional treatment to reduce the risk of TUR syndrome, such as blood transfusion, intravenous diuretics, and saline infusion. It is generally recommended that surgery should be performed under regional anesthesia when there is an increased risk of TUR syndrome, as this enables early detection of gross changes in mental status, but this is not universally accepted [16]. TUR syndrome can have many causes and the clinical manifestations may be vague, making early detection difficult. It is therefore important to identify the risk factors for TUR syndrome to increase vigilance among medical and nursing staff and enable early intervention.

This study is limited by its retrospective, observational design. However, the patient details and timing of blood tests were carefully evaluated using data recorded in the comprehensive preoperative and anesthetic records to ensure accuracy. A further prospective study with a larger study population should be conducted to verify our findings.

## Conclusions

In this study, preoperative estimation of prostate weight by ultrasonography could predict the development of clinical manifestations of TUR syndrome. When the preoperative estimated prostate weight is > 75 g, patients should be monitored closely and appropriate intervention should be planned.

### Competing interests

The authors declare that they have no competing interests.

### Authors' contributions

AF participated in the design and coordination of the study and helped to draft the manuscript. JN made substantial contributions to the conception and design of the study and the acquisition of data, and drafted the manuscript and tables. TS performed the statistical analyses and revised the manuscript critically for important intellectual content. TI made substantial contributions to the conception of the study and helped to correct the manuscript. TM made substantial contributions to the conception of the study and helped to draft the manuscript. All authors read and approved the final manuscript.

### Author details

[1]Department of Anesthesiology, Osaka Medical College, 2-7 Daigaku-machi, Takatsuki, Osaka 569-8686, Japan. [2]Department of Urology, Osaka Medical College, 2-7 Daigaku-machi, Takatsuki, Osaka 569-8686, Japan.

### References

1. Bhansali M, Patankar S, Dobhada S, Khaladkar S: **Management of large (>60 g) prostate gland: plasma kinetic superpulse (bipolar) versus conventional (monopolar) transurethral resection of the prostate.** *J Endourol* 2009, **23**:141–145.
2. Mebust WK, Holtgrewe HL, Cockett AT, Peters PC: **Transurethral prostatectomy: immediate and postoperative complications. A cooperative study of 13 participating institutions evaluating 3,885 patients.** *J Urol* 2002, **167**:999–1003.
3. Michielsen DP, Debacker T, De Boe V, Van Lersberghe C, Kaufman L, Braekman JG, Amy JJ, Keuppens FL: **Bipolar transurethral resection in saline–an alternative surgical treatment for bladder outlet obstruction?** *J Urol* 2007, **178**:2035–2039.
4. Hahn RG: **Fluid absorption in endoscopic surgery.** *Br J Anaesth* 2006, **96**:8–20.
5. Gravenstein D: **Transurethral resection of the prostate (TURP) syndrome: a review of the pathophysiology and management.** *Anesth Analg* 1997, **84**:438–446.
6. Nakahira J, Sawai T, Fujiwara A, Minami T: **Transurethral resection syndrome in elderly patients: a retrospective observational study.** *BMC Anesthesiology* 2014, **14**:30.
7. Watanabe H, Igari D, Tanahashi Y, Harada K, Saito M: **Measurements of size and weight of prostate by means of transrectal ultrasonotomography.** *Tohoku J Exp Med* 1974, **114**:277–285.
8. Naito Y, Miyamoto K, Maruyama K: **Preoperative volumetry of the prostate by transabdominal ultrasonography.** *Hinyokika Kiyo* 1987, **33**:1812–1817.
9. Hawary A, Mukhtar K, Sinclair A, Pearce I: **Transurethral resection of the prostate syndrome: almost gone but not forgotten.** *J Endourol* 2009, **23**:2013–2020.
10. Rassweiler J, Teber D, Kuntz R, Hofmann R: **Complications of transurethral resection of the prostate (TURP)–incidence, management, and prevention.** *Eur Urol* 2006, **50**:969–979.
11. Akata T, Yoshimura H, Matsumae Y, Shiokawa H, Fukumoto T, Kandabashi T, Yamaji T, Takahashi S: **Changes in serum Na + and blood hemoglobin levels during three types of transurethral procedures for the treatment of benign prostatic hypertrophy.** *Masui* 2004, **53**:638–644.
12. Nakahira J, Sawai T, Fujiwara A, Minami T: **Transurethral resection syndrome in elderly patients: a retrospective observational study.** *BMC Anesthesiol* 2014, **14**:30.
13. Hahn RG: **Intravesical pressure during irrigating fluid absorption in transurethral resection of the prostate.** *Scand J Urol Nephrol* 2000, **34**:102–108.
14. Olsson J, Hahn RG: **Simulated intraperitoneal absorption of irrigating fluid.** *Acta Obstet Gynecol Scand* 1995, **74**:707–713.
15. Yende S, Wunderink R: **An 87-year-old man with hypotension and confusion after cystoscopy.** *Chest* 1999, **115**:1449–1451.
16. Reeves MDS, Myles PS: **Does anaesthetic technique affect the outcome after transurethral resection of the prostate?** *BJU Int* 1999, **84**:982–986.

# 17

# How do stone attenuation and skin-to-stone distance in computed tomography influence the performance of shock wave lithotripsy in ureteral stone disease?

Gautier Müllhaupt[*], Daniel S. Engeler, Hans-Peter Schmid and Dominik Abt

**Abstract**

**Background:** Shock wave lithotripsy (SWL) is a noninvasive, safe, and efficient treatment option for ureteral stones. Depending on stone location and size, the overall stone-free rate (SFR) varies significantly. Failure of stone disintegration results in unnecessary exposure to shock waves and radiation and requires alternative treatment procedures, which increases medical costs. It is therefore important to identify predictors of treatment success or failure in patients who are potential candidates for SWL before treatment. Nowadays, noncontrast computed tomography (NCCT) provides reliable information on stone location, size, number, and total stone burden. The impact of additional information provided by NCCT, such as skin-to-stone distance (SSD) and mean attenuation value (MAV), on stone fragmentation in ureteral stone disease has hardly been investigated separately so far. Thus, the objective of this study was to assess the influence of stone attenuation, SSD and body mass index (BMI) on the outcome of SWL in ureteral stones.

**Methods:** We reviewed the medical records of 104 patients (80 men, 24 women) with ureteral stone disease treated consecutively at our institution with SWL between 2010 and 2013. MAV in Hounsfield Units (HU) and SSD were determined by analyzing noncontrast computed tomography images. Outcome of SWL was defined as successful (visible stone fragmentation on kidney, ureter, and bladder film (KUB)) or failed (absent fragmentation on KUB).

**Results:** Overall success of SWL was 50 % (52 patients). Median stone attenuation was 956.9 HU (range 495–1210.8) in the group with successful disintegration and 944.6 (range 237–1302) in the patients who had absent or insufficient fragmentation. Median SSD was 125 mm (range 81–165 mm) in the group treated successfully and 141 mm (range 108–172 mm) in the patients with treatment failure. Unlike MAV ($p = 0.37$), SSD ($p < 0.001$) and BMI ($p = 0.008$) significantly correlated with treatment outcome.

**Conclusion:** The choice of treatment for ureteral stones should be based on stone location and size as considered in the AUA and EAU guidelines on urinary stone disease. In ambiguous cases, SSD and BMI can be used to assist in the decision. In this study, MAV showed no correlation with fragmentation rate of SWL.

**Keywords:** Ureteral stones, Treatment outcome, Shock wave lithotripsy, Hounsfield Units, Skin-to-stone distance

* Correspondence: gautier.muellhaupt@kssg.ch
Department of Urology, Cantonal Hospital St. Gallen, Rorschacherstrasse 95,
9007 St. Gallen, Switzerland

## Background

Shock wave lithotripsy (SWL) is a noninvasive, safe, and efficient treatment option for ureteral stones. Depending on stone location and size, the overall stone-free rate (SFR) varies significantly, leading to corresponding recommendations in the guidelines of the American Urological Association and the European Association of Urology: For proximal ureteral stones <10 mm, SWL has a higher SFR than ureterorenoscopy (URS), while URS seems to be superior for stones >10 mm. For mid-ureteral stones, URS appears to be superior, with statistical limitations, because fewer patients have been investigated. For distal stones >10 mm, URS is the treatment of choice, while SWL and URS are options for small stones [1, 2]. Failure of stone disintegration results in unnecessary exposure to shock waves and radiation, further patient suffering, and requires alternative treatment procedures, which increases medical costs [3]. It is therefore important to identify predictors of treatment success or failure in patients who are potential candidates for SWL before treatment.

Radiographic assessment of the stone is required to decide on the best treatment. Nowadays, noncontrast computed tomography (NCCT) provides reliable information on stone location, size, number, and total stone burden, and is therefore recommended as the standard diagnostic tool in urinary stone disease [3, 4]. Moreover, several studies have shown an impact of mean attenuation value (MAV) on treatment success of SWL in kidney stones, leading to corresponding guideline recommendations [1, 2]. Despite the widespread use of NCCT, however, the impact of additional information provided by NCCT, such as skin-to-stone distance (SSD) and MAV, on stone fragmentation in ureteral stone disease has hardly been investigated separately so far [5–8]. Moreover, as limiting factors, three of the four studies reported on so far covered only one SWL session regardless of whether disintegration occurred or not, and treatment success was analyzed in all four studies at the earliest 2 weeks after SWL. The study by Ng et al. also included only proximal ureteral stones, and no real-time fluoroscopic screening was performed during treatment [7].

Thus, the objective of this study was to determine how additional information provided by NCCT and patient's physical constitution might influence fragmentation rate of SWL in ureteral stone disease.

Table 1 shows a summary of the literature.

## Methods

One hundred four patients treated consecutively with SWL for distal and proximal ureteral stones in our department between January 2010 and December 2013 were included in this retrospective study. Data analysis was conducted according to the declaration of Helsinki and approved by the Local Ethics Committee of St. Gallen (EKSG 15/055). Written informed consent for data analysis was obtained. NCCT was performed before treatment using a multidetector row helical CT scanner (Siemens, Definition Flash, Forchheim, Germany) with 30–460 mA, 120 kV and 2 mm collimation in every patient. As suggested in a study by Eisner et al. [9], stone size and Hounsfield Unit (HU) measurements were obtained in a standard bone window (window width-1,120 and window level-300). The image with the largest stone diameter was used to define maximum stone size. MAV was obtained by measuring the mean HU of defined regions of interest just smaller than the stone in magnified images without including adjacent soft tissue on each slice of the axial planes (Fig. 1). SSD was calculated as described by El Nahas et al. [3] and the distances at 0°, 45° and 90° were measured using radiographic calipers (Fig. 2). The average was calculated as the SSD. The measurements were performed analogous in prone position when targeting pelvic stones. The SSD was also measured and evaluated at an angle of 90° separately, as this seems to be the most important angle in the setting of the SLX-F2 (Storz Medical, Tägerwilen, Switzerland) which was used to perform SWL under sedoanalgesia.

If tolerated by the patient, up to 4,000 shocks (60–90/min) with an energy level of up to 8 according to the manufacturer's scale were delivered during each SWL session. The energy level 8 corresponded to 16.4 kV with the precise focus and 12.8 kV with the extended focus. In patients with pain resistant to analgesic treatment, the energy and number of shocks were reduced according to the patient's tolerance. Stones were targeted and fragmentation was monitored by biplanar fluoroscopy at regular intervals during treatment.

Patients were further evaluated by kidney, ureter, and bladder (KUB) film, renal ultrasound, and sieving of urine to assess fragmentation, the presence of renal dilatation and expulsion of ureteral stones the day after the respective session. In cases of missing or inadequate disintegration in KUB, SWL was repeated once or twice at intervals of 1 day. The clinical outcome was defined as successful (visible stone fragmentation on KUB) or failed (absent fragmentation on KUB) immediately after the last SWL session.

The correlation with and influence of a range of baseline characteristics on treatment outcome of SWL was examined: patient's age, gender, weight, and BMI; stone location and volume, MAV, SSD; use of alpha blockers; presence of ureteral stents. Both univariate (chi-square or Mann–Whitney U-tests for dichotomous or continuous variables) and multivariate (binary logistic regression) analyses were performed to define significant factors. ROC curves were used for the determination of the best cut-off values. All tests were two-sided and a

**Table 1** Review of the literature

| References | Year | Stone location | n All/Renal/Ureteral | Prediction of successful disintegration/treatment | | | Cut off MAV/SSD/BMI |
|---|---|---|---|---|---|---|---|
| | | | | Mean attenuation value (MAV) All/Renal/Ureter | SSD All/Renal/Ureter | BMI All/Renal/Ureter | |
| Joseph et al. [14] | 2002 | Renal | 30/30/- | Yes/Yes/- | -/-/- | No/No/- | Renal: 950 HU/-/- |
| Pareek et al. [6] | 2003 | Renal and ureteral | 50/20/30 | Yes/Yes/Yes | -/-/- | No/-/- | Ureteral: 900 HU/-/- |
| Wang et al. [15] | 2005 | Renal | 80/80/- | Yes/Yes/- | -/-/- | -/-/- | Renal: 900HU/-/- |
| Gupta et al. [16] | 2005 | Renal and proximal ureter | 108/89/19 | Yes/-/- | -/-/- | -/-/- | All: 750 HU/-/- |
| Yoshida et al. [17] | 2006 | Renal and proximal ureter | 56/25/31 | Yes/-/- | -/-/- | -/-/- | -/-/- |
| El Nahas et al. [3] | 2007 | Renal | 120/120/- | Yes/Yes/- | Yes/Yes/- | Yes/Yes/- | Renal: 1000HU/-/- |
| Perks et al. [11] | 2008 | Renal | 111/111/- | Yes/Yes/- | Yes/Yes/- | No/No/- | Renal: 900HU/9 cm/- |
| Ng et al. [7] | 2009 | Proximal ureter | 94/-/94 | Yes/-/Yes | Yes/-/Yes | No/-/No | Renal:593 HU/9.2 cm/- |
| Patel et al. [10] | 2009 | Renal | 83/83/- | No/No/- | Yes/Yes/- | -/-/- | Renal: -/10 cm/- |
| Wiesenthal et al. [5] | 2010 | Renal and ureteral | 422/218/204 | Yes/Yes/Yes | Yes/Yes/Yes | Yes/No/Yes | All: 900 HU/ 11 cm/- |
| Park et al. [12] | 2010 | Renal | 115/115/- | Yes/Yes/- | No/-/- | -/-/- | Renal: 863 HU/-/- |
| Shah et al. [18] | 2010 | Renal and proximal ureter | 99/71/28 | Yes/-/- | -/-/- | -/-/- | -/-/- |
| Tanaka et al. [13] | 2013 | Renal and ureteral | 75/27/48 | Yes/-/- | No/-/- | No/-/- | All: 780 HU/-/- |
| Celik et al. [8] | 2015 | Renal and ureteral | 254/123/131 | Yes/Yes/Yes | -/Yes/ | -/Yes/- | Renal: 750 HU/-/- |
| Nakasato et al. [19] | 2015 | Renal and ureteral | 260/92/168 | Yes/-/- | No/-/- | -/-/- | All: 815 HU/-/- |

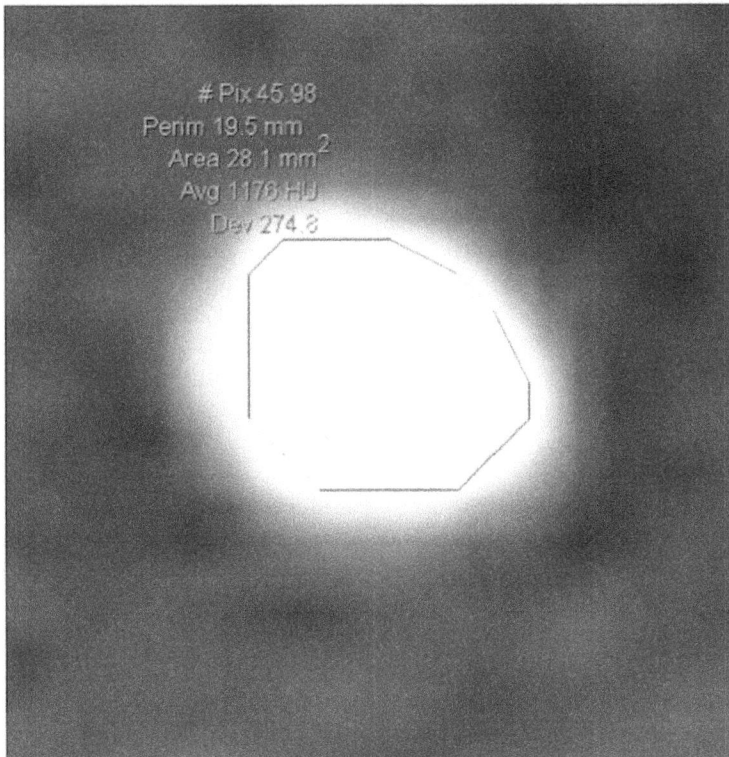

**Fig. 1** Defined regions of interest just smaller than the stone without including adjacent soft tissue

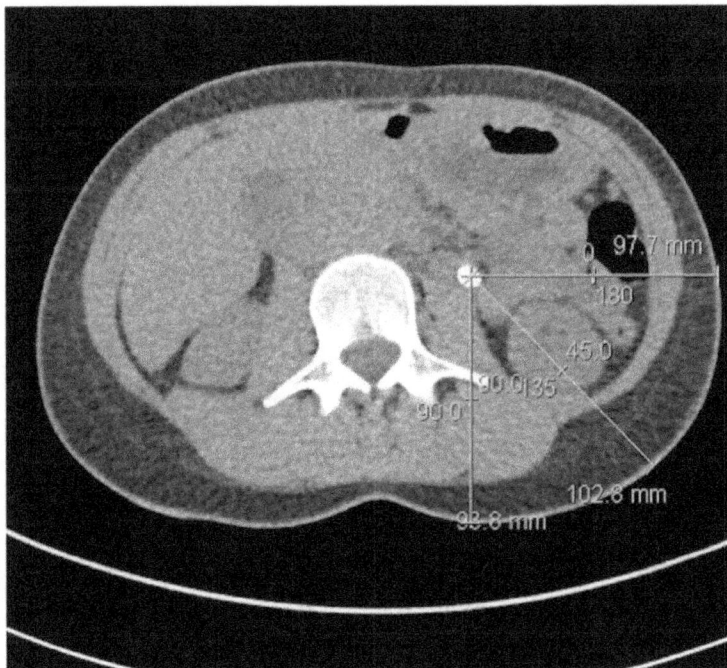

**Fig. 2** Skin-to-stone distance (SSD) was calculated by the measuring distances from Stone-to-skin at 0°, 45°, and 90° using radiographic calipers

p-value of <0.05 was necessary to reject the null-hypothesis. Statistical analyses were performed using IBM SPSS Statistics Version 22 (IBM Corp., New York, U.S.A.).

## Results

A total of 104 consecutive patients were included (24 women, 80 men), median age was 45.5 years (range 19–80 years). Median largest diameter of stones was 6 mm (range 2–15 mm) and median MAV 949.3 HU (range 237–1302 HU).

The stones were located in the proximal ureter in 73 (70.2 %) patients and the distal ureter in 31 (29.8 %). Median BMI was 26.2 (range 17.4–37.0), median SSD (0°/45°/90°) 131.5 mm (range 81–172 mm) and median SSD (90°) 119 mm (range 76–161 mm).

Stone fragmentation was visible in 52 (50 %) patients and was not visible in the remaining patients, of whom 49 (94.2 %) needed further treatment: 43 (82.7 %) by URS, 4 (7.7 %) by ureteral stent insertion, and 2 (3.8 %) by further cycles of SWL. The three patients who needed no further treatment showed spontaneous stone passage during the treatment with SWL without stone disintegration.

Of the 52 patients who showed good stone fragmentation, 13 (25 %) needed further treatment by URS (8 patients, 15.4 %,), ureteral stent insertion (1 patient, 1.9 %) or further cycles of SWL (4 patients, 7.7 %) because of impacted fragments or distal steinstrasse.

Median MAV was 956.9 HU (range 495–1210.8 HU) in patients with good stone fragmentation and was 944.6 HU (range 237–1302 HU) in patients showing no stone fragmentation and requiring further treatment. In univariate analysis, MAV showed no correlation with stone fragmentation ($p = 0.373$).

Median BMI, SSD (0°/45°/90°) and SSD (90°) in patients with good stone fragmentation were 25.5 (range 17.4–35.0), 125 mm (range 81–165 mm) and 114.5 mm (range 76–159 mm). In patients without stone fragmentation, median BMI, SSD (0°/45°/90°) and SSD (90°) were 27.1 (range 21.1–37.0), 141 mm (range 108–172 mm) and 130 (range 85–161). In univariate analysis, BMI ($p = 0.008$), SSD (0°/45°/90°) ($p < 0.001$) and SSD (90°) ($p < 0.001$) significantly correlated with stone fragmentation.

In addition, maximum energy delivered showed a significant correlation with disintegration outcome ($p = 0.015$). Median energy level was 6 (range 4–8) in patients with good stone fragmentation and 6.4 (range 5–8) in patients with no stone fragmentation.

The results of univariate analyses are summarized in Table 2.

According to multivariate analyses, SSD (90°) was a significant predictor for disintegration failure (regression coefficient: −0.046, standard error: 0.013, odds ratio 0.955, 95 % confidence interval: 0.930–0.980, p-value < 0.001). Moreover, maximum delivered energy tended to be lower in patients with successful disintegration than

**Table 2** Results of univariate analysis

| Characteristic | Successful disintegration | Unsuccessful disintegration | p-value |
|---|---|---|---|
| Number of patients (%) | 52 (50 %) | 52 (50 %) | - |
| Age, years (median, range) | 43.5 (19–80) | 47.5 (22–77) | 0.136 |
| Gender, M/F (N/%) | 35 (67.3 %)/17 (32.7 %) | 45 (86.5 %)/7 (13.5 %) | 0.035 |
| Weight, kg (median, range) | 73 (49–116) | 85 (58–120) | <0.001 |
| BMI, kg/m$^2$ (median, range) | 25.5 (17.4–35.0) | 27.1 (21.6–37.0) | 0.008 |
| Skin-to-stone distance, mm, mean of 0°, 45° and 90° (median, range) | 125 (81–165) | 141 (108–172) | <0.001 |
| Skin-to-stone distance, mm, 90° (median, range) | 114.5 (76–159) | 130 (85–161) | <0.001 |
| Mean attenuation value, HU (median, range) | 956.9 (495–1210.8) | 944.6 (237–1302) | 0.373 |
| Stone size, mm (median, range) | 7 (3–15) | 6 (2–12) | 0.071 |
| Location, proximal/distal (N, %) | 36 (69.2 %)/16 (30.8 %) | 37 (71.2 %)/15 (28.8 %) | 1.000 |
| SWL cycles (median, range) | 2 (1–3) | 2 (1–3) | 0.786 |
| Number of shockwaves (median, range) | 8000 (1000–12000) | 8000 (3000–14000) | 0.583 |
| Power/Intensity Level (median, range) | 6 (4–8) | 6.4 (5–8) | 0.015 |
| Ureteral stent in place (N, %) | 15 (28.8 %) | 13 (25 %) | 0.825 |
| Alpha-blocker (N, %) | 42 (80.8 %) | 38 (73.1 %) | 0.486 |
| Secondary procedures | | | |
| URS (N, %) | 8 (15.4 %) | 43 (82.7 %) | - |
| Ureteral stent (N, %) | 1 (1.9 %) | 4 (7.7 %) | - |
| SWL (N, %) | 4 (7.7 %) | 2 (3.8 %) | - |

in patients with disintegration failure without reaching statistical significance (regression coefficient: –0.528, standard error: 0.272, odds ratio 0.590, 95 % confidence interval: 0.346–1.004, p-value < 0.052). Weight and BMI of the patient were not included in the multivariate analysis because of multicollinearity with SSD.

The ROC curves for different parameters were analyzed to find the optimum cut-off values to predict disintegration failure (Fig. 3). The optimum cut-off point for SSD (90°) would be >11.9 cm (sensitivity 65.4 %, specificity 65.3 %), for patient weight >82.5 kg (sensitivity 65.4 %, specificity 71.4 %), and for BMI >25.9 kg/m$^2$ (sensitivity 69.2 %, specifity 55.1 %).

## Discussion

The results of this study show that SSD and BMI are significant predictors of the outcome of SWL. As described earlier by Patel et al. for kidney stones [10], we found no significant association between MAV and fragmentation rate of SWL for ureteral stones.

The use of NCCT for diagnosis of ureteral stones is well established and a common practice worldwide [7]. The method of measuring SSD in NCCT has been well described in the literature and there are only marginal differences between studies with regard to the method [3, 5–7, 10–13].

The method for determining MAV has been described inconsistently, however. For example, Joseph et al. [14] used a calculous pixel map of 100 attenuation values in a 10 x 10 matrix in unenhanced axial NCCT section, while Wiesenthal et al. [5] measured attenuation values using bone windows on the magnified, axial image of the stone in the maximum diameter where the elliptical region of interest incorporated the largest cross-sectional area of stone without including adjacent soft tissue. In our study, we determined MAV by measuring the mean HU of defined regions of interest just smaller than the stone in magnified images without including adjacent soft tissue on each slice of the axial planes (Fig. 1) with a standard bone window (window width-1,120 and window level-300) as suggested in the study by Eisner et al. [9]. We believe that this is the most accurate method of determining MAV. The inconsistent methods used in the literature might also explain the differing results that have been reported, so far (Table 2). In our opinion, image magnification for MAV measurement is very important because accurate stone margins can be identified using only adequately magnified images (Fig. 1). Thus, inclusion of adjacent soft tissue into measurement can be avoided. In addition, we measured all available slices of stones in axial planes to calculate MAV, which might prevent assumption of too high or low MAVs, as stones often consist of different components. The method of measuring MAV should be standardized to allow comparison of different datasets.

Concerning MAV, cut-off values between 750 and 1000 HU for renal calculi and between 750 and 900 HU in studies examining mixed ureteral and renal stones have

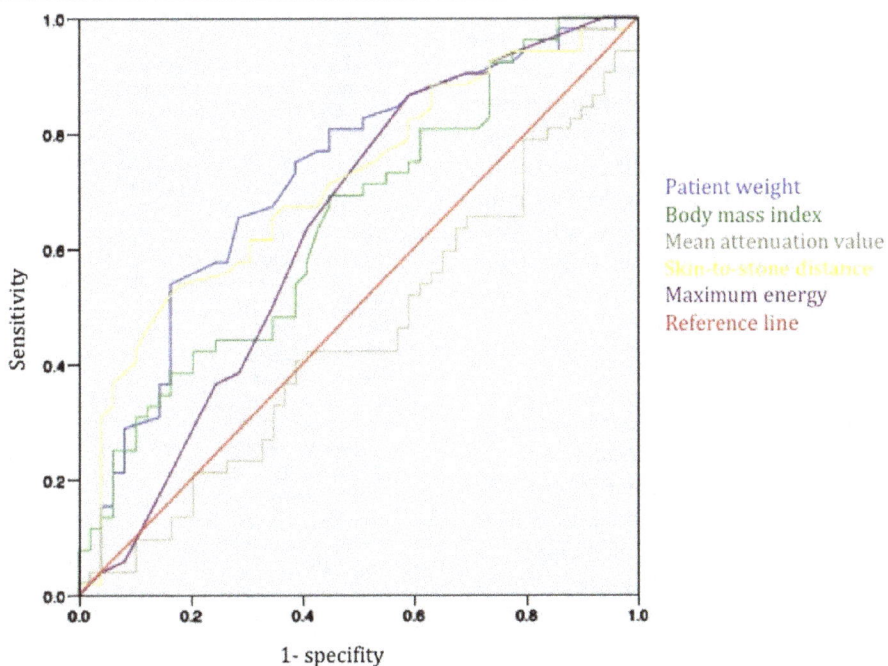

**Fig. 3** ROC curves

been suggested as predictors of SWL failure (Table 2). However, separate examination of cut-off values for ureteral stones has only been performed in two studies: Pareek et al. [6] suggested 900 HU as the cut-off value in their study of 30 ureteral stones, and Ng et al. [7] defined a very different threshold of 593 HU as a potential predictor of treatment success in a study in 94 patients with upper ureteral stones. Our study failed to show an association between MAV and the disintegration of ureteral stones using SWL.

SSD has been shown to be a significant predictor of the outcome of SWL in different studies on renal stones. The findings for BMI, however, have been inconsistent as illustrated in Table 2.

Only two studies have analyzed SSD as a predictor of SWL treatment success in ureteral stones separately [5, 7] and both showed that SSD was a significant predictor. In this context, Ng et al. [7] suggested an SSD cut-off of 9.2 cm as a predictor for SWL failure, but they studied only upper ureteral stones.

In our study, SSD (90°) emerged as an even stronger predictor of treatment success or failure than mean SSD, with a cut-off value of 11.9 cm for SWL failure, which might be because we had patients in the almost straight supine or prone position for treatment with SLX-F2.

Results for BMI as a predictor of stone disintegration with SWL are also contradictory [5, 7]. In our study, BMI and patient weight were significant predictors of SWL outcome with cut-off values of 25.9 kg/m$^2$ and 82.5 kg for SWL failure. Factors such as differences in body fat distribution between men and women, and age and race also have to be taken into consideration.

Possible limitations of our study are the retrospective design and assessment of disintegration outcome by KUB film and not by NCCT. Moreover, fragmentation rate instead of SFR was chosen to define treatment success or failure. We believed that this might represent the stone's response to SWL better, because SFR is influenced by other factors that might interfere with stone passage (e.g., ureteral diameter). On the other hand, stone disintegration on KUB does not inevitably lead to a successfully completed treatment.

## Conclusions

The choice of treatment for ureteral stones should be based on stone location and size as considered in the AUA and EAU guidelines on urinary stone disease. Patient preference also has to be taken into consideration. In ambiguous cases, SSD and BMI – in contrast to MAV - can be easily used for additional guidance. In this way, patients with a high risk of disintegration failure could be educated more precisely, unnecessary exposure to shock waves and radiation could be avoided and medical costs could be reduced.

## Abbrevations

SSD: Skin-to-stone distance; MAV: Mean attenuation value; HU: Hounsfield Units; SWL: Shock wave lithotripsy; BMI: Body mass index; AUA: American Urological Association; EAU: European Association of Urology; SFR: Stone-free rate; URS: Ureterorenoscopy; NCCT: Noncontrast computed tomography; CT: Computed tomography; kV: Kilovolt; KUB: Kidney, ureter, and bladder film; ROC: Receiver operating characteristic.

## Competing interests

The authors declare that they have no competing interests.

## Authors' contributions

GM: Conception, study design, acquisition of data, analysis and interpretation of data, manuscript drafting. DE: Analysis and interpretation of data, statistics, proofreading. HPS: Analysis and interpretation of data, proofreading. DA: Conception, study design, analysis and interpretation of data, proofreading. All authors read and approved the final manuscript.

## Acknowledgments

The authors thank Alistair Reeves for editing the manuscript. No funding has been obtained for this study.

## References

1.  Preminger GM, Tiselius HG, Assimos DG, Alken P, Buck C, Gallucci M, et al. 2007 Guideline for the management of ureteral calculi. J Urol. 2007;178:2418.
2.  Preminger GM, Tiselius HG, Assimos DG, Alken P, Buck C, Gallucci M, et al. 2007 Guideline for the management of ureteral calculi. Eur Urol. 2007;52:1610.
3.  El-Nahas AR, El-Assmy AM, Mansour O, Sheir KZ. A prospective multivariate analysis of factors predicting stone disintegration by extracorporeal shock wave lithotripsy: the value of high-resolution noncontrast computed tomography. Eur Urol. 2007;51:1688.
4.  Williams Jr JC, Kim SC, Zarse CA, McAteer JA, Lingeman JE. Progress in the use of helical CT for imaging urinary calculi. J Endourol. 2004;18:937.
5.  Wiesenthal JD, Ghiculete D, D'A Honey RJ, Pace KT. Evaluating the importance of mean stone density and skin-to-stone distance in predicting successful shock wave lithotripsy of renal and ureteric calculi. Urol Res. 2010;38:307.
6.  Pareek G, Armenakas NA, Fracchia JA. Hounsfield units on computerized tomography predict stone-free rates after extracorporeal shock wave lithotripsy. J Urol. 2003;169:1679.
7.  Ng CF, Siu DY, Wong A, Goggins W, Chan ES, Wong KT. Development of a scoring system from noncontrast computerized tomography measurements to improve the selection of upper ureteral stone for extracorporeal shock wave lithotripsy. J Urol. 2009;181:1151.
8.  Celik S, Bozkurt O, Kaya FG, Egriboyun S, Demir O, Secil M, et al. Evaluation of computed tomography findings for success prediction after extracorporeal shock wave lithotripsy for urinary tract stone disease. Int Urol Nephrol. 2015;47:69.
9.  Eisner BH, Kambadakone A, Monga M, Anderson JK, Thoreson AA, Lee H, et al. Computerized tomography magnified bone windows are superior to standard soft tissue windows for accurate measurement of stone size: an in vitro and clinical study. J Urol. 2009;181:1710.
10. Patel T, Kozakowski K, Hruby G, Gupta M. Skin to stone distance is an independent predictor of stone-free status following shockwave lithotripsy. J Endourol. 2009;23:1383.
11. Perks AE, Schuler TD, Lee J, Ghiculete D, Chung DG, D'A Honey RJ, et al. Stone attenuation and skin-to-stone distance on computed tomography predicts for stone fragmentation by shock wave lithotripsy. Urology. 2008;72:765.
12. Park YI, Yu JH, Sung LH, Noh CH, Chung JY. Evaluation of possible predictive variables for the outcome of shock wave lithotripsy of renal stones. Korean J Urol. 2010;51:713.
13. Tanaka M, Yokota E, Toyonaga Y, Shimizu F, Ishii Y, Fujime M, et al. Stone attenuation value and cross-sectional area on computed tomography predict the success of shock wave lithotripsy. Korean J Urol. 2013;54:454.

14. Joseph P, Mandal AK, Singh SK, Mandal P, Sankhwar SN, Sharma SK. Computerized tomography attenuation value of renal calculus: can it predict successful fragmentation of the calculus by extracorporeal shock wave lithotripsy? A preliminary study. J Urol. 2002;167:1968.
15. Wang LJ, Wong YC, Chuang CK, Chu SH, Chen CS, See LC, et al. Predictions of outcomes of renal stones after extracorporeal shock wave lithotripsy from stone characteristics determined by unenhanced helical computed tomography: a multivariate analysis. Eur Radiol. 2005;15:2238.
16. Gupta NP, Ansari MS, Kesarvani P, Kapoor A, Mukhopadhyay S. Role of computed tomography with no contrast medium enhancement in predicting the outcome of extracorporeal shock wave lithotripsy for urinary calculi. BJU Int. 2005;95:1285.
17. Yoshida S, Hayashi T, Ikeda J, Yoshinaga A, Ohno R, Ishii N, et al. Role of volume and attenuation value histogram of urinary stone on noncontrast helical computed tomography as predictor of fragility by extracorporeal shock wave lithotripsy. Urology. 2006;68:33.
18. Shah K, Kurien A, Mishra S, Ganpule A, Muthu V, Sabnis RB, et al. Predicting effectiveness of extracorporeal shockwave lithotripsy by stone attenuation value. J Endourol. 2010;24:1169.
19. Nakasato T, Morita J, Ogawa Y. Evaluation of Hounsfield Units as a predictive factor for the outcome of extracorporeal shock wave lithotripsy and stone composition. Urolithiasis. 2015;43:69.

# 18

# Study protocol: patient reported outcomes for bladder management strategies in spinal cord injury

Darshan P. Patel[1], Sara M. Lenherr[1], John T. Stoffel[2], Sean P. Elliott[3], Blayne Welk[4], Angela P. Presson[5], Amitabh Jha[6], Jeffrey Rosenbluth[6], and Jeremy B. Myers[1*] for the Neurogenic Bladder Research Group

## Abstract

**Background:** The majority of spinal cord injury (SCI) patients have urinary issues, such as incontinence, retention, and frequency. These problems place a significant burden on patients' physical health and quality of life (QoL). There are a wide variety of bladder management strategies available to patients with no clear guidelines on appropriate selection. Inappropriate bladder management can cause hospitalizations and serious complications, such as urosepsis and renal failure. Patients believe that both independence and ability to carry out daily activities are just as important as physical health in selecting the right bladder-management strategy but little is known about patient's QoL with different bladder managements. Our study's aim is to assess patient reported QoL measures with various bladder managements after SCI. This manuscript describes the approach, study design and common data elements for our central study.

**Methods:** This is a multi-institutional prospective cohort study comparing three different bladder-management strategies (clean intermittent catheterization, indwelling catheters, and surgery). Information collected from participants includes demographics, past medical and surgical history, injury characteristics, current and past bladder management, and SCI /bladder-related complications. Patient reported outcomes and QoL questionnaires were administered at enrollment and every 3 months for 1 year. Aims of this study protocol are: (1) to assess baseline QoL differences between the three different bladder-management strategies; (2) determine QoL impact when those using either form of catheter management undergo a surgery over the 1 year of follow-up among patients eligible for surgery; (3) assess the effects of changes in bladder management and complications on QoL over a 1-year longitudinal follow-up.

**Discussion:** By providing information about patient-reported outcomes associated with different bladder management strategies after SCI, and the impact of bladder management changes and complications on QoL, this study will provide essential information for shared decision-making and guide future investigation.

**Keywords:** Urinary bladder, Spinal cord injury, Patient reported outcomes, Quality of life, Incontinence, Bladder management

* Correspondence: Jeremy.myers@hsc.utah.edu
[1]Division of Urology, Department of Surgery, University of Utah Health Care, 30 North 1900 East, Room #3B420, Salt Lake City, UT 84132, USA
Full list of author information is available at the end of the article

# Background

Nearly 250,000 Americans live with a spinal cord injury (SCI) [1]. Approximately 74-80% of SCI individuals report some degree of bladder dysfunction within 1 year of injury [2–4]. Urinary dysfunction has a significant clinical, physical, and quality of life (QoL) burden in patients with SCI and neurogenic bladder. Common urinary symptoms, after SCI, include urinary retention, incontinence, and increased urinary frequency / urgency. Inappropriate bladder management can cause significant complications, including recurrent urinary tract infections (UTIs), urosepsis, and progressive renal failure due to high pressures within the bladder [5]. In addition to bladder dysfunction, SCI patients usually have physical limitations due to their injury, which may have a compound negative effect on their QoL [6, 7].

Multiple bladder management options are available for urinary issues in SCI patients including medications to reduce bladder spasticity and pressure, catheter based management (intermittent or permanent indwelling catheters), and reconstructive surgery to expand the bladder or bypass the bladder via a conduit or continent catheterizable pouch urinary diversion. The gold standard for management of bladder dysfunction includes clean intermittent catheterization (CIC) to empty the bladder (passing a temporary catheter periodically during the course of a day) and/or medications to reduce bladder spasticity and pressure. This strategy can significantly reduce urinary complications and related hospitalizations in patients who are able to tolerate the medications and perform urethral catheterizations. However, despite the well-recognized benefits to CIC, only 30% of SCI individuals who start CIC continue it over time and mostly patients transition to indwelling catheters (IDC), which is the management strategy with the highest complication rate [8–10]. The underlying reasons for this transition over time are not known but likely rooted in QoL issues, such as inconvenience, dependence on others, privacy, and incontinence between catheterizations [4, 11].

Most studies evaluating treatment options for neurogenic bladder focus on clinical outcome measures, such as the number of incontinent episodes in a day or the number of urinary tract infections in a year. The impact of these clinical parameters on patient-centered outcomes such as QoL is unclear. Additionally, there are some disparities in clinical and patient-centered outcomes for different bladder management strategies with some studies indicating a preference for IDC over CIC [8, 12]. Bladder management affects an individual's daily experience with SCI and is the second most common topic that SCI patients want to address when seen by a healthcare provider. Therefore, in order to provide more patient-centered care, it is critical to define patient reported outcomes and QoL in order to target issues that are important to patients in future studies.

One of the greatest knowledge gaps for bladder management strategies in SCI exists for reconstructive bladder surgery, such as bladder augmentation cystoplasty or urinary diversion. In our review of the literature, there were only 4 studies with a median sample size of 21 that assessed patient reported outcomes using non-validated instruments following urinary diversion in neurogenic bladder patients [13]. Closing this knowledge gap is important because these procedures are major surgeries and performed often in patients with sub-optimal medical health. In addition to deficits in patient reported outcomes with different bladder managements, there is also very little known about how complications, such as those associated with indwelling catheters, adversely affect patient QoL. Most published studies are cross-sectional or measure QoL before and after an intervention with little long-term follow-up.

The primary aim (*aim 1*) of our study it to determine baseline patient reported QoL with three different bladder management strategies (CIC, IDC, and surgery) in SCI. The secondary aim (*aim 2*) is to assess the comparative effectiveness of CIC/IDC versus surgery in terms of QoL over the 1 year of follow-up among patients eligible for surgery. The tertiary aim (*aim 3*) of our study is to determine, during longitudinal follow-up, how changes in bladder management and urinary tract complications affect patient reported outcomes and QoL. The overall goal of the study is to gain critical knowledge in this area to facilitate shared decision making surrounding bladder management after SCI and guide future patient-centered investigation.

# Methods/Design

## Study design

This study is a multi-institutional prospective cohort study of patient reported outcomes of adult patients with acquired SCI comparing 3 different bladder management methods (CIC, IDC, and reconstructive surgery).

## Study location

The three study locations are the Universities of Michigan, Minnesota, and Utah, which all have dedicated SCI treatment centers and urologic specialty clinics for neurogenic bladder management. Institutional review board approval was obtained from each study site before beginning the study.

## Study population and recruitment

Inclusion and exclusion criteria are listed in Table 1. To meet eligibility criteria, a patient must have SCI and neurogenic lower urinary tract symptoms. Study inclusion is also limited to patients with acquired etiologies

**Table 1** Study inclusion and exclusion criteria for patients with spinal cord injury

Inclusion criteria:

- Age ≥ 18 years
- Ability to effectively communicate in English
- Ability to provide informed consent
- Willing to participate and answer 5 sets of questionnaires over 1-year.
- Acquired SCI – traumatic, spinal cord stroke, malignancy (not active), surgical injury, transverse myelitis.

Exclusion criteria:

- Congenital SCI – cerebral palsy, spina bifida, caudal regression, sacral agenesis.
- Progressive SCI – multiple sclerosis, active malignancy, progressive neurologic diseases leading to SCI

of SCI, such as trauma, tumor without current progressive malignancy, spinal cord stroke, vascular bleed such as an arterio-venous malformation, transverse myelitis without progression to multiple sclerosis, and post-surgical / procedural complications. Any level of SCI, including those with cauda equina, are eligible to participate in the study. Exclusion criteria are progressive spinal disorders (e.g. multiple sclerosis, active malignancy, other progressive neurologic or neuromuscular diseases), as well as congenital forms of SCI (myelomeningocele, spina bifida, cerebral palsy, etc.).

A priori recruitment goals based on power calculations was 900-1300 total participants. Participants will be recruited over a 1-year period and followed for an additional year. Recruitment will occur at multiple settings for each university. These settings include: urology clinics, physical medicine and rehabilitation SCI clinics, physical therapy centers, inpatient rehabilitation hospital, and chronic SCI residential facilities. Other settings for local recruitment include SCI-oriented informational seminars, and other SCI-oriented activities. In addition to local in-person recruitment, the study will be available for remote enrollment via a web-based portal. Participants in the United States and Canada may fill out a screening eligibility form on a website created for promotion of bladder research and information (NBRG.org). If eligible, interested participants will be contacted by a research coordinator from 1 of the 3 study centers. The study will be advertised via social media (Twitter and Facebook) and on SCI advocacy groups websites. In addition, experts in the field on neurogenic bladder will be contacted and asked to advertise and promote the study to patients they see in a clinical setting.

### Patients as research team participants

One key to patient-centered research is engagement of patient and clinical "stakeholders." Stakeholders are individuals with personal and or professional insight into the disease process or interventions being studied. This study involves stakeholders in all aspects of the research process in order to assure that the research design, implementation, and dissemination of the results are relevant to clinicians, patients, and caregivers dealing with the SCI on a day-to-day basis. We will assemble a team of people living with SCI to create a Patient Advisory Group, which will provide input regarding the following parameters: meaningfulness of research questions, important characteristics of study participants, comparators, major outcomes, monitor the study progress, ease of questionnaire administration, advocate change in study design where needed, and suggest implementation plans for dissemination of relevant findings.

### Study aims
#### Aim 1

To compare cross-sectional patient reported outcome measures and QoL for 3 different bladder management methods (1) CIC, (2) IDC, and (3) reconstructive surgery. We will use the two bladder-specific instruments from the Spinal Cord Injury Quality of Life (SCI-QoL) panel and Neurogenic Bladder Symptom Score (NBSS) for this purpose.

#### Aim 2

To determine the comparative effectiveness of CIC/IDC versus surgery in terms of QoL (using the two bladder-specific SCI-QoL instruments and the NBSS) over 1-year of follow-up. This analysis will be conducted in a causal inference framework among the patients who have not previously had surgery but are eligible for surgery.

#### Aim 3

To measure the effect of bladder management changes and urinary complications on patient reported bladder management outcomes and QoL (using the two bladder-specific SCI-QoL instruments and the NBSS). Longitudinal collection of these instruments will allow analysis of participants who have either of these events during the course of the study.

### Study procedures

The study procedures are summarized in Fig. 1. Upon enrollment participants will undergo an interview with a trained study coordinator gathering information including demographics, SCI injury specifics, pertinent past medical and surgical history, past and current bladder management, SCI-related complications, and urologic follow-up over time. If acute rehabilitation location is known, records will be obtained and SCI injury specifics and management will be confirmed. After the enrollment interview participants will answer a panel of questionnaires designed to assess many aspects of patient reported bladder outcomes and QoL. These questionnaires were

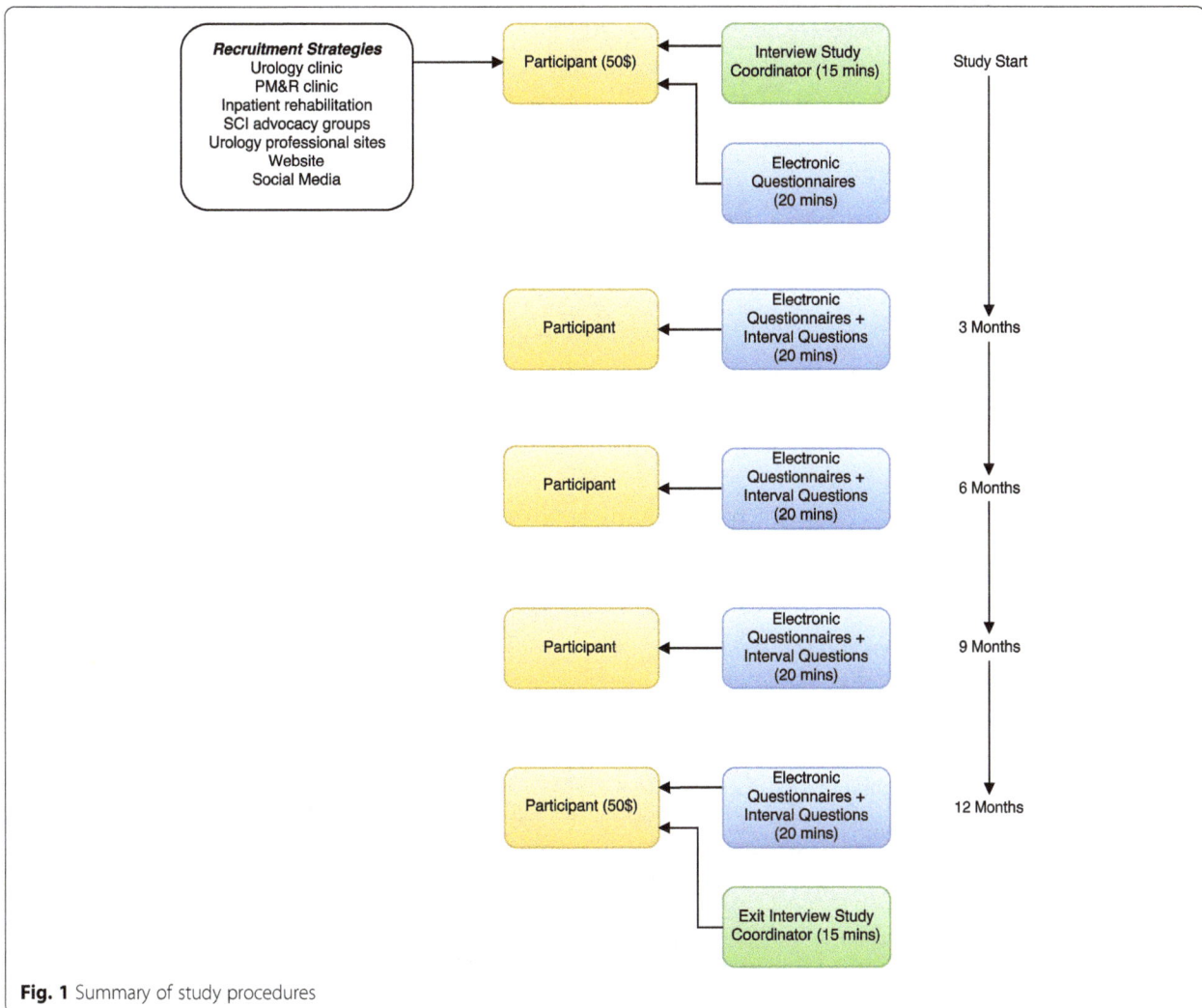

**Fig. 1** Summary of study procedures

deemed relevant by investigators and the Patient Advisory Panel. Every three months for the next 12 months after enrollment, the same panel of questions will be electronically sent to the participants, along with non-validated questions about changes in bladder management or urologic complications occurring in the intervening 3 months.

Longitudinal follow-up will occur for 12 months. A subject can potentially switch bladder-management strategy group during the course of the follow-up or experience a urologic complication. Figure 2 illustrates possible scenarios using 3 example patients. QoL data will not be collected within 3 months of a major surgery (bladder augmentation, urinary diversion), however, other interventions such as first-time Onabotulinum toxin A injection will be assessed at the next scheduled 3-month interval after the intervention. Urinary complications will be assessed in a similar fashion. These complications will include but are not limited to: admission for UTI/pyelonephritis, urinary stone episode, any urological

complication (orchitis, gross hematuria, etc.), need for surgical treatment to treat complications of previous surgery. We estimate that switching bladder-management strategy (for example, participant 1 in Fig. 2) could happen for approximately 10-15% of patients based upon the experience of the research team.

After the enrollment interview, patients will complete the panel of questionnaires on an electronic tablet or via a web-based platform accessible from any location with internet access. A study coordinator will be available if they need assistance with electronic questionnaire completion either in person or over the phone. All electronic questionnaires will be administered via the secure and Health Insurance Portability and Accountability Act (HIPAA)-compliant Assessment Center[SM] platform (www.assessmentcenter.net). This online data collection portal supports repeated administrations of the same questionnaires at pre-determined time points, real-time monitoring of questionnaire completion and data integrity analysis. Participants will be electronically prompted

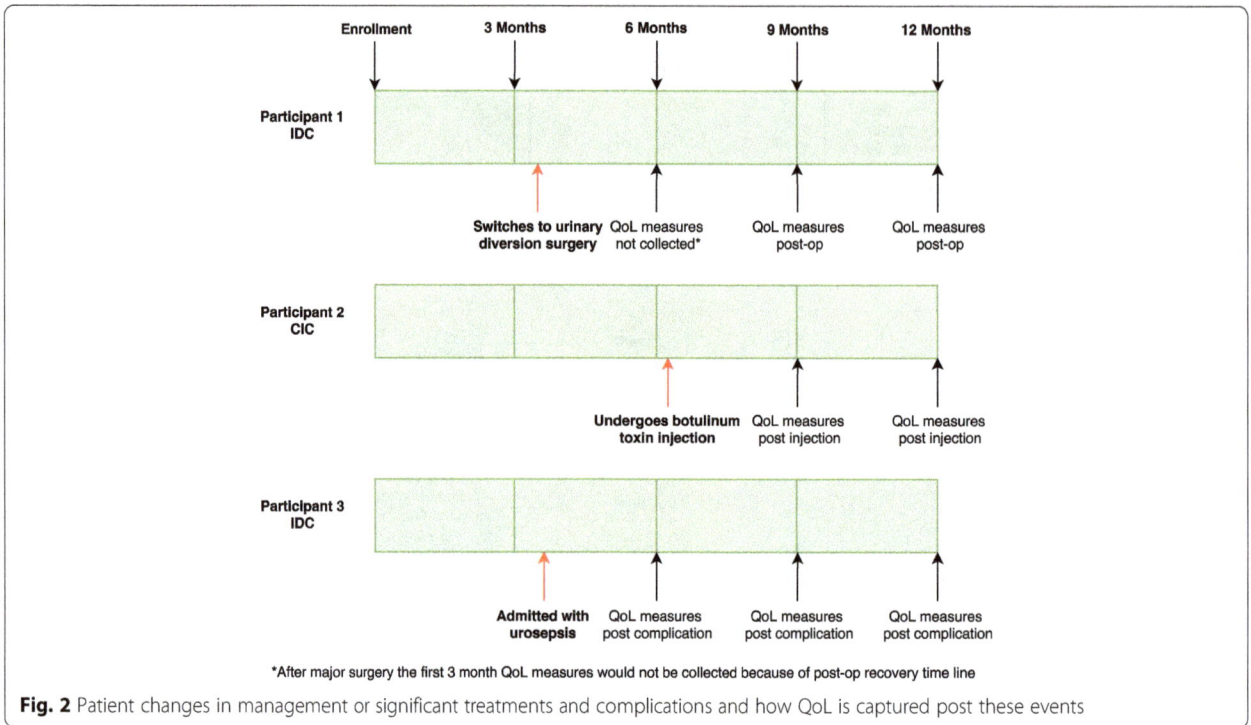

**Fig. 2** Patient changes in management or significant treatments and complications and how QoL is captured post these events

to complete their next due questionnaires 15-days prior to their next 3-month questionnaire due-date and for 15-days afterwards. Research coordinators will routinely monitor completion and those that are near past-due will be sent e-mail and/or phone reminders requesting their completion of the set of questionnaires to improve adherence. With successful completion of the first panel of questionnaires, participants will be provided with $50 gift card to the preferred retailor of their choice (e.g. Amazon, Walmart, etc.). An additional $50 gift card will be given to participants after completion of 1 year of follow-up questionnaires. As mentioned above, at each 3-month questionnaire administration, participants will also receive non-validated questions about interval changes in their bladder management or urologic complications. Changes and complications will therefore be tracked over time. Clarifications needed based on these interval responses will be followed-up with a phone call from a research assistant. In addition, at the end of 12-months a telephone administered exit interview with a research assistant will be performed which will confirm if there are any additional changes in bladder management or urinary complications over the course of the study. A Likert 15-point scale will be given to participants assessing the impact from these 'events' over the course of the year from "a very great deal worse" to "a very great deal better".

### Outcome instruments

A full list of patient-reported outcomes and QoL measures is summarized in Table 2.

**Table 2** Patient reported outcome measures used for the study

Bladder specific:
- Neurogenic Bladder Symptom Score
- SCI-QoL
  - Bladder management difficulties
  - Bladder complications

General QoL:
- Modified SF-12

Psychosocial:
- SCI-QoL
  - Pain interference
  - Independence
  - Positive affect and well-being
  - Satisfaction with social roles and activities

Other:
- Likert pain scale
- Autonomic dysreflexia
- SCI-QoL
  - Basic mobility
  - Fine motor
  - Self-care
- Bowel function
  - Neurogenic Bowel Dysfunction Score
  - SCI-QoL – Bowel management difficulties

### Bladder-specific measurements

The bladder-specific instruments from the SCI-QoL measurement system and the NBSS are the outcome measures used for all aims of this study. The SCI-QoL measurement system is a validated, comprehensive patient-reported outcome measurement item bank panel, which consists of 19 item banks including two item banks related to complications and consequences of bladder management ("Bladder Complications"), as well as feelings about bladder related limitations and function ("Bladder Management Difficulties") [14]. SCI-QoL instruments uses item response theory and computerized adaptive testing using the Assessment Center[SM] platform. Computer adaptive testing utilizes participant responses to guide the administration of only select, pertinent questions drawn from a larger item bank. For example, when chronically ill patients with limited functioning responds that they can't get out of bed without help, they are not next asked if they can jog a mile. Instead the participant is asked more narrowed questions relevant to their mobility level, such as "Can you brush your hair or open a jar?" A final calibrated score is produced for each health domain to provide an individual's QoL or function score. Computer adaptive testing minimizes floor and ceiling effects and allows accurate assessment over a wide range of function and symptoms while minimizing participant burden and maximizing patient relevance.

The NBSS is a 24-item validated instrument with three domains, as well as one question about global satisfaction with urinary function. The three domains of the NBSS are incontinence, storage and voiding, and urinary complications. The NBSS was developed and validated in a diverse group of neurogenic bladder patients, including those with SCI, multiple sclerosis, and congenital neurogenic bladder. This instrument incorporates self-reported urinary complications such as urinary tract infections, kidney and bladder stones, and pain associated with urination or catheter use. The questionnaire emphasizes function and consequences rather than feelings and social limitations.

### General QoL measurements

The Short Form-12 (SF-12) from the Medical Outcomes Study will be used to asses general QoL. The SF-12 is a generic QoL instrument used very commonly and has been modified for people that utilize wheelchairs and have SCI [15]. There is considerable population-level normative data using the SF-12 that is available for comparison with study populations of interests (39, 40).

### Psychosocial measurements

Patient Advisory Group and other clinical stakeholders provided guidance on selection of other measures of non-bladder related psychosocial functioning, which we thought would potentially influence how participants would report their bladder function. For example, we postulated that a person who was depressed with SCI might report much worse feelings about bladder function than someone who was not depressed. The final selected psychosocial measures encompass the following areas: independence, pain interference with life, satisfaction with social participation and roles, and positive affect and well-being [16]. These instruments are all SCI-QoL item banks and administered with computer adaptive testing via the Assessment Center[SM] platform.

### Other measurements of physical function

Spinal cord injury affects many other aspects of physical function and all of these in turn have the potential for affecting how a patient reports their bladder function and related QoL. For instance, if a patient has severe bowel dysfunction they may also report worse bladder dysfunction. In an effort to capture other physical limitations and dysfunction associated with SCI and evaluate the relationship to bladder satisfaction, we asked participants about a variety of other physical functioning. These areas of physical function included: autonomic dysreflexia, pain level, ability for self-care, mobility, fine motor function, and bowel dysfunction. These questionnaires include (1) autonomic dysreflexia questions based on a longer validated Autonomic Dysfunction Following Spinal Cord Injury (ADFSCI) instrument [17], (2) a 0-10 point Likert pain scale, (3) the validated Neurogenic Bowel Dysfunction Score (NBD) [18], (4) three functional–index physical function banks from SCI-QoL (Basic mobility, Fine motor, Self-care), [14, 19], and (5) the SCI-QOL bowel management difficulties computer adaptive item bank.

### Statistical analyses and outcomes

#### Primary outcome

The primary outcomes are the total scores from the following instruments: SCI-QoL Bladder Management Difficulties, SCI-QoL Bladder Complications, and the NBSS. These will be compared between different management groups (CIC, IDC, and reconstructive surgery) in *aim 1*, between CIC/IDC versus surgery among those eligible for surgery in *aim 2*, and before and after changes in bladder management or complications in *aim 3*. Non-eligible candidates for surgery include patients whose risk of an unfavorable outcome is higher than average.

#### Secondary outcomes

The secondary outcomes include the NBSS subdomains of (1) Incontinence, (2) Storage and voiding, (3) Complications, and the NBSS single global question about satisfaction with urinary system function. Secondary outcomes will undergo the same comparisons and modeling frameworks used for primary outcomes.

**Aim 1** To address the question comparing QoL related to CIC, IDC and surgery at baseline, we will compare bladder management strategy with our primary and secondary outcomes in both univariable and multivariable linear regression models. Multivariable models will adjust for age, sex, years since injury, complete injury, pain, education level, and severity of bowel dysfunction. Models will be constructed within paraplegic and tetraplegic patients, as the relationship between QoL and bladder management strategy differs across these injury types.

**Aim 2** To address Aim 2, comparing the effectiveness of CIC/IDC bladder management with surgery in terms of longitudinally collected QoL data, we first subset our data to patients that could theoretically be randomized to either maintaining CIC/IDC bladder management or receiving surgical treatment. Thus we will exclude patients who have previously had surgery. We plan to estimate the causal effect of surgical treatment at any point during the 1-year assessment period of our study compared to continuation of CIC/IDC throughout this period. Because the treatment will be administered at different times for different patients, and because confounding will be time dependent, standard methods using regression analysis or propensity scores for treatments at a fixed time are not applicable. Instead, we will apply inverse probability weighting under a marginal structural model (MSM) to evaluate the comparative effectiveness of surgery versus CIC/IDC among patients who are candidates for surgery. Specifically, we will compare mean levels of patient outcomes at the final 12-month time point between patients who have received surgery during the 1 year assessment period versus patients who continued CIC/IDC management, controlling for time-dependent confounding by using stabilized weights. The main time-dependent confounders include complications and SCI-QoL and NBSS – as these variables may indicate a need or desire for surgery, be influenced by surgery, and potentially affect patient-reported outcomes at the final time point. The final stabilized weights are the product of stabilized inverse probability of treatment weights (IPTW), which account for confounding, and inverse probability of censored weights (IPCW), which account for loss-to-follow-up [20]. The product of IPTW and IPCW is the subject-specific weight used in the MSM to adjust for time-dependent confounding. Applying the stabilized weights essentially generates a pseudo-population under which subjects are randomly assigned to treatment and

have complete follow-up information under the assumption that the measured covariates fully account for confounding. In this pseudo-population we will estimate the average causal effect of surgical treatment during the 1-year study period using regression analyses with an indicator variable for surgery during the study period as the predictor variable while adjusting for the baseline covariates. We will use this model to report the comparative effectiveness of surgery in terms of the average difference in SCI-QoL and NBSS scores between the two groups, along with 95% confidence intervals. Additional analyses will estimate the average causal effect of receiving the surgical treatment at varying times prior to the 12-month outcome assessment.

We will plan to report the covariate summaries for the CIC/IDC and surgery groups at baseline and at each follow-up time point (3, 6, 9, and 12 months) for the time-varying measures. Fixed-time covariates will include: age, sex, years since injury at baseline, complete injury, pain, education level, and severity of bowel dysfunction. Time-varying covariates will include complications, SCI-QoL, NBSS, and the measurement time point. Complications will be included in the stabilized weights at all time points (baseline, 3, 6, 9, and 12 months). SCI-QoL and NBSS will be included at all time points < 12 m, and they will serve as outcomes (in their respective MSMs) at the final 12-month time point.

Multiple imputation will be used to impute missing data. Baseline and follow-up factors beyond the variables being analyzed will be incorporated into the imputation model to account for dependence of the missing data mechanism on other measured factors. We will apply the method of data augmentation using Markov Chain Monte Carlo (MCMC) to generate imputed values [21, 22].

**Aim 3** To assess the effects of changes in bladder management strategy and complications on QoL, we will take a descriptive approach due to the potentially limited sample size. We expect that 10-15% of patients will change bladder management strategy. Among those who change bladder management strategy, we will compare the impact of this change on QoL outcomes using linear mixed effects models with an indicator for first/s bladder management strategy, controlling for a few key covariates (age, sex, time since injury, complete/incomplete injury and parapalegic/tetrapalegic). Correlation of the QoL outcomes within subjects will be modeled with a compound symmetry covariance matrix. We will use a similar model framework to examine the effect of complications on QoL, where this analysis will be conducted within subjects who experienced a complication. We will test whether QoL differed before and after the complication occurred by including an indicator for first/s bladder management strategy, and controlling for the same key covariates.

## Determination of sample size

We designed our study to detect clinically important differences in QoL between the 3 bladder management strategy groups (1) CIC, (2) IDC, and (3) reconstructive surgery. Practically, we anticipated the ability to recruit approximately 900-1350 subjects over a 1-year time frame after accounting for a 10% loss to follow-up. We expected CIC to comprise about 24% of our sample, IDC to be about 41%, and reconstructive surgery to be about 34%. The primary bladder specific patient-reported outcome measures used to compare these groups are the two bladder-specific SCI-QoL instruments (Bladder Complications and Bladder Management Difficulties) and the NBSS. Our effect size calculations were based on a mixed models analysis of repeated measures data assuming a conservative correlation of 0.8 and an autoregressive order 1 AR(1) covariance structure between five repeat measures on the same subject. Assuming a standard deviation of 10 for both SCI-QoL and NBSS based on previous studies and a mean of 50 and 20 respectively, we would have 80% power at a Bonferroni-adjusted alpha level (0.05/3 = 0.017, for three pair-wise comparisons among our bladder management strategies) to detect the minimum differences presented in Table 3 [23, 24]. For the SCI-QoL bladder-specific instruments, we expect to detect differences in the overall score of about 4-5% or 3-4% for our minimum and maximum sample sizes, respectively. For the NBSS, we expect to detect score differences of about 10-12% or 8.5-10% for our minimum and maximum sample sizes, respectively.

## Ethics and dissemination

The following precautions will be taken to ensure subject privacy is protected: research and questionnaire completion will be conducted in private place; all discussion regarding involvement in the study and study related data collection will occur in private; collected information about participants will be limited to the amount necessary to achieve the aims of the study; no unneeded information will be collected or stored. This study is being performed in accordance with the World Medical Association Declaration of Helsinki and after approval from each sponsoring center's Institutional Review Boards [25]. This study has been registered at clinicaltrails.gov (https://clinicaltrials.gov/ct2/show/NCT02616081).

We plan to use several strategies to enhance rapid dissemination and implementation of our findings to improve patient-centered healthcare delivery and shared decision making for those with SCI. We have developed a project resource website founded by our research group, the Neurogenic Bladder Research Group (www.NBRG.org). The website is available for patient recruitment and will be used for rapid dissemination of findings. Throughout duration of the study, clinicians and patient partners will blog about their personal experience being involved in the project and provide research progress updates. Social media sites such Twitter© and Facebook© will be used to increase traffic to our website and bring global interest to our study and subsequent findings. This will be an integral aspect of the dissemination of the final results of our research. Once results for the study are available, an informational web special will be available on the (www.NBRG.org) website explaining the relevant findings and implications for patients, caregivers, clinicians, and researchers. Additionally, study participants will be emailed a link to this web special to review relevant findings in this study as a result of their participation. For clinicians and other stakeholders that follow the peer-reviewed literature, we will publish our findings in a diverse number of journals to reach urologists and physical medicine & rehabilitation specialists that would be interested in our findings.

## Discussion

Our study will address critical knowledge gaps in patient-centered outcomes for various bladder management strategies in SCI patients. This study is multi-centered, drawing participants from three large academic referral centers for SCI and complex urologic care. The use of open enrollment via the internet will augment our recruitment goals and help improve the generalizability of our findings. Additionally, our use of robust, validated instruments for assessment of patient reported outcomes and health related QoL strengthens our study. We believe that information about patient reported outcomes and QoL with common bladder management strategies after SCI, as well as the longitudinal collection of patient-reported outcomes with changes in bladder management and urinary specific complications will advance patient-centered care and shared decision-making.

## Trial status

The trial is in the recruiting phase at the time of manuscript submission.

**Table 3** Estimates of number of participants to detect differences in the SCI-QoL and the NBSS

| Questionnaire | Comparison groups | Detected differences n = 900 | Detected differences n = 1350 |
|---|---|---|---|
| SCI-QoL | IDC vs CIC | 2.34 (4.7%) | 1.91 (3.8%) |
| | IDC vs. surgery | 2.11 (4.2%) | 1.72 (3.4%) |
| | CIC vs. surgery | 2.42 (4.8%) | 1.98 (4.0%) |
| NBSS | IDC vs CIC | 2.34 (11.7%) | 1.91 (9.6%) |
| | IDC vs. surgery | 2.11 (10.6%) | 1.72 (8.6%) |
| | CIC vs. surgery | 2.42 (12.1%) | 1.98 (9.9%) |

*SCI-QoL* Spinal Cord Injury Quality of Life Scale, *NBSS* Neurogenic Bladder Symptom Score, *CIC* clean intermittent catheterization, *IDC* indwelling catheter

## Abbreviations

CI: Confidence interval; CIC: Clean intermittent catheterization; IDC: Indwelling catheter; NBSS: Neurogenic Bladder Symptom Score; QoL: Quality of life; SCI: Spinal cord injury; SCI-QoL: Spinal cord injury-quality of life questionnaire; SF-12: Short form 12; UTI: Urinary tract infection

## Acknowledgements

The authors would like to acknowledge our patient stakeholders (Ms. Elizabeth Fetter, Mr. Jason Hall, Ms. Kelsey Peterson, and Lynn Wolf) and our study coordinators for their contributions to this study.

## Funding

Patient Centered Outcomes Research Institute, PCORI/CER-1409-21,348. All statements in this report, including its findings and conclusions, are solely those of the authors and do not necessarily represent the views of PCORI.

## Authors' contributions

All authors participated in creating the study design. DPP and JBM drafted the manuscript. DPP, JTS, SPE, BW, APP, SML, JBM provided a critical revision of the manuscript. DPP, APP, and JBM obtained the funding of this study. All the authors read and approved the final manuscript.

## Competing interests

The authors declare that they have no competing interests.

## Author details

[1]Division of Urology, Department of Surgery, University of Utah Health Care, 30 North 1900 East, Room #3B420, Salt Lake City, UT 84132, USA. [2]Department of Urology, University of Michigan, Ann Arbor, Michigan, USA. [3]Department of Urology, University of Minnesota, Minneapolis, Minnesota, USA. [4]Divsion of Urology, University of Western Ontario, London, Ontario, Canada. [5]Divsion of Epidemiology, Department of Internal Medicine, University of Utah Health Care, Salt Lake City, Utah, USA. [6]Department of Physical Medicine and Rehabilitation, University of Utah Health Care, Salt Lake City, Utah, USA.

## References

1.  Sekhon LH, Fehlings MG. Epidemiology, demographics, and pathophysiology of acute spinal cord injury. Spine (Phila Pa 1976). 2001;26(24 Suppl):S2–12.
2.  Ku JH. The management of neurogenic bladder and quality of life in spinal cord injury. BJU Int. 2006;98(4):739–45. doi:10.1111/j.1464-410X.2006.06395.x.
3.  Ginsberg D. The epidemiology and pathophysiology of neurogenic bladder. Am J Manag Care. 2013;19(10 Suppl):s191–6.
4.  Manack A, Motsko SP, Haag-Molkenteller C, Dmochowski RR, Goehring EL Jr, Nguyen-Khoa BA, et al. Epidemiology and healthcare utilization of neurogenic bladder patients in a US claims database. Neurourol Urodyn. 2011;30(3):395–401. doi:10.1002/nau.21003.
5.  Gormley EA. Urologic complications of the neurogenic bladder. Urol Clin North Am. 2010;37(4):601–7. doi:10.1016/j.ucl.2010.07.002.
6.  de Seze M, Ruffion A, Denys P, Joseph PA, Perrouin-Verbe B. The neurogenic bladder in multiple sclerosis: review of the literature and proposal of management guidelines. Mult Scler (Houndmills, Basingstoke, England). 2007;13(7):915–28. doi:10.1177/1352458506075651.
7.  Tapia CI, Khalaf K, Berenson K, Globe D, Chancellor M, Carr LK. Health-related quality of life and economic impact of urinary incontinence due to detrusor overactivity associated with a neurologic condition: a systematic review. Health Qual Life Outcomes. 2013;11:13. doi:10.1186/1477-7525-11-13.
8.  Cameron AP, Wallner LP, Forchheimer MB, Clemens JQ, Dunn RL, Rodriguez G, et al. Medical and psychosocial complications associated with method of bladder management after traumatic spinal cord injury. Arch Phys Med Rehabil. 2011;92(3):449–56. doi:10.1016/j.apmr.2010.06.028.
9.  Cameron AP, Wallner LP, Tate DG, Sarma AV, Rodriguez GM, Clemens JQ. Bladder management after spinal cord injury in the United States 1972 to 2005. J Urol. 2010;184(1):213–7. doi:10.1016/j.juro.2010.03.008.
10.  Weld KJ, Wall BM, Mangold TA, Steere EL, Dmochowski RR. Influences on renal function in chronic spinal cord injured patients. J Urol. 2000;164(5):1490–3.
11.  Cameron AP, Clemens JQ, Latini JM, McGuire EJ. Combination drug therapy improves compliance of the neurogenic bladder. J Urol. 2009;182(3):1062–7. doi:10.1016/j.juro.2009.05.038.
12.  Patel DP, Elliott SP, Stoffel JT, Brant WO, Hotaling JM, Myers JB. Patient reported outcomes measures in neurogenic bladder and bowel: a systematic review of the current literature. Neurourol Urodyn. 2016;35(1):8–14. doi:10.1002/nau.22673.
13.  Patel DP, Elliott SP, Stoffel JT, Brant WO, Hotaling JM, Myers JB. Patient reported outcomes measures in neurogenic bladder and bowel: a systematic review of the current literature. Neurourol Urodyn. 2014; doi:10.1002/nau.22673.
14.  Tulsky DS, Kisala PA, Tate DG, Spungen AM, Kirshblum SC. Development and psychometric characteristics of the SCI-QOL bladder management difficulties and bowel management difficulties item banks and short forms and the SCI-QOL bladder complications scale. J Spinal Cord Med. 2015;38(3):288–302. doi:10.1179/2045772315y.0000000030.
15.  Ware J Jr, Kosinski M, Keller SD. A 12-item short-form health survey: construction of scales and preliminary tests of reliability and validity. Med Care. 1996;34(3):220–33.
16.  Tulsky DS, Kisala PA, Victorson D, Tate DG, Heinemann AW, Charlifue S, et al. Overview of the Spinal Cord Injury–Quality of Life (SCI-QOL) measurement system. J Spinal Cord Med. 2015;38(3):257–69. doi:10.1179/2045772315y.0000000023.
17.  Hubli M, Gee CM, Krassioukov AV. Refined assessment of blood pressure instability after spinal cord injury. Am J Hypertens. 2015;28(2):173–81. doi:10.1093/ajh/hpu122.
18.  Krogh K, Christensen P, Sabroe S, Laurberg S. Neurogenic bowel dysfunction score. Spinal Cord. 2006;44(10):625–31. doi:10.1038/sj.sc.3101887.
19.  Tulsky DS, Jette AM, Kisala PA, Kalpakjian C, Dijkers MP, Whiteneck G, et al. Spinal cord injury-functional index: item banks to measure physical functioning in individuals with spinal cord injury. Arch Phys Med Rehabil. 2012;93(10):1722–32. doi:10.1016/j.apmr.2012.05.007.
20.  Toh S, Hernan MA. Causal inference from longitudinal studies with baseline randomization. Int J Biostat. 2008;4(1):Article 22. doi:10.2202/1557-4679.1117.
21.  Schafer JL. Multiple imputation: a primer. Stat Methods Med Res. 1999;8(1):3–15. doi:10.1177/096228029900800102.
22.  DB R. Multiple Inputation for Nonresponsive in Surveys. New York: Wiley; 1987.
23.  Welk B, Morrow S, Madarasz W, Baverstock R, Macnab J, Sequeira K. The validity and reliability of the neurogenic bladder symptom score. J Urol. 2014;192(2):452–7. doi:10.1016/j.juro.2014.01.027.
24.  Cella D, Nowinski C, Peterman A, Victorson D, Miller D, Lai JS, et al. The neurology quality-of-life measurement initiative. Arch Phys Med Rehabil. 2011;92(10 Suppl):S28–36. doi:10.1016/j.apmr.2011.01.025.
25.  World Medical Assosciation. World Medical Association Declaration of Helsinki: ethical principles for medical research involving human subjects. JAMA. 2013;310(20):2191–4. doi:10.1001/jama.2013.281053.

# 19

# Unilateral congenital giant megaureter with renal dysplasia compressing contralateral ureter and causing bilateral hydronephrosis

Mingming Yu, Geng Ma, Zheng Ge, Rugang Lu, Yongji Deng and Yunfei Guo[*]

## Abstract

**Background:** Congenital giant megaureter (CGM) is uncommon in the pediatric population. The major clinical presentations are marked protruberances and abdominal cysts.

**Case presentation:** We reported a case of CGM with almost the whole left ureter dilation accompanied with a 1 cm stricture at the entrance of the bladder and renal dysplasia, immediately compressing the contralateral ureter and causing bilateral hydronephrosis for the first time. At one-stage of the operation, a left nephrostomy with a right ureterolysis were performed, and a poor left kidney function was found. Then, the left kidney and ureter were cut off by nephroureterectomy at the second-stage. Eventually, the follow-up showed that the patient recovered well by abdominal ultrasound.

**Conclusion:** Based on the findings of these reported literatures, CGM is rare. The physical and imaging examinations are essential for the diagnosis of CGM, and the appropriate treatment methods should be performed based on patients' specific condition.

**Keywords:** Congenital giant megaureter, Hydronephrosis, Renal dysplasia, Congenital megaureter

## Background

Congenital giant megaureter (CGM) is an extremely rare condition, which is defined as "the lumen of a ureter is congenitally, focally and segmentally dilated to more than 10 times of the normal diameter, in presence of normal bladder volume and function [1]." The first CGM was reported by Chaterjee SK [2] in 1964. Since then, a small number of patients with CGM have been reported and a PubMed search yielded less than 10 published case reports to date.

Herein, we reported an entirely dilated CGM accompanied with 1 cm stricture at the entrance of the bladder and renal dysplasia, thereby compressing the contra-

lateral ureter and causing bilateral hydronephrosis in a 3-year-old boy. In addition, we reviewed the epidemiology, pathogenesis, diagnosis and therapies of this rare condition by analyzing all previously reported cases.

## Case presentation

A 3-year-old boy presented to our hospital with a big abdominal circumference (Fig. 1) since he was born. He had no history of urinary tract infection or flank pain. The abdominal examination showed a defined cystic abdominal mass with a smooth surface measuring 15 × 10 cm. The abdominal ultrasound revealed a separated acoustic dark area on the left abdomen and bilateral hydronephrosis with upper ureter dilatation on the right abdomen. Similarly, abdominal computed tomography (CT) scan demonstrated a giant ureter on the left side and right hydronephrosis with the whole dilatation of

* Correspondence: yunfeiguo_yfg@163.com
Department of Urology, Nanjing Children's Hospital Affiliated to Nanjing Medical University, Nanjing, Jiangsu 210029, China

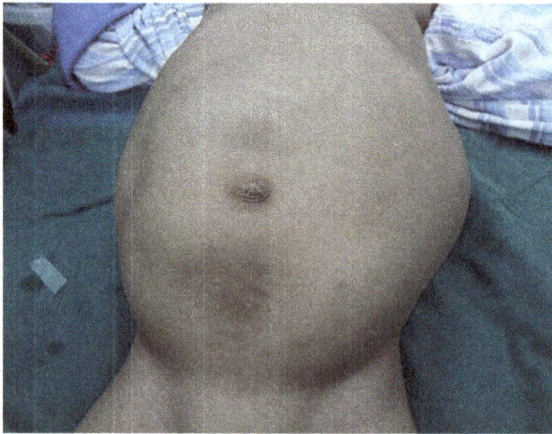

**Fig. 1** Physical examination shows a big abdominal circumference

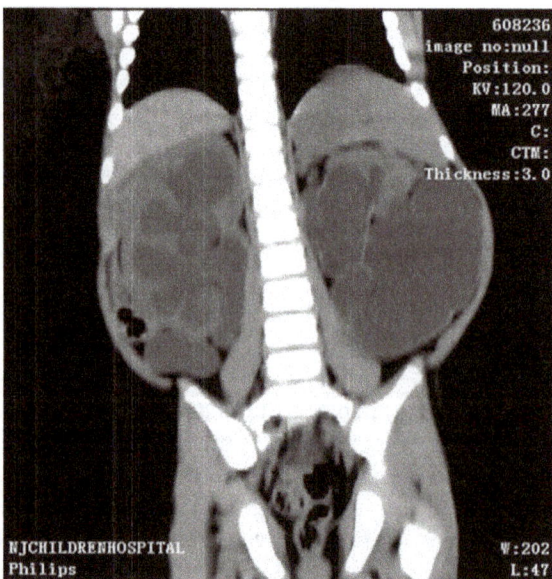

**Fig. 3** Contrast-enhanced computed tomography scan shows renal dysplasia with giant ureter on the left side and right hydronephrosis with the whole right ureter dilatation

right ureter (Fig. 2). Contrast-enhanced CT scan further showed renal dysplasia with a giant ureter (Fig. 3). In addition, a dynamic diethylene triamine pentaacetic acid (DPTA) radionuclide renogram showed no function in the left glomeruli and compensatory increase in the right glomeruli. On cystoscopy, the left ureteric orifice could not be found. Based on these examinations, a diagnosis of left CGM causing a malfunction of the left kidney and bilateral hydronephrosis was made.

At one-stage of the operation, the giant left ureter and the right ureter dilated about 5 cm from the entrance of the bladder (the submucosal segment of the ureter) were found in the deep right bladder. So we considered that the right ureter was compressed by the giant left ureter,

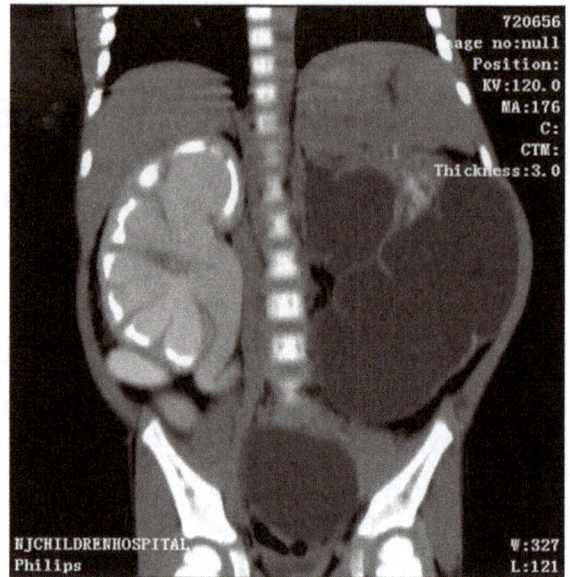

**Fig. 2** Abdominal computed tomography shows a giant ureter on the left side and right hydronephrosis with the whole right ureter dilatation

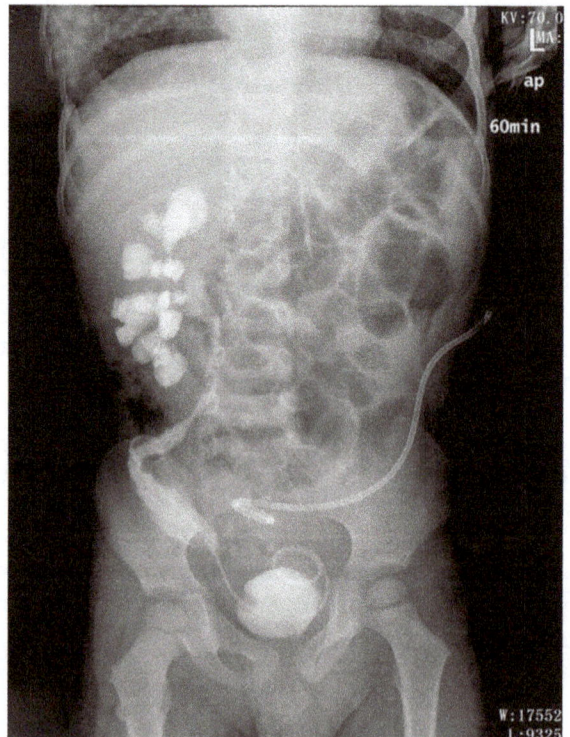

**Fig. 4** Intravenous pyelography reveals no images of the left kidney and ureter, and also shows the compressed right ureter

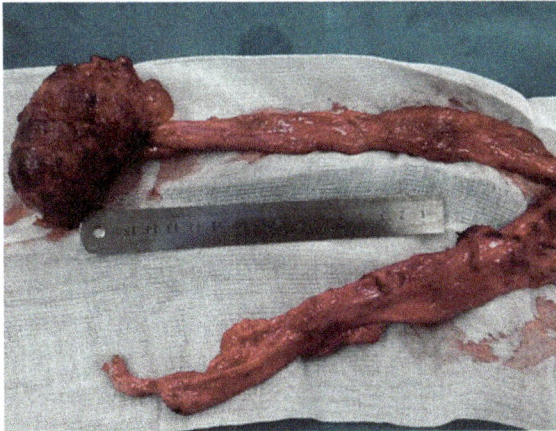

**Fig. 5** The dilated ureter is about 40 cm and we can observe the small left kidney with many vesicles on the surface and the stricture in the distal segment of the dilated ureter

and then a left nephrostomy with a right ureterolysis were performed. After the first operation, the liquid outflowing from the single J tube was about 10 mL per day. After the first operation for 19 days, a dynamic DPTA radionuclide renogram was performed again and revealed a serious decline in the function of left kidney. In addition, an intravenous pyelography showed no images of the left kidney and ureter (Fig. 4). These results indicated a poor left kidney function and we considered that the left kidney could not be kept any more. As a result, a second-stage operation was performed thirty days after the first operation. During the operation, we could see a dysplastic left kidney and an almost entirely dilated left ureter with only 1 cm stricture at the entrance of the bladder, then nephroureterectomy was performed through cutting off the left kidney and ureter close to the bladder (Fig. 5). The postoperative pathologic examination showed that the left kidney and ureter were similar to multicystic dysplastic kidney (Fig. 6). The patient recovered well and remarkably reduced right hydronephrosis was found by the follow-up

abdominal ultrasound (Fig. 7). The patient was observed to be asymptomatic after 2 years of follow-up.

## Discussion

CGM is extremely rare in the pediatric population. To the best of our knowledge, only 27 cases have been reported in the English literatures [1, 3–8] (Table 1). Among 27 patients with CGM, the ratio of women/men was approximately 1:1, indicating that there was no sex difference in CGM, while congenital megaureter occurred more often in men [9]. The megaureter often began from birth to pre-school age. There were 2 cases with CGM from birth, 6 cases before one year old, 8 cases from one to three years old, and 10 cases from four to eight years old. The oldest patient reported was 15 years old. Unlike congenital megaureter which might be observed bilaterally in about 20 % cases [10], all of the 27 patients with CGM were unilateral with 14 megaureter on the left side and 13 megaureter on the right side.

Currently, the pathogenesis of CGM or congenital megaureter is considered to be related to the expression of transforming growth factor β which might lead to a lack of post-natal muscle dysplasia [11, 12]. In the earlier study, Mackinnon et al. [13] put forward a theory that a lack of longitudinal muscle in the distal ureter led to the functional obstruction, which was accepted by many scholars. Then, Notley et al. [14] found the normal nerves distribution and collagen fiber hyperplasia in the muscular layer of the megaureters by the electron microscopy, which was considered as the major reason of the megaureter. In addition, Tokunaka et al. [15, 16] described a small subgroup of megaureters with muscle dysplasia which affected the dilated part of the ureter, and muscle dysplasia was thought as the primary cause leading to the dilatation. In recent years, most scholars believed that multiple factors contributed to the congenital megaureter.

The diagnosis of CGM was usually based on the history, the physical examinations and imaging examinations. In

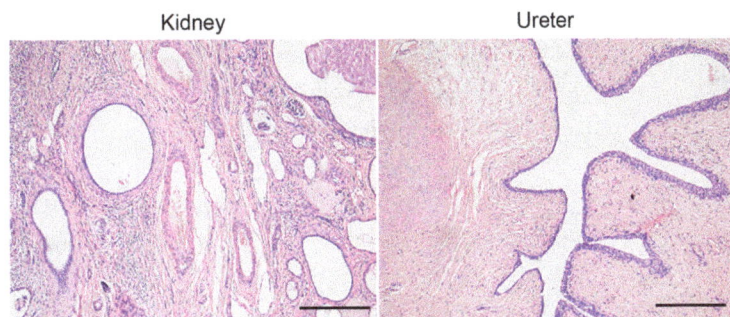

**Fig. 6** The postoperative pathologic examination shows the multicystic dysplastic kidney and ureter with fibroplasia. Bar = 100 ㎛

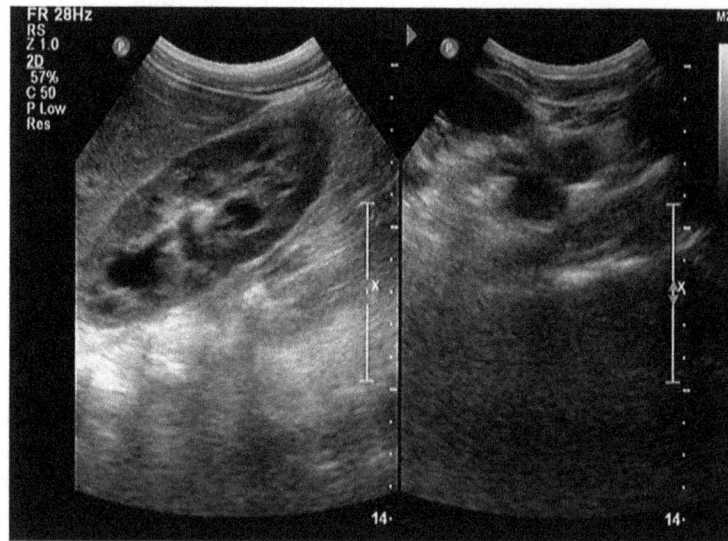

**Fig. 7** The follow-up abdominal ultrasound shows remarkably reduced right hydronephrosis

the present case, the diagnosis of CGM with the left giant ureter immediately compressing the contralateral ureter and causing bilateral hydronephrosis was made according to the physical examination and the imaging examination mainly including the abdominal ultrasound, the abdominal CT and the intravenous pyelography. Abdominal ultrasound was a basic methods to reveal the rough morphology of the kidney and ureter. Intravenous urography was the major diagnostic method, which could show the extent of the dilated ureter and renal pelvis, as well as the peristalsis and morphology of the ureter, thereby estimating the renal function. Besides, magnetic resonance urography (MRU) combined with urography could clearly reveal the features of megaureter, including the extent of the dilated ureter and renal pelvis, as well as the location of the narrow segment [17]. Therefore, MRU might be a good choice for infant patients.

The treatment of congenital megaureter is controversial. Upadhyay et al. [18] proposed an early surgical therapy, while Chertin et al. [19] suggested a conservative treatment temporarily for most patients. Compared with congenital megaureter, the treatment of CGM is specific. Ureteroureterostomy following the excision of the dilated segment or ureteral re-implantation was effective for patients with segmental dilation and the preserved renal function; however, for the patients with the whole dilated ureter and poor renal function, nephroureterectomy might be a good choice [3–5]. Noteworthily, during nephroureterectomy, it was essential to protect the compressed contralateral ureter and kidney [6].

## Conclusion

This study described an unilateral CGM with renal dysplasia compressing contralateral ureter and causing

**Table 1** Case reports on congenital giant megaureter

| Author, year | The number of cases | Age | Treatments | Follow-up | Outcomes |
|---|---|---|---|---|---|
| Huang [1], 1987 | 21 | Ranged from 2 months to 8 years | Nephrectomy/heminephrectomy and resection of the giant megaureter | - | Nineteen patients: free of urinary symptoms; One girl: died |
| | | | | | One boy: poorly recovered |
| Chiesa et al. [3], 2001 | 1 | 1-day-old | Nephroureterectomy | Four years | Uneventful with normal right renal function, a normal bladder and urethra |
| Ramaswamy et al. [4], 1995 | 1 | 2-year-old | Ureteroureterostomy. | - | Uneventful |
| Saurabh et al. [5], 2010 | 1 | 7-year-old | Surgical exploration was planned | - | - |
| Khattar et al. [6], 2009 | 1 | 15-year-old | Nephroureterectomy. | One year | Recovered well |
| Goto et al. [7], 2010 | 1 | 1-day-old | Ureteroureterostomy | Eighteen months | Experienced two febrile urinary tract infection, and no obstruction in the right upper urinary tract |
| Annigeri et al. [8], 2012 | 1 | 20-day-old | Nephroureterectomy. | Nine months | Uneventful |

bilateral hydronephrosis in a 3-year-old boy. Based on the findings of these reported literatures, CGM is rare. The physical examinations and imaging examinations are essential for the precise diagnosis of CGM, and the appropriate treatment methods such as nephrostomy, ureterolysis, ureteroureterostomy and nephroureterectomy, should be performed based on patients' specific condition. However, further studies on the pathogenesis of CGM are recommended.

## Consent

Written informed consent was obtained from the patient's parents for publication of this case report and any accompanying images.

### Abbreviations

CGM: Congenital giant megaureter; CT: Computed tomography; DPTA: Diethylene triamine pentaacetic acid; DRF: Differential renal function; MRU: Magnetic resonance urography.

### Competing interests

The authors declare that they have no competing interests.

### Authors' contributions

MY participated in the design of this study, GM performed the statistical analysis. ZG carried out the study, together with RL, and collected important background information. YG drafted the manuscript. YD conceived of this study, and participated in the design and helped to draft the manuscript. All authors read and approved the final manuscript.

### Acknowledgments

The authors thank the patient and her parents for allowing us to publish this case report.

## References

1. Huang C-J. Congenital giant megaureter. J Pediatr Surg. 1987;22:235–9.
2. Chatterjee S. Giant megaureter. Br J Urol. 1964;36:406–12.
3. Lelli-Chiesa P, Cupaioli M, Rossi C, Dòmini M, Angelone A. Congenital giant megaureter: first neonatal case. J Pediatr Surg. 2001;36:944–5.
4. Ramaswamy S, Bhatnagar V, Mitra D, Gupta A. Congenital segmental giant megaureter. J Pediatr Surg. 1995;30:123–4.
5. Saurabh G, Lahoti B, Geetika P. Giant megaureter presenting as cystic abdominal mass. Saudi J Kidney Dis Transplant. 2010;21:160.
6. Khattar N, Dorairajan LN, Kumar S, Pal BC, Elangovan S, Nayak P. Giant obstructive megaureter causing contralateral ureteral obstruction and hydronephrosis: a first-time report. Urology. 2009;74:1306–8.
7. Goto H, Kanematsu A, Yoshimura K, Miyazaki Y, Koyama T, Yorifuji T, et al. Preoperative diagnosis of congenital segmental giant megaureter presenting as a fetal abdominal mass. J Pediatr Surg. 2010;45:269–71.
8. Annigeri VM, Hegde HV, Patil PB, Halgeri AB, Rao PR. Congenital giant megaureter with duplex kidney presenting as abdominal lump in a neonate. J Indian Assoc of Pediatric Surg. 2012;17:168.
9. Wood B, Ben-Ami T, Teele R, Rabinowitz R. Ureterovesical obstruction and megaloureter: diagnosis by real-time US. Radiology. 1985;156:79–81.
10. Hemal A, Ansari M, Doddamani D, Gupta N. Symptomatic and complicated adult and adolescent primary obstructive megaureter—indications for surgery: analysis, outcome, and follow-up. Urology. 2003;61:703–7.
11. Öztürk E, Burgu B, Gülpınar Ö, Soygür T. 647 Effects of transforming growth factor on the developing embryonic ureter: An in-vitro megaureter model in mice. Eur Urol Suppl. 2013;1, e647.
12. Nicotina P, Romeo C, Arena F, Romeo G. Segmental up-regulation of transforming growth factor-β in the pathogenesis of primary megaureter. An immunocytochemical study. Br J Urol. 1997;80:946–9.
13. Mackinnon K, Foote J, Wiglesworth F, Blennerhassett J. The pathology of the adynamic distal ureteral segment. J Urol. 1970;103:134–7.
14. Notley RG. Electron microscopy of the primary obstructive megaureter. Br J Urol. 1972;44:229–34.
15. Tokunaka S, Koyanagi T. Morphologic study of primary nonreflux megaureters with particular emphasis on the role of ureteral sheath and ureteral dysplasia. J Urol. 1982;128:399–402.
16. Tokunaka S, Gotoh T, Koyanagi T, Miyabe N. Muscle dysplasia in megaureters. J Urol. 1984;131:383–90.
17. T-r L, X-k D, T-l H. Magnetic Resonance Urography and X-ray Urography Findings of Congenital Megaureter. Chin Med Sci J. 2011;26:103–8.
18. Upadhyay J, Shekarriz B, Fleming P, Gonzalez R, Barthold JS. Ureteral reimplantation in infancy: evaluation of long-term voiding function. J Urol. 1999;162:1209–12.
19. Chertin B, Pollack A, Koulikov D, Rabinowitz R, Shen O, Hain D. Long-term follow up of antenatally diagnosed megaureters. J Pediatr Urol. 2008;4:188–91.

# 20

# Acute bacterial prostatitis and abscess formation

Dong Sup Lee[1], Hyun-Sop Choe[1], Hee Youn Kim[1], Sun Wook Kim[2], Sang Rak Bae[3], Byung Il Yoon[4] and Seung-Ju Lee[1*]

## Abstract

**Background:** The purpose of this study was to identify risk factors for abscess formation in acute bacterial prostatitis, and to compare treatment outcomes between abscess group and non-abscess group.

**Methods:** This is a multicenter, retrospective cohort study. All patients suspected of having an acute prostatic infection underwent computed tomography or transrectal ultrasonography to discriminate acute prostatic abscesses from acute prostatitis without abscess formation.

**Results:** A total of 31 prostate abscesses were reviewed among 142 patients with acute prostatitis. Univariate analysis revealed that symptom duration, diabetes mellitus and voiding disturbance were predisposing factors for abscess formation in acute prostatitis. However, diabetes mellitus was not related to prostate abscess in multivariate analysis. Patients with abscesses <20 mm in size did not undergo surgery and were cured without any complications. In contrast, patients with abscesses >20 mm who underwent transurethral resection had a shorter duration of antibiotic treatment than did those who did not have surgery. Regardless of surgical treatment, both the length of hospital stay and antibiotic treatment were longer in patients with prostatic abscesses than they were in those without abscesses. However, the incidence of septic shock was not different between the two groups. A wide spectrum of microorganisms was responsible for prostate abscesses. In contrast, *Escherichia coli* was the predominant organism responsible for acute prostatitis without abscess.

**Conclusion:** Imaging studies should be considered when patients with acute prostatitis have delayed treatment and signs of voiding disturbance. Early diagnosis is beneficial because prostatic abscesses require prolonged treatment protocols, or even require surgical drainage. Surgical drainage procedures such as transurethral resection of the prostate were not necessary in all patients with prostate abscesses. However, surgical intervention may have potential merits that reduce the antibiotic exposure period and enhance voiding function in patients with prostatic abscess.

**Keywords:** Prostate, Abscess, Prostatitis, Transurethral resection of prostate

## Background

In general, abscesses form as a result of an inflammatory process that arises from an infection. Therefore, it is reasonable to assume that a prostate abscess develops from a prostatic infection. However, to the best of our knowledge, there have been no reports comparing acute prostatitis with and without abscesses. Prostate abscess is a rare condition. Only a few reports of its diagnosis and treatment have been described over several decades [1–4]. Several groups have suggested that indwelling catheters, infravesical obstruction, instrumentation of the lower urinary tract, diabetes mellitus (DM), liver disease, and prostate biopsy are predisposing factors of prostate abscess [5, 6]. These risk factors are reasonable, but not yet supported by evidence. Patients with prostate abscess must be watched closely, as they may experience a high mortality rate if adequate and proper and timely treatment does not occur [7]. However, compared to acute prostatitis without abscess, outcomes of acute prostatitis with abscess are unclear. Here, we present data from 142 acute bacterial prostatic infections and compare acute bacterial prostatitis with and without abscess.

* Correspondence: lee.seungju@gmail.com; bbangbbangi@naver.com
[1]Department of Urology, St. Vincent's Hospital, The Catholic University of Korea, College of Medicine, 93-6 Ji-dong Paldal-gu, Suwon 442-723, South Korea
Full list of author information is available at the end of the article

## Methods

### Data collection

This study is a retrospective, multicenter cohort study. Chart review for each patient was done. Distinguishable individual information was thoroughly removed during data collection. Data were gathered from four teaching hospitals with 600–1000 beds in the capital region of Korea (Seoul and Gyeonggi) using a web-based electronic system. Data were shared among all of the involved institutions. A central office managed all electronically recorded data.

### Study population and design

Any male patient between 20 and 80 years old who presented between January 2012 and December 2014 was eligible for the study. Patients were considered to have acute prostate infection if they met the following criteria: (i) one or more recent symptoms and signs such as voiding disturbance, dysuria, urgency, frequency, perineal pain, suprapubic pain or tenderness during digital rectal exam; (ii) fever (temperature of tympanic membrane >37.8 °C, [8]); and (iii) ≥5 white blood cells per high-power field in the urine. All included patients had undergone computed tomography (CT) or transrectal ultrasonography (TRUS). Such imaging studies were used to determine the presence or absence of an abscess. Successive cultures from the same patient were excluded to avoid data duplication during the treatment period. Patients with recurrent prostatitis were also excluded because the condition could negatively or positively influence susceptibility data. In order to access voiding function, uroflowmetry or post-void residual urine were checked in non-catheterized patients. Underlying diseases were reviewed based on patient medical records.

The sensitive automatic MicroScan identification system (Baxter Diagnostics, Inc., MicroScan, West Sacramento, California, USA) was used to identify causative bacteria. Minimal inhibitory concentrations (MICs) were measured using the microbroth dilution method. The following antibiotics were used to measure MICs: ampicillin, amoxicillin/clavulanic acid, cephalothin, cefoxitin, cefotaxime, ceftazidime, ciprofloxacin, imipenem, piperacillin, piperacillin/tazobactam and co-trimoxazole. A Sensitive/Intermediate/Resistant (SIR) interpretation was used for simple description and easy comparison of the data. We applied the standard Clinical and Laboratory Standards Institute guidelines to establish the MIC breakpoints.

### Statistical analysis

Student's $t$-tests or Mann–Whitney U tests were used to compare continuous variables between the two groups. The Chi-square test or Fisher's exact test was also used to perform univariate analysis of binominal variables. The logistic regression test was used for multivariate analysis. Each statistical method is also summarized beneath the corresponding table.

## Results

One hundred forty-two patients with acute prostatitis were enrolled, 31 of these showed prostatic abscess. Of all of the 142 patients, 101 were admitted to the urology department or department of infectious medicine from the emergency department and 41 patients were admitted to the urology department from outpatient clinics. 101 patients underwent CT scans in the emergency department. Among these 101 patients, there were 22 prostatic abscesses without other associated abscesses, two prostatic abscesses with liver abscesses, one prostatic abscess with a renal abscess, one prostatic abscess with a buttock abscess and one renal abscess without a prostatic abscess. 37 of 41 patients admitted from outpatient clinics underwent TRUS when their fever subsided. Based on this imaging study, three prostate abscesses were diagnosed. The remaining four patients underwent CT scanning because of persistent fever; this imaging diagnosed two prostate abscesses without metastatic abscess foci, and one liver abscess without a prostate abscess. Therefore, a total of 31 prostate abscesses were diagnosed and analyzed among a total of 142 acute bacterial prostatitis cases. The baseline patient demographic characteristics are summarized in Table 1.

In this study, the symptom duration and voiding disturbance with low Qmax (<5 ml/sec) or high residual urine (>100 ml) were associated with abscess formation in acute bacterial prostatitis. Two of 17 prostate abscess patients with voiding problems had urethral stricture. The size of the prostate tended to be larger in acute prostatitis patients with abscesses than in those without abscesses, although not significantly. Over half of the patients in the abscess group (51.6 %) had DM, while 28.8 % of non-abscess patients had DM ($p = 0.03$, $OR = 2.633$). Other underlying medical diseases were not associated with the presence of prostate abscess. Catheterization also did not exert an influence on abscess formation in this study. In multivariate analysis, symptom duration and voiding disturbances were predisposing factors for abscess formation in acute prostatitis (Table 2).

Twenty-six patients (83.8 %) with acute prostatitis with abscesses eventually underwent suprapubic cystostomy. 14 patients with prostate abscess (45.2 %) had transurethral resection of prostate (TUR-P) during the treatment period (Fig. 1). Among those 14 patients, one with a liver abscess simultaneously underwent percutaneous drainage for liver abscess. Only one patient among 15 patients who had prostate abscess larger than 20 mm in maximal diameter, did not have any procedures, and eventually died two days after admission. 16 patients with abscesses less than 20 mm in size were treated conservatively (Fig. 2a and b). Among the 30 survivors with prostatic abscesses, only one patient who

**Table 1** Demographic characteristics in 142 acute febrile prostatic infections

| | With abscess (n = 31) | Without abscess (n = 111) | Statistical results |
|---|---|---|---|
| **Underlying factors** | | | |
| Age (years)† | 62.23 ± 14.60 | 63.99 ± 14.27 | 0.546, 2.913, −7.524 ~ 3.994 |
| BMI (Kg/m²)† | 23.93 ± 4.04 | 24.05 ± 3.79 | 0.887, 0.827, −1.756 ~ 1.521 |
| PSA (ng/ml)† | 15.95 ± 11.46 | 20.76 ± 19.17 | 0.200, 3.730, −12.181 ~ 2.571 |
| Prostate size (cc)† | 47.73 ± 19.25 | 40.80 ± 17.53 | 0.063, 3.694, −0.377 ~ 14.242 |
| Abscess size (mm) | 22.03 ± 11.69 | NA | |
| | <10 mm: 4; 10 ~ 20 mm: 12; 20 ~ 30 mm: 8; >30 mm: 7 | | |
| Other abscess foci | 4; 2 liver abscesses, 1 renal abscess, 1 buttock abscess | 2; 1 liver abscess, 1 renal abscess | NA |
| Symptom duration† | 7.81 ± 5.42 | 3.04 ± 2.57 | <0.001, 0.691, 3.404 ~ 6.136 |
| **Underlying diseases** | | | |
| Diabetes mellitus‡ | 16/31 | 32/111 | 0.030, 2.633, 1.165 ~ 5.951 |
| Hypertension‡ | 11/31 | 49/111 | 0.418, 0.696, 0.305 ~ 1.589 |
| Heart disease‡ | 4/31 | 23/104 | 0.316, 0.522, 0.166 ~ 1.644 |
| Neurological deficit‡ | 10/31 | 31/111 | 0.658, 1.229, 0.520 ~ 2.903 |
| Chronic kidney disease* | 4/31 | 16/111 | 1.000, 0.880, 0.271 ~ 2.851 |
| Chronic lung disease* | 2/31 | 11/111 | 0.734, 0.627, 0.131 ~ 2.991 |
| Liver cirrhosis* | 7/31 | 15/111 | 0.261, 1.867, 0.685 ~ 5.087 |
| Previous hospitalizations‡ | 8/31 | 16/111 | 0.174, 2.065, 0.788 ~ 5.411 |
| Urological procedures* | 3/31 3 cystoscopy | 10/111 4 cystoscopy 4 prostate biopsy 2 urodynamic study | 1.000, 1.082, 0.279 ~ 4.201 0.176, 2.866, 0.606 ~ 13.553 NA NA |
| Long term catheterization* | 2/31 | 12/111 | 0.735, 0.569, 0.120 ~ 2.689 |
| Recent catheterization* | 5/31 | 8/111 | 0.158, 2.476, 0.748 ~ 8.198 |
| Voiding disturbance (Qmax < 5 or PVR > 100)‡ | 15/31 | 15/111 | <0.001, 6.000, 2.464 ~ 14.612 |
| **Treatment outcomes** | | | |
| Septic shock* | 3/31 | 3/111 | 0.118, 3.857, 0.738 ~ 20.152 |
| Death | 1/31 | 1/111 | 0.390, 3.667, 0.223 ~ 60.360 |
| Recurrence | 1/31 | 3/111 | 1.000, 1.189, 0.119 ~ 11.848 |
| Treatment duration† | 40.96 ± 10.61 | 26.98 ± 9.43 | <0.001, 2.111, 9.802 ~ 18.158 |
| With TUR-P (n = 13)[a] | 32.31 ± 9.34 | | 0.001†† |
| Without TUR-P (n = 13)[b] | 40.85 ± 7.94 | | |
| Admission duration† | 12.38 ± 6.59 | 6.69 ± 2.92 | <0.001, 1.321, 2.978 ~ 8.403 |
| With TUR-P (n = 13)[a] | 10.23 ± 2.55 | | 0.650†† |
| Without TUR-P (n = 13)[b] | 11.08 ± 9.32 | | |
| Follow-up duration† | 216.0 ± 69.92 | 202.11 ± 59.01 | 0.302, 13.391, −12.602 ~ 40.378 |

†: These continuous values are expressed as means ± standard deviations and student t-tests were performed (statistical data include p-values, standard errors and 95 % confidence intervals, respectively)

‡,*: Statistical evaluation for the nominal parameters was performed using the Chi-squared test‡ or Fisher's exact test* (statistical data include p-values, odds ratios and 95 % confidence intervals, respectively.)

††: p-values between 'a' and 'b' were evaluated using the Mann–Whitney U test. Note that all cases (n = 13) treated by TUR-P had abscesses >20 mm in size
Among the 142 cases, 6 cases with metastatic abscesses (1 patient underwent TUR-P) and 2 fatal cases were excluded when comparing the treatment duration, admission duration and follow-up duration

Abbreviations: BMI body mass index; PSA prostate specific antigen; Qmax (ml/sec) maximum urinary flow rate; PVR (ml) post-void residual; TUR-P transurethral resection of prostate

**Table 2** Multivariate analysis of risk factors for abscess formation in acute bacterial prostatitis

|  | $p$-value | OR | 95 % CI |
| --- | --- | --- | --- |
| Voiding disturbance | 0.041 | 2.749 | 1.551 ~ 12.333 |
| Diabetes mellitus | 0.153 | 2.064 | 0.764 ~ 5.575 |
| Symptom duration | <0.001 | 1.343 | 1.166-1.548 |

Statistical analysis was performed using logistic regression test

had been treated conservatively developed a recurrence within 3 months. This patient eventually underwent transurethral resection of prostate.

Six patients had additional abscess at distant sites. Among the three cases of liver abscesses, two resulted from *K. pneumoniae* infection, while the causative organism was not identified from the third. Most cases of acute prostatitis without abscess resulted from infections with *E. coli*. In contrast, various organisms were detected in cases of acute prostatitis with abscess (Table 3). S. aureus was significantly related to abscess formation ($p = 0.03$, OR = 12.222 by Fisher exact test). Squamous cell cancer was identified in one case of acute prostatitis with abscess.

In general, the treatment period with antibiotics was longer in cases of prostate abscess than in those without abscess, regardless of the surgical intervention. It is promising that patients who underwent TUR-P required shorter antibiotic treatment than did patients treated conservatively, despite the fact that the surgery group had larger prostate abscesses than did the non-surgery group (Table 1). There was no difference between prostate abscess and acute

prostatitis without abscess with regard to the incidence of septic shock.

It was difficult to compare the susceptibility of *E. coli*, *K. pneumoniae* and *P. aeruginosa* between the two groups because of the small numbers of each respective isolate in abscess group. Bacteria were detected in 120 of the 142 urinary specimens. Among these, *E. coli* was isolated in 78 specimens (65.0 %), and *K. pneumoniae* in 14 cases (11.7 %). Therefore, *E. coli* and *K. pneumoniae* consisted of 76.7 % of acute prostatitis cases in this study. Antimicrobial susceptibilities (%) of the 78 *E. coli* cases to cefoxitin (second generation cephalosporins; cefamycins), cefotaxime (third-generation cephalosporins) and ciprofloxacin (fluoroquinolones) were 75/78 (96.2), 64/78 (82.1) and 63/78 (80.8), respectively. Those of the 14 *K. pneumoniae* cases to cefoxitin, cefotaxime and ciprofloxacin were 14/14 (100.0), 14/14 (100.0) and 13/14 (92.9), respectively. Antimicrobial susceptibility results in detail were presented in Table 4. The susceptibilities of *P. aeruginosa* infection to third generation cephalosporins and to fluoroquinolones were lower than 80 % in both abscess and non-abscess group. *P. aeruginosa* infection was related to previous urological procedures (by Fisher exact test, $p = 0.002$, OR = 13.889, 2.971 < 95 % CI < 64.927).

## Discussion

One previous report described that approximately 6 % of prostatic abscesses develop in patients during the follow-up period after acute prostatitis [9]. However, prostatic abscess are often found in patients who do not improve with initial antibiotic therapy [6, 10]. Therefore, without routine

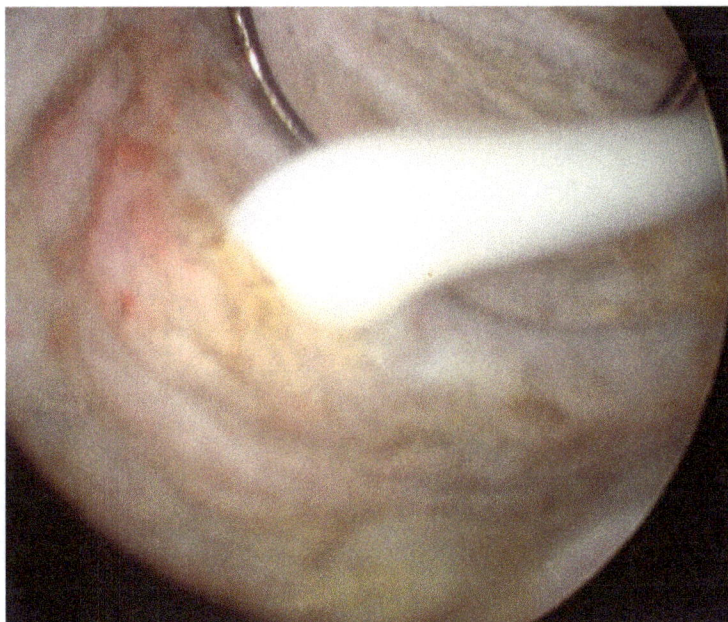

**Fig. 1** Abscess drainage with transurethral resection of the prostate

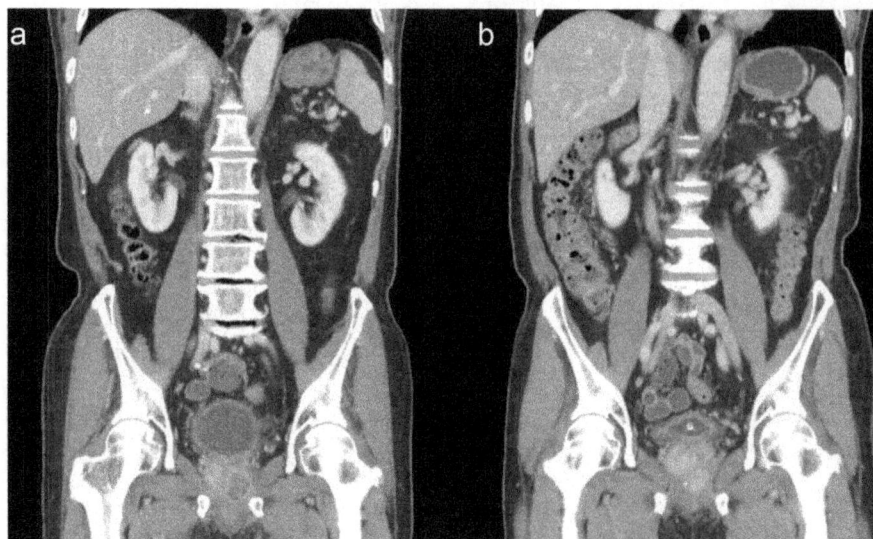

**Fig. 2** Medical treatment of prostate abscess. **a**: Before treatment (at diagnosis): an approximately 20-mm-sized abscess was identified in the left lobe of the prostate gland, **b**: After treatment (follow-up at 4 weeks): a cystostomy catheter was inserted into the urinary bladder. The previous abscess pocket was disappeared

imaging study, a prostate abscess present initially may be missed rather than developing from acute prostatitis during the follow-up period. In our 111 cases of confirmed acute prostatitis without abscess, abscess formation was not identified during the treatment period. Routine imaging studies such as CT or TRUS should be considered in cases of acute prostatitis for this reason, especially in patients with long-term symptom duration and voiding disturbances. Such imaging will allow physicians to anticipate a treatment method for an abscess, since these abscesses may require drainage [3, 7]. Ludwig et al. found that fluctuation during the digital rectal

**Table 3** Microorganisms isolated from 142 urinary specimens

| | With Abscess n (%) | Notes | Without abscess n (%) | Notes |
|---|---|---|---|---|
| E. coli | 7 (26.9) | 1 renal abscess | 71 (74.7) | 1 renal abscess, 1 death |
| K. pneumoniae | 6 (23.1) | 1 liver abscess | 8 (8.4) | 1 liver abscess |
| P. aeruginosa | 4 (15.4) | | 4 (4.2) | |
| P. mirabilis | 1 (3.8) | | 1 (1.1) | |
| K. oxytoca | 1 (3.8) | | 1 (1.1) | |
| Enterobacter aerogens | 1 (3.8) | 1 Death | 2 (2.1) | |
| Enterobacter clocae | 0 (0.0) | | 1 (1.1) | |
| Morganella morganii | 1 (3.8) | | 1 (1.1) | |
| Serratia marcescens | 0 (0.0) | | 1 (1.1) | |
| Citrobacter freudii | 0 (0.0) | | 1 (1.1) | |
| S. aureus | 3 (11.5) | 1 buttock abscess, 1 squamous cell carcinoma | 1 (1.1) | |
| E. faecalis | 1 (3.8) | | 1 (1.1) | |
| E. faecium | 0 (0.0) | | 1 (1.1) | 1 Death |
| Other GPC | 1 (3.8) | | 1 (1.1) | |
| Positive culture | 26 | | 95 | |
| Negative culture | 5 | 1 Liver abscess | 16 | |

The percentage of each microorganism against positive culture is presented in parentheses

**Table 4** Antimicrobial susceptibility of *E. coli*, *K. pneumoniae* and *P. aeruginosa* infections

| | With abscess | | | Without abscess | | |
|---|---|---|---|---|---|---|
| | *E. coli* (n (%)) | *K. pneumoniae* (n (%)) | *P. aeruginosa* (n (%)) | *E. coli* (n (%)) | *K. pneumoniae* (n (%)) | *P. aeruginosa* (n (%)) |
| Amikacin | S 7/7 (100.0) | S 6/6 (100.0) | S 3/4 (75.0) | S 71/71 (100.0) | S 8/8 (100.0) | S 4/4 (100.0) |
| | I 0/7 | I 0/6 | I 0/4 | I 0/71 | I 0/8 | I 0/4 |
| | R 0/7 | R 0/6 | R ¼ | R 0/71 | R 0/8 | R 0/4 |
| Amoxicillin | S 4/7 (57.1) | S 0/6 (0.0) | NA | S 31/71 (43.7) | S 0/8 (0.0) | NA |
| | I 0/7 | I 0/6 | | I 0/71 | I 0/8 | |
| | R3/7 | R 6/6 | | R 40/71 | R 8/8 | |
| Amoxicillin/clavulanic acid | S 5/7 (71.4) | S 6/6 (100.0) | NA | S 48/71 (67.6) | S 8/8 (100.0) | NA |
| | I 2/7 | I 0/6 | | I 17/71 | I 0/8 | |
| | R 0/7 | R 0/6 | | R 6/71 | R 0/8 | |
| Aztreonam | S 5/7 (71.4) | S 6/6 (100.0) | S 1/4 (25.0) | S 65/71 (91.5) | S 8/8 (100.0) | S 2/4 (50.0) |
| | I 0/7 | I 0/6 | I 1/4 | I 0/74 | I 0/8 | I 1/4 |
| | R 2/7 | R 0/6 | R 2/4 | R 6/74 | R 0/8 | R 1/4 |
| Cefazolin | S 5/7 (71.4) | S 6/6 (100.0) | NA | S 54/71 (76.1) | S 8/8 (100.0) | NA |
| | I 0/7 | I 0/6 | | I 0/71 | I 0/8 | |
| | R 2/7 | R 0/6 | | R 17/71 | R 0/8 | |
| Cefepime | S 5/7 (71.4) | S 6/6 (100.0) | S 3/4 (75.0) | S 67/71 (94.4) | S 8/8 (100.0) | S 3/4 (75.0) |
| | I 0/7 | I 0/6 | I 0/4 | I 0/71 | I 0/8 | I 1/4 |
| | R 2/7 | R 0/6 | R ¼ | R 4/71 | R 0/8 | R 0/4 |
| Cefotaxime | S 5/7 (71.4) | S 6/6 (100.0) | S 0/4 (0.0) | S 59/71 (83.1) | S 8/8 (100.0) | S 0/4 (0.0) |
| | I 0/7 | I 0/6 | I 0/4 | I 0/71 | I 0/8 | I 0/4 |
| | R 2/7 | R 0/6 | R 4/4 | R 12/71 | R 0/8 | R 4/4 |
| Cefoxitin | S 7/7 (100.0) | S 6/6 (100.0) | NA | S 68/71 (95.8) | S 8/8 (100.0) | NA |
| | I 0/0 | I 0/6 | | I 2/71 | I 0/8 | |
| | R 0/0 | R 0/6 | | R 1/71 | R 0/8 | |
| Ceftazidime | S 5/7 (71.4) | S 6/6 (100.0) | S 3/4 (75.0) | S 68/71 (95.8) | S 8/8 (100.0) | S 4/4 (100.0) |
| | I 0/7 | I 0/6 | I 0/4 | I 0/74 | I 0/8 | I 0/4 |
| | R 2/7 | R 0/6 | R 1/4 | R 3/71 | R 0/8 | R 0/4 |
| Ciprofloxacin | S 5/7 (71.4) | S 6/6 (100.0) | S 3/4 (75.0) | S 58/71 (81.7) | S 7/8 (87.5) | S 3/4 (75.0) |
| | I 0/7 | I 0/6 | I 0/4 | I 0/71 | I 0/8 | I 0/4 |
| | R 2/7 | R 0/6 | R 1/4 | R 13/71 | R 1/8 | R 1/4 |
| Imipenem | S 7/7 (100.0) | S 6/6 (100.0) | S 4/4 (100.0) | S 71/71 (100.0) | S 8/8 (100.0) | S 4/4 (100.0) |
| | I 0/0 | I 0/6 | I 0/4 | I 0/71 | I 0/8 | I 0/4 |
| | R 0/0 | R 0/6 | R 0/4 | R 0/71 | R 0/8 | R 0/4 |
| Piperacillin/tazobactam | S 7/7 (100.0) | S 6/6 (100.0) | S 2/4 (50.0) | S 68/71 (95.8) | S 7/8 (87.5) | S 4/4 (100.0) |
| | I 0/0 | I 0/6 | I 1/4 | I 1/71 | I 1/8 | I 0/4 |
| | R 0/0 | R 0/6 | R 1/4 | R 2/71 | R 0/8 | R 0/4 |
| Cotrimoxazole | S 5/7 (71.4) | S 6/6 (100.0) | S 0/4 (0.0) | S 56/71 (78.9) | S 6/8 (75.0) | S 0/4 (0.0) |
| | I 0/7 | I 0/6 | I 0/4 | I 0/71 | I 0/8 | I 0/4 |
| | R 2/7 | R 0/6 | R 4/4 | R 15/71 | R 2/8 | R 4/4 |

Susceptible categories (S/I/R: Sensitive/Intermediate/Resistant)

exam was present in 83.3 % of prostate abscesses. The group agreed that additional imaging is necessary to avoid missing a diagnosis of prostate abscess [2].

DM was a predisposing factor for abscess formation in univariate analysis. Studies of prostate abscesses commonly emphasize that DM is the most important predisposing medical condition [2, 3, 11]. However, diabetes by itself was not a risk factor for prostate abscess in multivariate analysis in the present study. DM is undoubtedly a serious condition that increases the risk of infection with uro-pathogens [12, 13]. However, its role in the development of prostatic abscess remains unclear and requires further investigation. Voiding disturbance was a significant risk factor for prostate abscess in the present study. Therefore, physicians should monitor voiding status in patients with acute prostatitis. In doing so, a physician can decide whether or not to perform a urinary diversion, such as suprapubic cystostomy, or to conduct imaging for the early diagnosis of a prostate abscess.

Abscess drainage with transurethral resection of prostate (TUR-P) was done in 45.2 % (14/31) of patients with prostatic abscess. The other 55.8 % of patients with abscesses only required medical treatment. We excluded confounding factors including one patient death, and 4 patients with other abscess foci when comparing the TUR-P group and medical treatment group in 31 abscesses. With regard to the length of hospital stay, it seems that medical treatment was non-inferior to surgical procedures in the treatment of prostatic abscesses. If we did not perform TUR-P in patient with prostate abscess over 20 mm, hospital stay might be longer in abscess patients. The duration of antibiotic treatment was longer in the medical treatment group (Table 1) than it was in the surgical group despite the cases treated with TUR-P had larger size of abscess pockets than the medical cases. Because TUR-P group and medical treatment group have different sizes of prostate abscess, and relevant cases in prostate abscess ($n = 26$) were small for comparison between TUR-P ($n = 13$) and medical treatment ($n = 13$), comparing treatment outcomes in 26 prostate abscesses may have potentially less clinically significant in the present study. However, considering there are wide concerns of antibiotic resistance in the community, minimizing the duration of exposure to antibiotics is an important issue. Furthermore, voiding disturbances were reflected in a large proportion of patients with prostate abscesses according to the present study. So, patients who underwent TUR-P might have an advantage. Therefore, TUR-P should be recommended to patients with prostate abscesses, although surgical procedures are not necessary for relatively small abscesses.

Regardless of the surgical procedure, the presence of a prostatic abscess did not increase the risk of septic shock during treatment. In our experience, patients with prostate abscesses require long-term antibiotic treatment and potentially surgery depending on abscess size. However, abscess formation may not exert an influence on the prognosis, such as septic shock or death, under the assumption that they were treated appropriately.

The vast majority of acute prostatitis were infected by gram negative bacteria. Regardless of the presence of an abscess, the selection of empirical antibiotics with cefoxitin, cefotaxime or ciprofloxacin would be appropriate in patients with acute prostatitis who have not undergone urological procedure (s) in Korea. Nevertheless, clinicians should be ready to adjust the antibiotic regimen according to susceptibility data, especially in the case of prostate abscess. This is because unexpected microorganisms are more likely to be isolated in acute prostatitis with abscess than in those without abscess.

This study has limitations. It is a retrospective, multicentre chart review in design which has potential biases associated with it, however designing a randomised control trial comparing treatment outcome in 2 groups of equally matched patients with prostatic abscess is not feasible given the rarity, severity of the disease and heterogeneity of management for this condition throughout the urological community.

## Conclusions

Ulleryd et al. concluded that [14] routine radiological exams are dispensable in men with febrile urinary tract infection. However, it would be wise to perform imaging studies in patients who are suspected to have acute prostatitis when their symptom duration is relatively long, or any evidence of voiding disturbance. Acute prostatitis with abscess requires long-term antibiotic treatment, and sometimes even surgical drainage. Surgical procedures such as TUR-P in patients with prostatic abscesses are advantageous because they reduce the period of antibiotic treatment and may improve voiding symptoms. A wide range of microorganisms may be detected in prostatitis with abscess. Therefore, physicians should perform urine culture prior to administering empirical antibiotics. These cultures should be repeated, if possible, during treatment. With appropriate treatment, the prognosis of acute prostatitis with and without abscess would not differ.

**Abbreviations**
CT, computed tomography; DM, diabetes mellitus; TRUS, transrectal ultrasonography; TUR-P, transurethral resection of prostate

**Acknowledgements**
The authors would like to thank In-ae Park for his/her assistance in gathering and sorting data from the multicenter network system.

**Funding**
Noting to declare.

**Authors' contributions**
Study design was done by DSL and SJL, acquisition of data was done by HSC, HYK, SWK, SRB and BIY, analysis and interpretation of data was performed by DSL, HSC and HYK, drafting of manuscript was done by DSL, and all authors read and approved the final manuscript.

**Competing interests**

The authors declare that they have no competing interests.

**Author details**

[1]Department of Urology, St. Vincent's Hospital, The Catholic University of Korea, College of Medicine, 93-6 Ji-dong Paldal-gu, Suwon 442-723, South Korea. [2]Department of Urology, Yeouido St. Mary's Hospital, The Catholic University of Korea, College of Medicine, Seoul, South Korea. [3]Department of Urology, Uijeongbu St. Mary's Hospital, The Catholic University of Korea, College of Medicine, Uijeongbu, South Korea. [4]Department of Urology, International St. Mary's Hospital, Catholic Kwandong University, Incheon, South Korea.

**References**

1. Granados EA, Riley G, Salvador J, et al. Prostatic abscess: Diagnosis and treatment. J Urol. 1992;148(1):80–2.
2. Ludwig M, Schroeder-Printzen I, Schiefer HG, Weidner W. Diagnosis and therapeutic management of 18 patients with prostatic abscess. Urology. 1999;53(2):340–5.
3. Jang K, Lee DH, Lee SH, Chung BH. Treatment of prostatic abscess: case collection and comparison of treatment methods. Korean J Urol. 2012; 53(12):860–4.
4. Elshal AM, Abdelhalim A, Barakat TS, Shaaban AA, Nabeeh A, Ibrahiem E-H. Prostatic abscess: Objective assessment of the treatment approach in the absence of guidelines. Arab J Urol. 2014;12(4):262–8.
5. Trauzzi SJ, Kay CJ, Kaufman DG, Lowe FC. Management of prostatic abscess in patients with human immunodeficiency syndrome. Urology. 1994;43(5): 629–33.
6. Brede CM, Shoskes DA. The etiology and management of acute prostatitis. Nat Rev Urol. 2011;8(4):207–12.
7. Aravantinos E, Kalogeras N, Zygoulakis N, Kakkas G, Anagnostou T, Melekos M. Ultrasound-guided transrectal placement of a drainage tube as therapeutic management of patients with prostatic abscess. J Endourol. 2008;22(8):1751–4.
8. Sund-Levander M, Forsberg C, Wahren LK, Forsberg W. Normal oral, rectal, tympanic and axillary body temperature in adult men and women: a systematic literature review. Scand J Caring Sci. 2002;16(2):122–8.
9. Ha US, Kim ME, Kim CS, Shim BS, Han CH, Lee SD, Cho YH. Acute bacterial prostatitis in Korea: clinical outcome, including symptoms, management, microbiology and course of disease. Int J Antimicrob Agents. 2008;31 Suppl 1: S96–S101.
10. Davidson KC, Garlow WB, Brewer J. Computerized tomography of prostatic and periurethral abscesses: 2 case reports. J Urol. 1986;135:1257–8.
11. Tiwari P, Pal DK, Tripathi A, Kumar S, Vijay M, Goel A, Sharma P, Dutta A, Kundu AK. Prostatic abscess: diagnosis and management in the modern antibiotic era. Saudi J Kidney Dis Transpl. 2011;22(2):298–301.
12. Nitzan O, Elias M, Chazan B, Saliba W. Urinary tract infections in patients with type 2 diabetes mellitus: review of prevalence, diagnosis, and management. Diabetes Metab Syndr Obes. 2015;8:129–36.
13. Muller LM, Gorter KJ, Hak E, Goudzwaard WL, Schellevis FG, Hoepelman AI, Rutten GE. Increased risk of common infections in patients with type 1 and type 2 diabetes mellitus. Clin Infect Dis. 2005;41(3):281–8.
14. Ulleryd P. Febrile urinary tract infection in men. Int J Antimicrob Agents. 2003;22(2003):S89–93.

# 21

# Different expression of B7-H3 in the caput, corpus, and cauda of the epididymis in mouse

Kai Li[1†], Xuedong Wei[1†], Guangbo Zhang[2], Miao Li[1], Xuefeng Zhang[1], Chenhao Zhou[1], Jianquan Hou[1*] and Hexing Yuan[1*]

## Abstract

**Background:** B7-H3, a member of the B7 family of the Ig superfamily of proteins, has been detected in the epididymis, which is a storage organ related to sperm maturation. However, the characteristics of its expression in different regions of the epididymis remain unknown. Our aim was to investigate the expression of B7-H3 in the caput, corpus, and cauda of the epididymis.

**Methods:** We extracted epididymis specimens from adult male C57BL/6 mice. The expression of B7-H3 was then measured with immunohistochemistry, enzyme-linked immunosorbent assay (ELISA) and western blotting.

**Results:** B7-H3 protein was predominantly detected on the membrane and in the cytoplasm of the principal cells in the epididymis. Moreover, the level of B7-H3 in the corpus of the mouse epididymis was significantly higher than that in the caput ($p < 0.05$) or the cauda of the epididymis ($P < 0.05$). However, there was no remarkable difference in the level of B7-H3 between the caput and the cauda ($p > 0.05$).

**Conclusions:** The caput, corpus, and cauda of the mouse epididymis all expressed B7-H3 protein. However, the levels of B7-H3 were different in the three regions of the epididymis.

**Keywords:** B7-H3, Caput, Corpus, Cauda, Epididymis, Sperm maturation, Mouse

## Background

The epididymis is a storage organ of sperm and is related to male fertility. From proximal to distal, the epididymis is divided into caput, corpus, and cauda regions. This conventional division has been widely used in studies on the biological functions of the epididymis, including studies of gene expression, protein secretion, and many aspects of sperm maturation [1]. The epididymis provides a specific environment which plays an essential role in promoting the final maturation of sperm [2]. It can take sperm a few days to weeks to travel throughout the epididymis. During this time almost all of sperm gradually acquire natural fertilizing ability – including progressive motility, the ability to undergo capacitation and hyperactivation [3]. The epididymal epithelium has the functions of secretion and absorption. At least 66% of identified proteins can be secreted into the epididymal fluid [4]. A series of interactions between sperm and some specific proteins present in the epididymal fluid are believed to contribute to the final maturation of sperm [5].

B7-H3, also known as CD276, a novel member of the B7 immunoregulatory family, was initially identified from a human dendritic cell cDNA library in 2001 [6]. It is a 316-amino acid (aa) type I transmembrane glycoprotein [7]. This protein also exists in a soluble form. A study by our group reported that soluble B7-H3 could be detected in expressed prostatic secretions of the healthy donors and patients with chronic prostatitis [8]. Several studies have indicated that B7-H3 protein is expressed in dendritic cells, the heart and kidneys [9] as well as genital tissues, such as prostate, testis, and epididymis [10]. In the current study, B7-H3 is mainly thought to have a significant role in the immune system. Initial experiments reported that

* Correspondence: xf192@163.com; YHXurology@163.com
†Equal contributors
[1]Department of Urology, The First Affiliated Hospital of Soochow University, NO.188 Shizi Road, Suzhou 215006, Jiangsu, China
Full list of author information is available at the end of the article

B7-H3 might upregulate T cell activation [10] and promote T cell proliferation, as well as cytokine production [9, 11]. However, some subsequent studies showed that B7-H3 had a negative regulatory function in T cell -mediated immune responses both in vitro and in vivo [12, 13]. Moreover, some recent reports provided novel insights into the nonimmunological role of B7-H3 protein. Sun et al. suggested that B7-H3 could inhibit the expression of vascular endothelial growth factor (VEGF) [14], while Xu et al. found that the stimulation of B7-H3 could promote the differentiation of human marrow stromal cells (hMSCs) into osteoblasts [15]. Furthermore, B7-H3 is also expressed in fibroblast-like synoviocytes and other fibroblasts [16]. Consequently, the biological functions of B7-H3 remain unclear.

Suh et al. discovered that B7-H3 was expressed in the epididymis [10]. Additionally, a previous study by our group showed that in vitro, B7-H3 could promote sperm progressive motility [17]. Due to these findings, we focused on: (1) whether B7-H3 is expressed in all regions of the mouse epididymis, and (2) whether the levels of B7-H3 expressed in the caput, corpus, and cauda of the mouse epididymis are different.

## Methods

### Animals and samples collection

The experimental protocol was approved by the animal ethics committee of Soochow University. All procedures in the project were executed based on the guidelines for animal experiments. Male C57BL/6 mice for this research were purchased from Suzhou sealop match Biological Technology Co. Ltd. All of these mice were at ten weeks of age. All mice were kept in mesh bottom cages, and the room temperature was maintained at 22–25 °C. All mice had free access to water and food. The epididymis tissues were obtained fresh from twelve mice, which were randomly divided into three groups according to Johnston et al.[18]. Each epididymis was then segmented into caput, corpus, and cauda regions for ELISA (Fig. 1). Samples from ten mice were used in western blotting for each independent experiment. For immunohistochemical staining three mice had their epididymides extracted.

### Immunohistochemistry

The protocol of immunohistochemical staining was performed according to Li et al. [19]. Briefly, the paraffin -embedded epididymis tissues were cut into sections of 4 μm. The sections were dewaxed in xylene and rehydrated in a graded dilution of ethanol solutions, followed by heating the sections at 100 °C for 30 min in citrate solution. Endogenous peroxidase activity was blocked with 0.3% hydrogen peroxide for 20 min and washed with phosphate–buffered saline(PBS). Then, these sections were blocked with 5% BSA and incubated with B7-H3 antibody (dilution 1:200, Proteintech, China), overnight at 4 °C. These sections were then washed with PBS, and horseradish peroxidase -conjugated goat anti -rabbit IgG antibody was used as secondary antibody. Finally, the sections were counterstained with hematoxylin.

### ELISA

During preparation, each tissue sample was collected, divided into three regions (Fig. 1) and weighted using the same method. Each region was cut into pieces of 1 mm$^3$ and digested with IV collagenase for about 1 h (hour) at 37 °C. Then, the samples were prepared with PBS and homogenized in cell lysis buffer containing a protease inhibitor produced at our laboratory. After incubation on ice for 30 min (minutes), the homogenate was centrifuged at 14000 X gravity for 20 min at 4 °C and the supernatant was collected for ELISA assay. We used enzyme-linked immunosorbent assay kits, produced by Suzhou Bi Liya Biotechnology Co. Ltd, to measure B7-H3 in the caput, corpus, and cauda of the epididymis. These assay kits are specific for mouse B7-H3 at 1.0 ng/ml

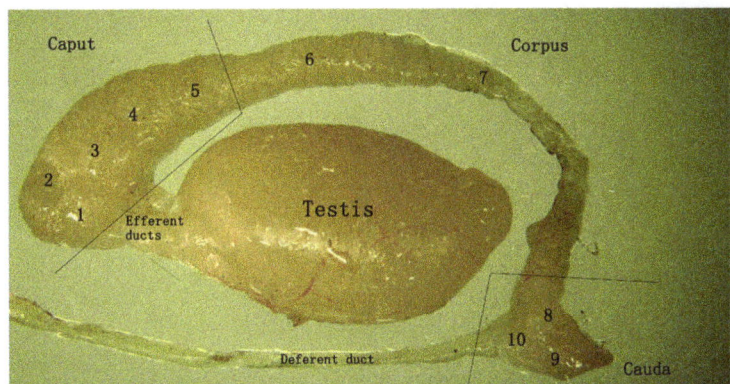

**Fig. 1** Mouse testis and epididymis. The epididymis was subdivided into 10 segments (1–10): 1–5, caput; 6–7, corpus; 8–10, cauda

minimum detectable dose. The procedures were performed as recommended by the manufacturer. Assays were read at 450 nm in a Thermo Multiskan Mk3 microplate reader (Labsystems, Helsinki, Finland). We used a standard curve to determine B7-H3 concentration.

### Western blotting

Ten mice for each independent experiment were randomly selected for Western blotting. All epididymis tissues were dissected and homogenized in cell lysis buffer containing protease inhibitors. After homogenization and centrifugation, the supernatant was collected for Western blotting. The proteins were then extracted in 6 x SDS–PAGE sample loading buffer. The proteins were then separated by 10% SDS-PAGE and transferred to a 0.45 mm PVDF membrane for approximately 300 mA for 90 min. After transfer, the membrane was blocked in 5% fat-free milk/1xTBS/0.1%Tween for 1 h at room temperature, and incubated with B7-H3 antibody (dilution 1:1000, Lianke, China) and GAPDH antibody (dilution 1:1000, Sigma) overnight at 4 °C. The membrane was then incubated with the secondary antibody of horseradish peroxidase -conjugated goat anti-rabbit IgG antibody (dilution 1:10,000, Lianke, China) for 1 h at room temperature. The blots were visualized using the BeyoECL Plus substrate system (Beyotime, China). Equal protein loading was confirmed by measurement of GAPDH.

### Statistical analysis

Data are shown as means ± standard deviation, and all statistical analyses were performed using GraphPad Prism 5.0. The Students $t$-test was used for between-group comparisons. Values with $P < 0.05$ were considered to indicate statistically significant differences.

### Results

#### Segmentation of the mouse epididymis

The epididymis was subdivided into ten segments (Fig. 1) by a method used previously [18]. Large epididymal regions (caput, corpus, cauda) were used in this study. We extracted the epididymis specimens carefully with the help of a dissecting microscope. Slight variations between epididymides with respect to the shape and size of specific segments were identified. However, three large regions were identified precisely and consistently.

#### Localization of B7-H3 in mouse epididymis

Immunohistochemical staining (Fig. 2) showed that B7-H3 staining was positive both on the membrane and in the cytoplasm of the principal cells in mouse epididymides from all regions. Moreover, the immunopositive signals of B7-H3 in the corpus were the highest of all three regions of the epididymis.

#### Different levels of B7-H3 in the three regions of the epididymis

As shown in Fig. 3, the levels of B7-H3 in the caput, corpus, and cauda of the epididymis were different. The level of B7-H3 protein in the corpus of the epididymis was significantly higher than that in the caput ($24.121 \pm 2.275$ versus $19.268 \pm 1.583$ ng/ml, $P < 0.05$) and in the cauda ($24.121 \pm 2.275$ versus $18.712 \pm 0.088$ ng/ml, $P < 0.05$) of the epididymis. However, there was no obvious difference in the levels of B7-H3 between the caput and the cauda of the epididymis ($19.268 \pm 1.583$ versus $18.712 \pm 0.088$ ng/ml, $P = 0.5764$). These results were consistent with the Western blotting data (Fig. 4).

### Discussion

At present, research on the role of B7-H3 protein has become a subject of great interest. However, most studies on B7-H3 have focused only on its immunological function. Very few studies have investigated the effects of this protein in the male reproductive field. The mammalian epididymis is the site of post-testicular sperm maturation and storage [20]. To date, large epididymal regions (caput, corpus, cauda) have been used in most studies on protein expression [18]. Each region of the epididymis contributes to the maturation, transport, concentration, or storage of sperm [21]. However, reports about the expression of B7-H3 are rare. As such, the questions of whether B7-H3 is expressed in all regions of the mouse epididymis and

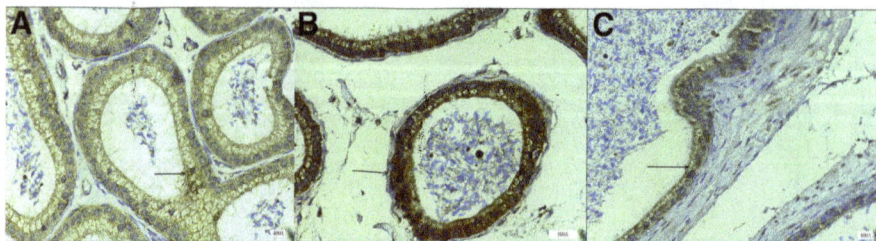

**Fig. 2** B7-H3 protein detected by Immunohistochemistry. **a** Section from the caput of the epididymis (magnification: [**a**] ×400); **b** Section from the corpus of the epididymis(magnification: [**b**] ×400); **c** Section from the cauda of the epididymis (magnification:[**c**] ×400). *Black arrows* indicate immunopositive epididymis epithelial cells

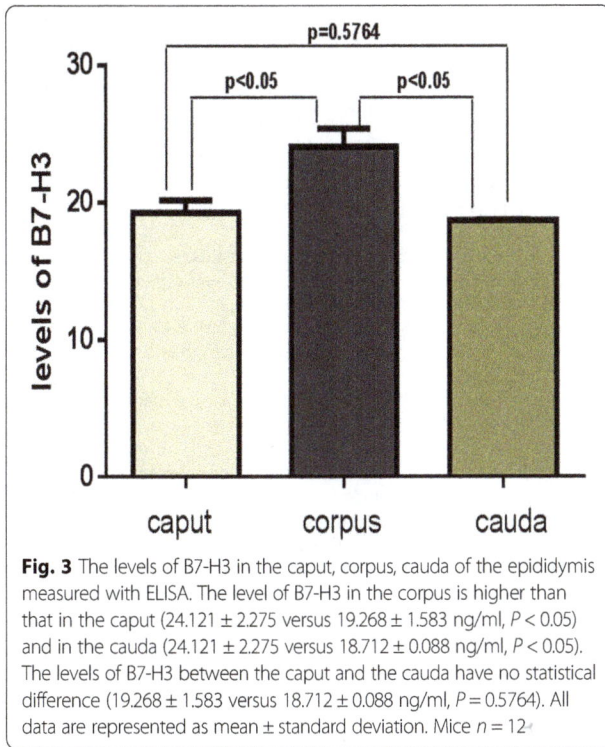

**Fig. 3** The levels of B7-H3 in the caput, corpus, cauda of the epididymis measured with ELISA. The level of B7-H3 in the corpus is higher than that in the caput ($24.121 \pm 2.275$ versus $19.268 \pm 1.583$ ng/ml, $P < 0.05$) and in the cauda ($24.121 \pm 2.275$ versus $18.712 \pm 0.088$ ng/ml, $P < 0.05$). The levels of B7-H3 between the caput and the cauda have no statistical difference ($19.268 \pm 1.583$ versus $18.712 \pm 0.088$ ng/ml, $P = 0.5764$). All data are represented as mean $\pm$ standard deviation. Mice $n = 12$

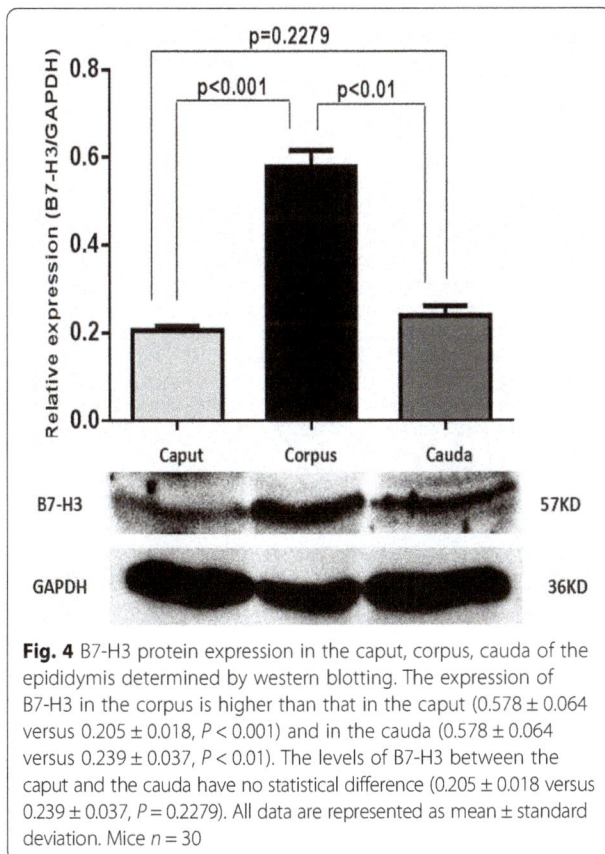

**Fig. 4** B7-H3 protein expression in the caput, corpus, cauda of the epididymis determined by western blotting. The expression of B7-H3 in the corpus is higher than that in the caput ($0.578 \pm 0.064$ versus $0.205 \pm 0.018$, $P < 0.001$) and in the cauda ($0.578 \pm 0.064$ versus $0.239 \pm 0.037$, $P < 0.01$). The levels of B7-H3 between the caput and the cauda have no statistical difference ($0.205 \pm 0.018$ versus $0.239 \pm 0.037$, $P = 0.2279$). All data are represented as mean $\pm$ standard deviation. Mice $n = 30$

whether the levels of B7-H3 are different in all regions are interesting.

In this study, we examined the expression of B7-H3 in the different regions of the epididymis. Immunohistochemical staining (Fig. 2) revealed that B7-H3 protein could be detected in the caput, corpus, and cauda of the epididymis, and it was mainly located on the membrane and in the cytoplasm of the principal cells in the epididymis epithelium. Andonian et al. [22] reported that the principal cells were active in the synthesis of proteins which would be secreted into the lumen of the epididymis in a merocrine manner. It is now widely recognized that sperm maturation in the epididymis mainly results from sequential interactions with proteins secreted by the epididymal epithelium [3]. Moreover, our previous study found that seminal B7-H3 could promote sperm progressive motility and sperm concentrations are related to the seminal B7-H3 level [17]. A putative receptor for B7-H3 was also detected on the surface of sperm by our group [17]. These findings provide the basis for our hypothesis that B7-H3 can be secreted into the epididymal fluid by principal cells to contribute to epididymal sperm maturation after binding to a putative receptor on the surface of the sperm.

In addition, we determined the B7-H3 levels in the caput, corpus, and cauda of the epididymis by ELISA (Fig. 3) and western blotting (Fig. 4). Our results showed that the level of B7-H3 in the corpus of the epididymis was significantly higher than that in the caput and in the cauda of the epididymis. However, the differences in the B7-H3 levels between the caput and the cauda of the epididymis were not statistically significant. A previous study reported that the composition of the epididymal fluid protein changed continuously throughout the epididymal duct [3]. Moreover, Jelinsky et al. indicated that regional differences of the epididymis were vital to establish the luminal environment, which was required for sperm maturation [1]. As such, another hypothesis highlighted by this research is that the different levels of B7-H3 found across the three regions of the epididymis may be necessary for epididymal sperm maturation.

This study demonstrated for the first time that the levels of B7-H3 expressed in three regions of the epididymis were different. We acknowledge that our study represents preliminary results and that further experiments are needed to confirm our findings. There are also some further limitations of our study. First, all the data in this study were generated from mouse epididymides because it is difficult to obtain epididymis tissues from healthy humans. Second, despite the fact that we found that B7-H3 was expressed in all regions of mouse epididymis, the present study did not investigate its biological functions in these locations. Therefore, our future work will include exploring the effects of B7-H3 on sperm maturation in epididymis and the related mechanism.

## Conclusions

Our study demonstrated that B7-H3 was expressed in the caput, corpus, and cauda of the epididymis. However, the levels of B7-H3 expressed in three regions of the epididymis were different, which may be important for sperm maturation in the epididymis.

## Abbreviations

ELISA: Enzyme-linked immunosorbent assay; hMSCs: Human marrow stromalb cells; PBS: Phosphate–buffered saline; VEGF: Vascular endothelial growth factor

## Acknowledgements

Not applicable.

## Funding

This work was supported by grants from the National Natural Science Foundation of China (Grant No.81300537) and, Science and Technology Development Program of Suzhou (Grant No.SYS201453).

## Authors'contributions

KL and XW designed the study, experiments, data analysis, and drafted the manuscript. GZ contributed to the design of the study, experiments and data analysis. ML and CZ contributed the experiments. HY and JH conceived of and designed the study and supervised the work. All authors read and approved the final manuscript.

## Authors' information

Hexing Yuan and Jianquan Hou are the corresponding authors. Kai Li and Xuedong Wei have contributed equally to this study and are considered to be co-first authors.

## Competing interests

The authors declare that they have no competing interests.

## Author details

[1]Department of Urology, The First Affiliated Hospital of Soochow University, NO.188 Shizi Road, Suzhou 215006, Jiangsu, China. [2]The Institute of Clinical Immunology, The First Affiliated Hospital of Soochow University, NO. 708 Renmin Road, Suzhou 215006, China.

## References

1. Jelinsky SA, Turner TT, Bang HJ, Finger JN, Solarz MK, Wilson E, et al. The Rat epididymal transcriptome: comparison of segmental gene expression in the Rat and mouse epididymides. Biol Reprod. 2007;76(4):561–70.
2. Dacheux J, Dacheux F, Druart X. Epididymal protein markers and fertility. Anim Reprod Sci. 2016;169:76–87.
3. Guyonnet B, Dacheux F, Dacheux JL, Gatti JL. The epididymal transcriptome and proteome provide some insights into New epididymal regulations. J Androl. 2011;32(6):651–64.
4. Belleannée C, Labas V, Teixeira-Gomes A, Gatti JL, Dacheux J, Dacheux F. Identification of luminal and secreted proteins in bull epididymis. J Proteomics. 2011;74(1):59–78.
5. Dacheux J, Castella S, Gatti JL, Dacheux F. Epididymal cell secretory activities and the role of proteins in boar sperm maturation. Theriogenology. 2005;63(2):319–41.
6. Yuan H, Wei X, Zhang G, Li C, Zhang X, Hou J. B7-H3 over expression in prostate cancer promotes tumor cell progression. J Urol. 2011;186(3):1093–9.
7. Wang L, Kang F, Shan B. B7-H3-mediated tumor immunology: friend or foe? Int J Cancer. 2014;134(12):2764–71.
8. Wei X, Zhang G, Yuan H, Ding X, Li S, Zhang X, et al. Detection and quantitation of soluble B7-H3 in expressed prostatic secretions: a novel marker in patients with chronic prostatitis. J Urol. 2011;185(2):532–7.
9. Chapoval AI, Ni J, Lau JS, Wilcox RA, Flies DB, Liu D, et al. B7-H3: a costimulatory molecule for T cell activation and IFN-gamma production. Nat Immunol. 2001;2(3):269–74.
10. Suh WK, Wang SX, Jheon AH, Moreno L, Yoshinaga SK, Ganss B, et al. The immune regulatory protein B7-H3 promotes osteoblast differentiation and bone mineralization. Proc Natl Acad Sci U S A. 2004;101(35):12969–73.
11. Lupu C, Eisenbach C, Kuefner M, Schmidt J, Lupu A, Stremmel W, et al. An orthotopic colon cancer model for studying the B7-H3 antitumor effect in vivo. J Gastrointest Surg. 2006;10(5):635–45.
12. Suh W, Gajewska BU, Okada H, Gronski MA, Bertram EM, Dawicki W, et al. The B7 family member B7-H3 preferentially down-regulates T helper type 1–mediated immune responses. Nat Immunol. 2003;4(9):899–906.
13. Ling V, Wu PW, Spaulding V, Kieleczawa J, Luxenberg D, Carreno BM, et al. Duplication of primate and rodent B7-H3 immunoglobulin V- and C-like domains: divergent history of functional redundancy and exon loss. Genomics. 2003;82(3):365–77.
14. Sun J, Guo YD, Li XN, Zhang YQ, Gu L, Wu PP, et al. B7-H3 expression in breast cancer and upregulation of VEGF through gene silence. Onco Targets Ther. 2014;7:1979–86.
15. Xu L, Zhang G, Zhou Y, Chen Y, Xu W, Wu S, et al. Stimulation of B7-H3 (CD276) directs the differentiation of human marrow stromal cells to osteoblasts. Immunobiology. 2011;216(12):1311–7.
16. Tran CN, Thacker SG, Louie DM, Oliver J, White PT, Endres JL, et al. Interactions of T cells with fibroblast-like synoviocytes: role of the B7 family costimulatory ligand B7-H3. J Immunol. 2008;180(5):2989–98.
17. Wei X, Li Z, Zhang G, Yuan H, Lv J, Jiang Y, et al. B7-H3 Promoted Sperm Motility in Humans. Urology. 2014;83(2):324–30.
18. Johnston DS. The mouse epididymal transcriptome: transcriptional profiling of segmental gene expression in the epididymis [J]. Biol Reprod. 2005; 73(3):404–13.
19. Li M, Zhang G, Zhang X, Lv G, Wei X, Yuan H, et al. Overexpression of B7-H3 in CD14+ monocytes is associated with renal cell carcinoma progression. Med Oncol. 2014;31(12):349.
20. Robaire B, Hinton B. The epididymis: from molecules to clinical practice. New York: Kluwer Academic/Plenum Publishers; 2002.
21. Robaire B. Efferent ducts, epididymis, and vas deferens: structure, functions and their regulation. In: Knobil E, Neil J, editors. Physiology of reproduction, vol. 1. New York: Raven; 1988. p. 999–1080.
22. Andonian S, Hermo L. Cell- and region-rpecific localization of lysosomal and secretory proteins and endocytic receptors in epithelial cells of the cauda epididymidis and vas deferens of the adult rat. J Androl. 1999;20(3):415–29.

# 22

# Performance of 5-aminolevulinic-acid-based photodynamic diagnosis for radical prostatectomy

Hideo Fukuhara[1], Keiji Inoue[1*], Atsushi Kurabayashi[2], Mutsuo Furihata[2] and Taro Shuin[1]

## Abstract

**Background:** The aim of this study was to investigate whether we could detect positive surgical margins during open and laparoscopic radical prostatectomy by 5-aminolevulinic acid (ALA) photodynamic diagnosis (PDD) and mapping of red fluorescence in human prostate cancer cells.

**Methods:** All 52 patients were diagnosed with prostate cancer by biopsy. They had a positive core in the apex or highly suspicious positive margins. Open and laparoscopic radical prostatectomy was performed in 18 and 34 cases, respectively. One gram of ALA solution was given intraoperatively, orally through a stomach tube. An endoscopic PDD system, including a D-Light C, CCU Tricam SLII/3CCD CH Tricam-P PDD, and HOPKINS II Straight Forward Telescope 0°, was used. The D-Light C light source was equipped with a band-pass filter. The CCU Tricam SLII/3CCD CHTricam-P PDD video camera system was equipped with a long-pass filter. The laparoscopy optic component was equipped with a yellow long-pass filter.

**Results:** One of the 52 patients had a red-fluorescent-positive margin of the excised whole prostate and the positive surgical margin was histologically confirmed. In the section of excised prostate, we obtained 141 biopsied samples. The sensitivity and specificity were 75.0 % and 87.3 %, respectively.

**Conclusions:** Intraoperative ALA-PDD is feasible. However, heat degeneration and length of positive surgical margin have crucial influences on red fluorescence. In future, a randomized clinical trial should be carried out.

## Background

The number of new prostate cancer cases in Japan has shown a consistent increase due to widespread acceptance of prostate-specific antigen (PSA) mass screening. The number of prostate cancer cases in Japan reached ~42,000 in 2006 [1]. Radical prostatectomy for localized prostate cancer is a highly effective standard treatment modality. However, the rate of positive surgical margins for radical prostatectomy was reported to be 14–26 % [2–5]. Positive surgical margins in prostate cancer are a significant risk factor for biochemical recurrence and lead to unfavorable prognosis [6–9].

5-Aminolevulinic acid (ALA) is a naturally occurring metabolite that is a precursor of porphyrin in heme biosynthesis. Exogenous ALA leads to accumulation of the potent photosensitizer protoporphyrin (Pp)IX in mitochondria. PpIX is known to accumulate more in malignant and proliferating tissues than in normal tissues [10–14]. In this way, PpIX selectively accumulates at a significant level in tumor cells. PpIX is an effective photosensitizer and fluorescent substance in heme biosynthesis.

5-ALA-mediated photodynamic diagnosis (PDD) is used widely in various cancers, including bladder cancer. If we could adapt this technique to PDD during radical prostatectomy, we could improve the rate of positive surgical margins. Zaak et al. and Adam et al. reported the feasibility of intraoperative ALA-PDD for the detection of positive surgical margins [15, 16].

In this study, we focused on two aspects. The first was to investigate the feasibility of intraoperative ALA-PDD for the detection of positive surgical margins. The second was to demonstrate the predominant accumulation of PpIX in human prostate cancer cells compared to normal prostate cells by the use of ALA-PDD on the divided surface of excised prostate. Thus, we investigated the feasibility of intraoperative PDD using 5-ALA in prostate cancer.

* Correspondence: keiji@kochi-u.ac.jp
[1]Department of Urology, Kochi Medical School, Kohasu, Oko, Nankoku, Kochi 783-8505, Japan
Full list of author information is available at the end of the article

## Methods

### Patients

Intraoperative ALA-PDD with radical prostatectomy was approved by the Ethical Committee of Kochi Medical School, Japan in January 2008. We enrolled 52 patients with histologically confirmed adenocarcinoma-type prostate cancer in the Department of Urology, Kochi Medical School Hospital between February 2009 and August 2012. All patients were informed about the potential efficacy and adverse events, such as skin photosensitivity, transient elevation of serum aspartate aminotransferase (AST) and alanine aminotransferase (ALT), nausea, and vomiting. All patients gave written informed consent. The 52 patients had a median age of 67.1 years (range, 56–76 years), initial PSA level of 7.71 ng/ml (range, 0.008–76 ng/ml), and histologically confirmed adenocarcinoma of the prostate apex (positive core rate 31.4 %; range, 8.3–75 %), according to the general rules for clinical and histological studies on prostate cancer, or an expected ≥25 % probability of extraprostatic extension (25.9 %; range, 3–59 %) defined by the Japan PC table (Preoperative nomogram developed for clinically localized prostate cancer in Japan) [17]. Patients were stratified according to the D'Amico classification into low-, intermediate- and high-risk groups. Twenty-eight patients were categorized as low risk, 13 as intermediate risk, and 11 as high risk. All 52 patients underwent radical prostatectomy; 10 received preoperative deprivation therapy; 34 underwent endoscopic retroperitoneal radical prostatectomy; and 18 underwent open retroperitoneal radical prostatectomy according to the technique described by Walsh [18]. The patient characteristics are shown in Table 1.

### Administration of 5-ALA

We administered ALA as a photosensitizer for ALA-PDD. ALA hydrochloride (COSMO BIO, Tokyo, Japan) was dissolved in 50 ml 5 % glucose solution. One gram of ALA solution was given intraoperatively, orally through a stomach tube.

### System of PDD

An endoscopic PDD system (Karl Storz, Tuttlingen, Germany), including a D-Light C, CCU Tricam SLII/3CCD CH Tricam-P PDD, and HOPKINS II Straight Forward Telescope 0°, was used. The light source, D-Light C (300 W xenon arc lamp), was equipped with a band-pass filter designed to transmit blue light (excitation wavelength, 375–445 nm; for excitation of fluorescence). The video camera system, CCU Tricam SLII/3CCD CHTricam-P PDD, was equipped with a long-pass filter designed to block blue light (for observation of fluorescence; fluorescence emission wavelength, 600–740 nm). The laparoscopy optic component was equipped with a yellow long-pass filter to reduce blue excitation light

**Table 1** Patients' characteristics

| Object | 2009/2–2012/9 | |
|---|---|---|
| | 52cases of prostate with operation | |
| | (Open: 18 cases, Laparoscopic: 34 cases) | |
| Age: average (range) (years old) | 67.1 (56–76) | |
| Initial PSA (range) (ng/ml) | 9.76 (3.07–86.69) | |
| Pre-op PSA (range) (ng/ml) | 7.71 (0.008–42.57) | |
| Pre-op MAB (+/−) (cases) | 10/42 | |
| Apex (biopsy) (+/−) (cases) | 17/35 | |
| Probability of EPE (%) in Japan PC table | 25.9 (3–59) | |
| Clinical stage (cases) | cT1c | 34 |
| | 2a | 9 |
| | 2b | 7 |
| | 3a | 2 |
| | N, M | 0 |
| Gleason score | 2–6 | 30 |
| in biopsy specimen (cases) | 7 | 12 |
| | 8–10 | 10 |

and enhance the fluorescence color contrast. The light source can be instantly switched between white light mode for conventional observation and blue light mode for fluorescence handled by a camera controller.

### Intraoperative procedure

In open radical prostatectomy, we placed the PDD laparoscope into the surgical field under general anesthesia and observed the surgical margins using the white and blue light modes. Blue light illuminated the surgical margins of the urethral, bladder, and rectal side, and enabled observation of the status of red fluorescence in the darkened operating room. To avoid unnecessary tissue removal, only the fluorescence-positive region was biopsied, for ethical reasons. When the fluorescence-positive region was close to a surrounding organ, such as the urethral sphincter and rectum wall, the region was removed as completely as possible with attention being paid to functional preservation of the surrounding organ. We sampled red-fluorescence-positive specimens and compared them with the pathological results.

### Examination of excised prostate

Soon after harvesting the whole prostate, we also performed laparoscopic PDD to detect red-fluorescence-positive surgical margins (base, apex, lateral, and rectal side). If a red-fluorescence-positive area was observed in the surgical margin of excised whole prostate, this area was biopsied by cold-cup for pathological examination. Subsequently, we divided the excised prostate in the median direction. The divided surface of excised prostate was also subjected to PDD. We separated the divided surface into four areas, and one specimen that was fluorescence-positive or -negative was biopsied by cold-cup in each area. The fluorescence intensity in each specimen was roughly divided into four categories (none, weak, moderate and strong), which was previously used in a clinical study on brain tumors performed by Miyoshi et al. [19]. The histological results were determined by two pathological specialists without knowledge of the results of fluorescence intensity.

## Statistical analysis

The diagnostic accuracy of the divided surface in excised prostate was calculated on the basis of comparison between fluorescence intensity and pathological results according to general rules for clinical and pathological studies on prostate cancer.

## Results

### PDD inside surgical margin

All 52 patients underwent retropubic radical prostatectomy and PDD. Eighteen patients underwent open radical prostatectomy and 34 underwent laparoscopic radical prostatectomy. There were no red-fluorescence-positive and pathologically positive surgical margins inside the surgical margin in either the laparoscopic or open surgery group.

### PDD in excised whole prostate

Soon after harvesting the prostate, we performed PDD on the surgical margins of the excised whole prostate. One case (Case 1 in Table 2) demonstrated a red-fluorescence-positive surgical margin of the excised whole prostate on the basal side. Pathologically, this area was classified as

Gleason score 6 adenocarcinoma (Fig. 1a). In this case with a red-fluorescence-positive surgical margin, the linear length of the positive surgical margin was 8.2 mm, without heat degeneration (Fig. 2a). However, another two cases had a pathological positive surgical margin with no red fluorescence. The first case showed heat degeneration of the surgical margin, with a 7-mm-long positive surgical margin (Case 3 in Fig. 2a, Table 2). In the second case, the positive surgical margin was only 1.5 mm long, without heat degeneration (Case 2 in Fig. 2a, Table 2). Three cases diagnosed as extraprostatic extension had no red fluorescence. In these cases, tumor cells were not present on the surface of the prostate. In fact, tumor cells were covered with prostatic capsule or peripheral fat tissue (Fig. 2b, Table 2). Ultimately, the rate of false negativity was 3.8 % in total. After examination of surgical margins, we divided the excised prostate from 29 cases and biopsied each area by cold-cup with PDD. We obtained 141 biopsied samples in all. Fluorescence positivity was found in 31 samples, while pathological positivity was found in 20 samples (Fig. 1b). The overall sensitivity and specificity were 75.0 % and 87.3 %, respectively (Table 3).

## Discussion

The number of new cases of prostate cancer detected by PSA screening is increasing every year; in particular, the number of low-risk cases with an indication for surgery. Radical prostatectomy is the gold standard therapy for prostate cancer in low-risk patients. The purpose of radical prostatectomy is to remove the whole cancerous prostate. However, positive surgical margins after radical prostatectomy were detected in 14–26 % of cases [2–5]. A histologically positive surgical margin is a major risk factor for biochemical recurrence and disease progression after radical prostatectomy. It was shown that positive surgical margins were associated with a 2.6-fold

**Table 2** Individual results of positive surgical margin and extraprostatic extension

| No | Operation | MAB | Preop PSA (ng/ml) | Probability of EPE (%) | D'amico classification | pT stage | Gleason score | Fluorescence intensity | Margin status | Heat Degeneration (pathological) | Linear length of surgical margin (mm) |
|---|---|---|---|---|---|---|---|---|---|---|---|
| 1 | open | none | 5.8 | 19 | low | 2b | 4 + 5 | moderate | positive surgical margin | - | 8.2 |
| 2 | open | none | 42.57 | 27 | high | 3b | 5 + 4 | none | positive surgical margin | + | 1.5 |
| 3 | Laparoscopy | none | 21.15 | 59 | intermediate | 3a | 4 + 3 | none | positive surgical margin | - | 7.0 |
| 4 | Laparoscopy | none | 6.87 | 30 | low | 3b | 3 + 4 | none | Extraprostatic extension | - | 1.2 |
| 5 | Laparoscopy | none | 11.93 | 21 | high | 3a | 4 + 5 | none | Extraprostatic extension | - | 2.0 |
| 6 | Laparoscopy | none | 21.15 | 59 | intermediate | 3a | 4 + 3 | none | Extraprostatic extension | - | 3.3 |

*MAB*, Maximum androgen blockade, *EPE*; Extraprostatic extension

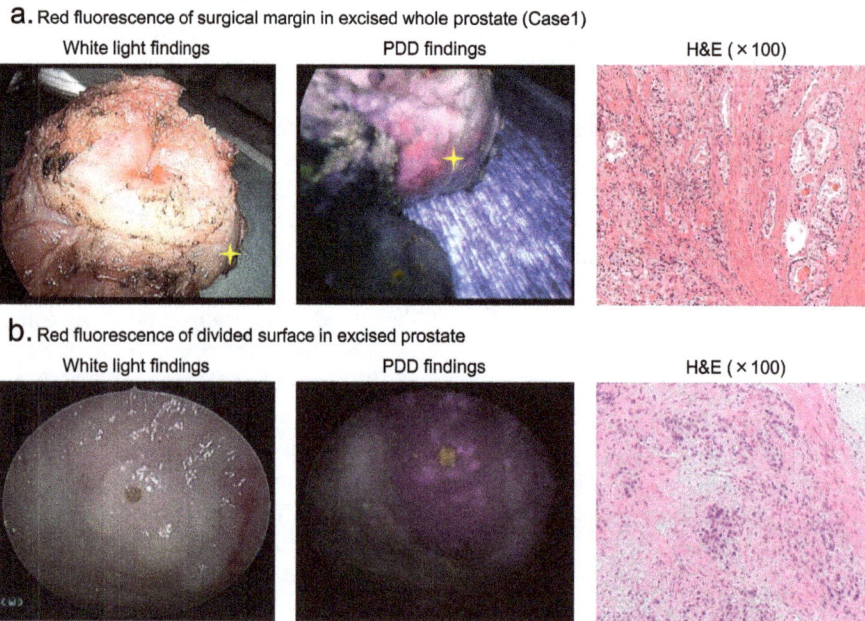

**Fig. 1** PDD finding in surgical margin and divided surface of excised prostate. **a**. Fluorescence-positive area of excised whole prostate was detected at the surgical margin in the base side (Gleason score 6). **b**. Longitudinal section in divided surface of excised prostate showed fluorescence-positive area in the transitional zone (Gleason score 7)

increased unadjusted risk of prostate-cancer-specific mortality [hazard ratio (HR) 2.55, 95 % confidence interval (CI) 2.02–3.21], and remained an independent predictor of prostate-cancer-specific mortality on multivariate analysis (HR 1.70, 95 % CI 1.32–2.18) in 65,633 patients who underwent radical prostatectomy for prostate cancer [20].

Overall, we believe it is important to reduce positive surgical margins for cancer control.

Kriegmair et al. published the first report about the feasibility of ALA-PDD for bladder cancer in 1996 [21]. Subsequently, Hungerhunber et al. reported a greater number of cases and demonstrated the feasibility of ALA-PDD [22].

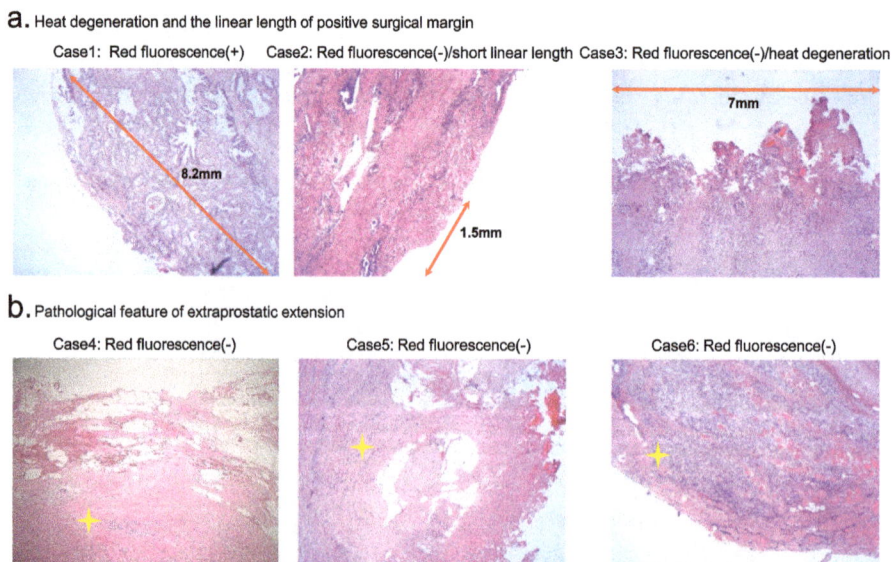

**Fig. 2** Association between pathological finding and red fluorescence in positive surgical margin and extraprostatic extension. **a**. In a case of heat degeneration and short linear length (<3 mm) of positive surgical margin, red fluorescence was not observed. **b**. All 3 cases of extraprostatic extension had no red fluorescence with tissue covering the tumor cells

**Table 3** Diagnostic accuracy of PDD in excised whole prostate and divided surface of excised prostate

| The surgical margin status of excised whole prostate | |
|---|---|
| Red fluorescence positive surgical margin | 1 |
| Pathologically positive surgical margin | 3 |
| Pathologically extraprostatic extension | 3 |
| Pathological result of divided surface in excised prostate | |
| Biopsy specimens in divided surface (samples) | 141 |
| Pathology results in divided surface (samples) | |
| Normal | 121 |
| Adenocarcinoma | 20 |
| Gleason score 2-6 | 9 |
| 7 | 6 |
| 8-10 | 5 |
| Diagnostic Accuracy of PDD in divided surface of excised prostate | |
| Positive fluorescence (samples/rate (%)) | 31/22.0 |
| Prediction accuracy (%) | 48.4 |
| Sensitivity (%) | 75.0 |
| Specificity (%) | 87.3 |

Zaak et al. reported the first experience of intraoperative ALA-PDD for prostate cancer in 2008 [15], and revealed its feasibility for detecting positive surgical margins. Adam et al. and Ganzer et al. revealed the diagnostic accuracy, with overall sensitivity and specificity of 56–75 % and 88.2–91.6 %, respectively [16, 23]. The present study showed that one case had a red-fluorescence surgical margin of the excised whole prostate and a histologically confirmed positive surgical margin of Gleason score 6. Heat degeneration using an electrical device and the length of the positive surgical margin have a crucial influence on ALA-PDD. Heat degeneration leads to damage of intracellular PpIX, so we could not detect red fluorescence. Besides these factors, we could not detect red fluorescence in a case with a short positive surgical margin because the total amount of PpIX in the tumor cells was small. In a case with an 8.2-mm-long positive surgical margin, we could detect red fluorescence, but not in a case with a 1.5-mm margin. Therefore, it is possible that a positive surgical margin length <3 mm makes it difficult to detect red fluorescence in ALA-PDD. In cases of extraprostatic extension, the tumor cells were not exposed on the surface of the prostate and were covered with prostatic capsule or peripheral fat tissue. The penetration of blue light was low at 0.2 mm [24]. Blue light has difficulty penetrating deeply into tissue and has a direct effect only on the surface of tissue. Therefore, it is difficult to detect red fluorescence on extraprostatic extension. In conclusion, heat degeneration by an electric device and

short linear length of positive surgical margin constitute limiting factors for ALA-PDD.

PDD of the divided surface of excised prostate could detect prostate cancer cells with a high degree of accuracy. We have previously shown *in vitro* accumulation of ALA-mediated PpIX in prostate cancer cell lines [25]. In the present study of the divided surface, we could clinically identify red-fluorescence emission in human prostate cancer cells and predominant accumulation of PpIX in cancerous tissue. In contrast, we could not detect red-fluorescence emission in normal prostate tissue. In terms of the diagnostic accuracy of PDD in bladder cancer, the overall sensitivity and specificity were 93.4 % and 58.9 %, respectively [26]. Meanwhile, sensitivity and specificity were 75.0 % and 87.3 %, respectively, in the divided surface of prostate. In terms of the prognostic accuracy of prostate cancer, there were lower sensitivity and higher specificity than for bladder cancer. Thus, the diagnostic accuracy of PDD varies according to the type of cancer. In addition, false-positive findings in prostate cancer were observed in basal hyperplasia with chronic inflammation similar to bladder cancer. Considering the location of prostate cancerogenesis, the capsule of the prostate has little effect on basal hyperplasia and chronic inflammation. Therefore, false-positive findings have no significant effect on intraoperative PDD.

This study showed preliminary results of intraoperative ALA-PDD in radical prostatectomy. We conclude that intraoperative ALA-PDD is feasible, but our study was limited by clinical stage and heat degeneration. In the future, a randomized trial should be carried out.

## Conclusions

Intraoperative ALA-PDD for prostate cancer is helpful in assessing the presence of residual tumor in the surgical margins. Clearly, future randomized studies are needed to examine high-risk prostate cancer patients.

**Abbreviations**
ALA: Aminolevulinic acid; PDD: Photodynamic diagnosis; PpIX: Protoporphyrin IX; PSA: Prostate-specific antigen.

**Competing interests**
The authors declare that they have no competing interests.

**Authors' contributions**
TS designed and contributed to this study. HF and KI made substantial contributions to the conception and design of the study and acquisition of data, and drafted the manuscript and figures/tables. AK and MF performed the pathological review. All authors read and approved the final manuscript.

**Acknowledgments**
This work was supported by the Department of Urology, Kochi Medical School.

**Author details**
[1]Department of Urology, Kochi Medical School, Kohasu, Oko, Nankoku, Kochi 783-8505, Japan. [2]Department of Pathology, Kochi Medical School, Kohasu, Oko, Nankoku, Kochi 783-8505, Japan.

**References**

1.  Matsuda T, Marugame T, Kamo K, Katanoda K, Ajiki W, Sobue T, et al. Cancer incidence and incidence rate in Japan in 2006: based on data from 15 population-based cancer registries in monitoring of cancer incidence in Japan (MCIJ) project. Jpn J Clin Oncol. 2009;42:139–47.

2.  Blute ML, Bostwick DG, Bergstralh EJ, Slezak JM, Martin SK, Amling CL, et al. Anatomic site-specific positive margins in organ-confined prostate cancer and its impact on outcome after radical prostatectomy. Urology. 1997;50:733–9.

3.  Terakawa T, Miyake H, Tanaka K, Takanaka A, Inoue T, Fujisawa M. Surgical margin status of open versus laparoscopic radical prostatectomy specimens. Int J Urol. 2008;15:704–8.

4.  Sasaki H, Miki J, Kimura T, Sanuki K, Miki K, Takahashi H, et al. Lateral view dissection of the prostate-urethral junction to reduce positive apical margin in laparoscopic radical prostatectomy. Int J Urol. 2009;16:664–9.

5.  Stephenson A, Wood DP, Kattan MW, Klein EA, Scardino PT, Eastham JA, et al. Location, extent of positive surgical margins do not improve accuracy of predicting prostate cancer recurrence after radical prostatectomy. J Urol. 2009;182:1357–63.

6.  Yossepowitch O, Bjartell A, Eastham JA, Graefen M, Guilloneau BD, Karakiewicz PI, et al. Positive surgical margins in radical prostatectomy: outlining the problem and its long-term consequences. Eur Urol. 2009;55:87–99.

7.  Hull GW, Rabbani F, Abbas F, Wheeler TM, Kattan MW, Scardino PT. Cancer control with radical prostatectomy alone in 1000 consecutive patients. J Urol. 2002;167:528–34.

8.  D'amico AV, Whittington R, Malkowicz SB, Cote K, Loffredo M. Biochemical outcome after radical prostatectomy or external beam radiation therapy for patients with clinically localized prostate carcinoma in the prostate specific antigen era. Cancer. 2002;95:281–6.

9.  Cheng L, Darson MF, Bergstralh EJ, Slezak J, Meyers RP, Bostwick DG, et al. Correlation of margin status and extraprostatic extension with progression of prostate carcinoma. Cancer. 1999;86:1775–82.

10. Filbeck T, Rossler W, Knuechel R, Straub M, Kiel HJ, Wieland WF. Clinical results of the transurethral resection and evaluation of superficial bladder carcinomas by means of fluorescence diagnosis after intravesical instillation of 5-aminolevulinic acid. J Endourol. 1999;13:117–21.

11. Koening F, McGovern FJ, Larne R, Enquist H, Schomacker KT, Deutsch TF. Diagnosis of bladder carcinoma using protoporphyrin IX fluorescence induced by 5-aminolevulinic acid. BJU Int. 1999;83:129–35.

12. Kreigmair M, Baumgartner R, Knuchel R, Stepp H, Hofstadter F, Hofstertter A. Detection of early bladder cancer by 5-aminolevulinic acid induced phorphyrin fluorescence. J Urol. 1996;155:105–9.

13. ZaaK D, Hungerhuber E, Schneede P, Stepp H, Frimberger D. Role of 5-aminolevulinic acid in the detection of urothelial premalignant lesions. Cancer. 2002;95:1234–8.

14. Steinbach P, Weingandt H, Baumgartner R, Kreigmair M, Hofstadter F, Knuchel R. Cellular fluorescence of the endogenous photosensitizer protoporphyrin IX following exposure to 5-aminolevulinic acid. Photochem Photobiol. 1995;62:887–95.

15. Zaak D, Sroka R, Khoder W, Adam C, Trischler S, Karl A, et al. Photodynamic diagnosis of prostate cancer using 5-aminolevulinic acid-first clinical experiences. Urology. 2008;72:345–8.

16. Adam C, Salmon G, Walter S, Zaak D, Khoder W, Becker A, et al. Photodynamic diagnosis using 5-aminolevulinic acid for the detection of positive surgical margins during radical prostatectomy in patients with carcinoma of the prostate: A multicenter, prospective, phase 2 trial of a diagnostic procedure. Eur Urol. 2009;55:1281–8.

17. Naito S, Kuroiwa K, Kinukawa N, Goto K, Koga H, Ogawa O, et al. Validation of Partin tables and development of a preoperative nomogram for Japanese patients with clinically localized prostate cancer using 2005 international society of urological pathology consensus on Gleason grading: Data from the clinicopathological research group for localized prostate cancer. J Urol. 2008;180:904–10.

18. Walsh PC. Anatomic radical prostatectomy: evolution of the surgical technique. J Urol. 1998;160:2418–24.

19. Miyoshi N, Ogasawara T, Ogawa T, Sano K, Kaneko S. Anapplication of fluorescence analysis of metabolized protoporphyrin IX (PpIX) in a tumor tissue administrated with 5-aminolevulinic acid (5-ALA). Jap Soc Laser Med. 2002;23:81–8.

20. Wright JL, Dalkin BL, True LD, Ellis WJ, Stanford JL, Lin DW, et al. Positive surgical margins at radical prostatectomy predict prostate cancer specific mortality. J Urol. 2010;183:2213–8.

21. Kreigmair M, Baumgartner R, Knuechel R, Steinbach P, Ehsam A, Lumper W, et al. Fluorescence photodetection of neoplastic urothelial lesions following intravesical instillation of 5-aminolevulinic acid. Urology. 1994;44:836–41.

22. Hungerhuber E, Stepp H, Kreigmair M, Stief C, Hofstetter A, Hartmann A, et al. Seven year's experience with 5-aminolevulinic acid in detection of transitional cell carcinoma of the bladder. Urology. 2007;69:260–4.

23. Ganzer R, Blana A, Denzinger S, Wieland WF, Adam C, Becker A, et al. Intraoperative photodynnmic evaluation of surgical margins during endoscopic extraprostatic radical prostatectomy with the use of 5-aminolevulinic acid. J Endourol. 2009;23:1387–94.

24. Honda N, Ishii K, Terada T, Nanjyo T, Awazu K. Determination of tumor tissue optical properties during and after photodynamic therapy using inverse Monte Carlo method and double integrating sphere between 350 and 1000nm. J Biomed Opt. 2011;16:058003-1-7.

25. Fukuhara H, Inoue K, Kurabayashi A, Furihata M, Fujita H, Utsumi K, et al. The inhibition of ferrochelatase enhances 5-aminolevulinic acid-based photodynamic action for prostate cancer. Photodiagnosis photodyn Ther. 2013;10:399–409.

26. Inoue K, Fukuhara H, Shimamoto T, Kamada M, Iiyama T, Miyamura M, et al. Comparision between intravesical and oral administration of 5-aminolevulinic acid in the clinical benefit of photodynamic diagnosis for nonmuscle invasive bladder cancer. Cancer. 2012;118:1062–74.

# Association of lower urinary tract symptoms and OAB severity with quality of life and mental health in China, Taiwan and South Korea

Kyu-Sung Lee[1], Tag Keun Yoo[2*], Limin Liao[3], Jianye Wang[4], Yao-Chi Chuang[5], Shih-Ping Liu[6], Romeo Chu[7,8] and Budiwan Sumarsono[7]

## Abstract

**Background:** Lower urinary tract symptoms (LUTS) and overactive bladder (OAB) symptoms have a substantial effect on quality of life (QoL). We report QoL and mental health results from a LUTS prevalence study in three Asian countries.

**Methods:** A cross-sectional, population-representative, internet-based study among individuals aged ≥40 years in China, Taiwan and South Korea. Instruments included: Overactive Bladder Symptom Score (OABSS); International Prostate Symptom Score (IPSS); other International Continence Society (ICS) symptom questions; health-related QoL 12-item short-form (HRQoL-SF12v2); Work Limitations Questionnaire (WLQ); Hospital Anxiety and Depression Scale (HADS). Presence of LUTS was determined according to ICS criteria, with three symptom groups (storage, voiding and post-micturition). Post-stratification weighting matched the age and sex population distribution per country. Initial data analyses were based on descriptive statistics. Significance testing undertaken post hoc included: independent-samples t-test (differences in HRQoL between sexes and between individuals with/without LUTS; relationship between HRQoL score and OABSS; differences in HADS anxiety and depression scores between individuals with/without LUTS; association between HADS anxiety/depression scores and OABSS), chi-square test (association between LUTS prevalence and workplace productivity) and analysis of variance (differences in HRQoL score and in HADS anxiety/depression scores between individuals with different symptom groups, association between HADS anxiety/depression scores and IPSS).

**Results:** In total, 8284 participants were included. HRQoL scores were significantly worse ($p < 0.001$) among individuals with versus without LUTS (ICS criteria): mean physical health domain scores were 61.1 (standard deviation [SD], 20.1) and 76.7 (17.0), respectively; corresponding mental health domain scores were 34.8 (12.7) and 43.7 (10.7). Workplace productivity was best among individuals without LUTS (difficulties reported by 2–3% of individuals), and worst in those with all three ICS symptom groups (difficulties reported by 29–38% of individuals; $p = 0.001$). Mean HADS scores showed significantly worse ($p < 0.001$) levels of anxiety and depression among individuals with versus without LUTS: anxiety, 6.5 (SD, 3.7) and 4.0 (3.3); corresponding mean depression scores were 6.8 (4.3) and 4.2 (3.6). Increasing OAB severity was also associated with decreasing HRQoL physical and mental health scores.

(Continued on next page)

* Correspondence: ytk5202@eulji.ac.kr
[2]Department of Urology, Nowon Eulji Medical Center, Eulji University School of Medicine, 68, Hangeulbiseok-ro, Nowon-gu, Seoul, Korea
Full list of author information is available at the end of the article

(Continued from previous page)

**Conclusion:** LUTS and increasing OAB severity are both associated with impaired QoL, reduced workplace productivity, and increased tendency towards anxiety and depression. These results highlight the need to ensure that individuals with LUTS receive appropriate, effective treatment.

**Keywords:** Asia, Epidemiology, Lower urinary tract symptoms, Mental health, Prevalence, Quality of life

## Background

Depending on definition, lower urinary tract symptoms (LUTS) are reported to affect over half of the world's adult population [1–4]. Although these symptoms are not life-threatening, associations with conditions such as obesity and type 2 diabetes have been reported [5] and they are often bothersome. The potential effects of LUTS are wide-ranging, from impairment of sleep and personal relationships to reductions in emotional well-being and workplace productivity [6]. Consequently, LUTS is associated with impaired quality of life (QoL) [7–9].

Studies from around the world have shown that the impact of LUTS on QoL may be manifested in overall QoL scores, either generic or disease-specific, as well as specific dimensions such as vitality, social functioning, physical activities and mental health [7–16]. The impact of moderate LUTS on QoL has been likened to that of diabetes, hypertension or cancer [12]. LUTS have also been shown in a variety of countries to be associated with increased rates of mental health issues, specifically depression and anxiety [5, 7, 9, 17]. The relationship between LUTS and depressive symptoms appears to be robust regardless of sex/ethnicity [18].

The substantial impact of LUTS on QoL reinforces the need for their treatment, and indicates the potential benefits of effective intervention. In addition, treatment of LUTS has been shown to improve QoL [19]. However, many patients with LUTS do not seek healthcare [20] and LUTS therapy may not be regarded as a high priority by primary care physicians [21].

We conducted a study to determine the prevalence of LUTS in the population aged ≥40 years in China, Taiwan and South Korea, using symptom definitions approved by the International Continence Society (ICS) in 2002 [22]. Here we report QoL and mental health results from the study.

## Methods

As the study methods are published in full elsewhere [23], they are described here in brief.

### Study design and population

We conducted a cross-sectional, population-representative internet-based study in China, Taiwan and South Korea.

Inclusion criteria were age ≥ 40 years, internet access and ability to read the local language. Pregnant women and individuals with a urinary tract infection during the previous month were excluded. The study was performed in compliance with the principles of the Declaration of Helsinki, Good Clinical Practice and the World Association for Social, Opinion and Market Research (ESOMAR) guidelines [24]. Informed consent was obtained from all participants.

Consumer survey panels were actively managed to ensure random sampling with representation of the target population in terms of age, sex and socioeconomic factors.

### Endpoints

Instruments in the study were validated in the local language and included the following: the International Prostate Symptom Score (IPSS) [25]; other ICS symptoms questions (related to splitting/spraying, hesitancy, terminal dribble, urgency); Overactive Bladder Symptom Score (OABSS) [26]; the 12-item short-form health survey for measuring health-related QoL (HRQoL-SF12v2; possible scores for mental health domain and physical health domain range from 0 to 100, with higher scores indicating better health) [27]; Work Limitations Questionnaire (WLQ) [28]; Hospital Anxiety and Depression Scale (HADS; total score for both anxiety and depression classified as normal, 0-7, borderline abnormal, 8-10, or abnormal, 11-21) [29]. Presence of LUTS was based on ICS criteria (presence of voiding, storage or post-micturition symptom[s] with frequency ≥ 1 in 5 times), with the exception that nocturia was defined as ≥2 episodes per night (ICS definition for nocturia is ≥1 episode per night; the higher threshold was chosen to avoid over-estimation) [22].

### Statistical analysis

A minimum sample size of 384 respondents per group was needed for estimating LUTS affecting 50% of patients within five percentage points. Five different age groups (40–44, 45–49, 50–54, 55–60 and >60 years) were planned for analysis, necessitating 1920 individuals per country. With an assumption that ~28% of data would be non-evaluable, a total population of 8000 study participants was planned (4000 in China, 2000 in Taiwan and 2000 in South Korea). The initial data analyses were based on descriptive statistics. Workplace productivity analyses excluded individuals who selected 'does not apply to my job' as a response. Post-stratification weighting was performed to match the age and sex distributions of the populations in the respective countries. All significance testing was undertaken post hoc. Predictors of HADS scores were identified by logistic regression. The independent-samples t-test was used for the following: differences in HRQoL scores between men and women; differences in HRQoL scores between individuals with or without LUTS according to ICS criteria; relationship between HRQoL score and severity of overactive bladder (OAB) according to the OABSS; differences in HADS anxiety and depression scores between individuals with or without LUTS according to ICS criteria; and the relationship between HADS anxiety and depression scores and OABSS. Associations between LUTS prevalence according to ICS criteria and workplace productivity were examined using the chi-square test. Analysis of variance (ANOVA) was used to assess differences in HRQoL score between individuals with different ICS symptom groups, and differences in HADS anxiety and depression scores between individuals with different ICS symptom groups. The relationships between HADS anxiety and depression scores and severity of OAB according to IPSS were also assessed by ANOVA.

## Results

The survey sample and response rate for each country has been reported previously [23]. The study included a total of 8284 participants, of whom 4136 were from China, 2068 from Taiwan and 2080 from South Korea. Table 1 shows demographic characteristics of the population.

HRQoL scores were lower (i.e. worse) among individuals with versus without LUTS according to ICS criteria (Fig. 1; $p < 0.001$ for both physical health domain and mental health domain). For the overall population with and without LUTS, the mean physical health domain scores were 61.1 (standard deviation [SD], 20.1) and 76.7 (17.0), respectively, and the mean mental health domain scores were 34.8 (12.7) and 43.7 (10.7). These differences were evident in all three countries. Men had higher (i.e. better) HRQoL scores than women, for both physical and mental health domains ($p < 0.001$ for both), but LUTS were associated with similar score reductions in both sexes. Individuals with all three ICS symptom groups had the lowest mean HRQoL scores (physical health domain: 52.3 [SD, 18.5]; mental health domain: 29.4 [11.5]; $p < 0.001$ for both domains versus all other ICS symptom group combinations), and the presence of two symptom groups was generally associated with lower HRQoL scores than one (Table 2). The presence of voiding and storage symptoms was associated with

**Table 1** Participants' demographic data. Table reproduced from Chapple et al. 2017 [23]

| | China (n = 4136) | Taiwan (n = 2068) | South Korea (n = 2080) | Overall (n = 8284) |
|---|---|---|---|---|
| Sex | | | | |
| Men | 50.3% | 48.6% | 47.6% | 49.2% |
| Women | 49.7% | 51.4% | 52.4% | 50.8% |
| Age group | | | | |
| 40–44 years | 19.9% | 15.6% | 16.9% | 18.1% |
| 45–49 years | 19.6% | 16.1% | 16.8% | 18.0% |
| 50–54 years | 15.3% | 16.3% | 16.3% | 15.8% |
| 55–59 years | 12.7% | 14.9% | 14.4% | 13.7% |
| ≥ 60 years | 32.6% | 37.1% | 35.6% | 34.4% |
| Education | | | | |
| High school or less | 28.0% | 39.3% | 30.3% | 31.4% |
| Some college | 28.4% | 23.7% | 3.4% | 20.9% |
| College degree/ college graduate | 40.2% | 28.2% | 57.0% | 41.4% |
| Postgraduate | 3.5% | 8.8% | 9.4% | 6.3% |
| Marital status | | | | |
| Single | 2.9% | 14.9% | 9.2% | 7.5% |
| Divorced | 1.5% | 5.2% | 4.0% | 3.0% |
| Married/living with partner | 91.7% | 72.8% | 81.6% | 84.5% |
| Widow/widower | 3.2% | 6.3% | 4.5% | 4.3% |
| Prefer not to answer | 0.8% | 0.7% | 0.7% | 0.7% |
| Work status | | | | |
| Homemaker | 2.6% | 12.0% | 22.4% | 9.9% |
| Retired | 28.7% | 16.9% | 6.0% | 20.1% |
| Student | 0.0% | 0.1% | 0.2% | 0.1% |
| Working, full-time | 62.6% | 60.0% | 53.9% | 59.8% |
| Working, part-time | 3.7% | 6.2% | 8.0% | 5.4% |
| Other work for pay | 0.4% | 0.8% | 3.2% | 1.2% |
| Other | 1.1% | 1.9% | 3.7% | 2.0% |
| Unemployed | 0.6% | 1.3% | 2.3% | 1.2% |
| Permanently disabled/cannot work due to ill health | 0.1% | 0.8% | 0.4% | 0.4% |

greater HRQoL impairment than any other pair of ICS symptom groups, with a mean physical health domain score of 58.4 (20.0) and a mean mental health domain score of 33.8 (13.2). Increasing severity of OAB, according to OABSS, was associated with decreasing HRQoL physical and mental health scores (Table 2; $p < 0.001$ for individuals with versus without OAB). These trends were similar in China, South Korea and Taiwan.

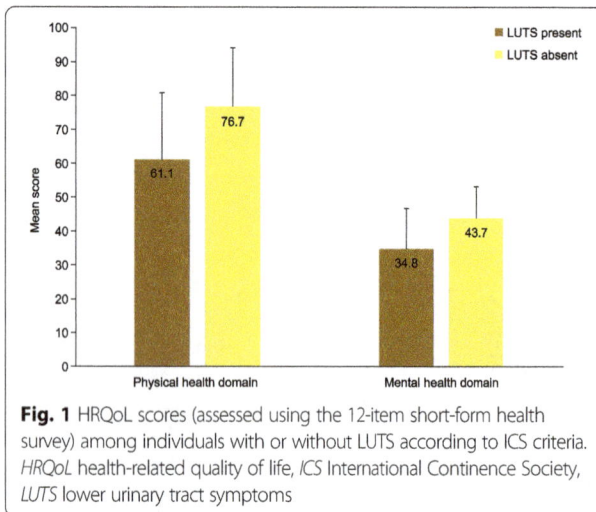

**Fig. 1** HRQoL scores (assessed using the 12-item short-form health survey) among individuals with or without LUTS according to ICS criteria. *HRQoL* health-related quality of life, *ICS* International Continence Society, *LUTS* lower urinary tract symptoms

The presence of LUTS according to ICS criteria was associated with statistically significantly impaired workplace productivity (Table 3; $p = 0.001$ for all eight domains, LUTS present versus LUTS absent). The best productivity was evident among individuals without LUTS, while productivity was worst in those with all three ICS symptom groups. Second worst results were obtained from individuals with voiding and storage symptoms. Compared with individuals without LUTS, productivity was least affected among individuals with only one ICS symptom group. The results showed a similar pattern across all eight items of the work limitations questionnaire. Impairment of workplace productivity (all

eight items) was shown to increase with increasing severity of OAB (Table 3; $p = 0.001$ for all eight domains, OAB present versus OAB absent).

Individuals with LUTS according to ICS criteria had higher (i.e. worse) scores for both anxiety and depression compared with those without LUTS (Fig. 2; $p < 0.001$ for men, women and both sexes together). The mean anxiety score for the population with LUTS was 6.5 (SD, 3.7), compared with 4.0 (3.3) for the population without LUTS. The corresponding mean depression scores were 6.8 (4.3) and 4.2 (3.6). Women had higher HADS scores than men ($p < 0.0001$ for both anxiety and depression), but the difference between individuals with versus without LUTS was similar in both sexes (Table 4). The highest (i.e. worst) HADS scores were observed among those with all three ICS symptom groups ($p < 0.001$ versus all other ICS symptom group combinations), with mean scores for anxiety and depression of 8.0 (3.6) and 8.2 (4.3), respectively. Individuals with two symptom groups generally had higher HADS scores than those with one symptom group. HADS scores were also higher among individuals with versus without OAB ($p < 0.0001$ for both anxiety and depression). HADS scores increased markedly with increasing OAB severity assessed by OABSS: mean anxiety scores for individuals with no versus severe OAB were 4.9 (3.5) and 11.5 (4.3); the corresponding depression scores were 5.1 (4.0) and 11.5 (5.1). In addition, statistically significant relationships were observed between HADS scores and IPSS-measured symptom severity (increased IPSS severity associated with

**Table 2** HRQoL by LUTS and OABSS

| | Physical health domain | | Mental health domain | |
| --- | --- | --- | --- | --- |
| | Mean score (standard deviation)[a] | p-value for comparison vs. No LUTS or No OAB | Mean score (standard deviation)[a] | p-value for comparison vs. No LUTS or No OAB |
| LUTS (ICS criteria) | | | | |
| No LUTS | 76.7 (17.0) | N/A | 43.7 (10.7) | N/A |
| Voiding Only | 71.5 (17.4) | <0.005 | 40.9 (10.9) | <0.005 |
| Storage Only | 68.2 (18.5) | <0.005 | 38.9 (12.0) | <0.005 |
| PM Only | 68.2 (18.0) | <0.005 | 38.6 (12.5) | <0.005 |
| Voiding + Storage | 58.4 (20.0) | <0.005 | 33.8 (13.2) | <0.005 |
| Voiding + PM | 68.8 (17.9) | <0.005 | 39 (12.0) | <0.005 |
| Storage + PM | 63.6 (19.0) | <0.005 | 36.2 (11.6) | <0.005 |
| Voiding + Storage + PM | 52.3 (18.5) | <0.005 | 29.4 (11.5) | <0.005 |
| OABSS | | | | |
| No OAB | 71.4 (18.7) | N/A | 40.8 (11.8) | N/A |
| Mild OAB | 58.6 (18.2) | <0.0005 | 33.3 (11.6) | <0.0005 |
| Moderate OAB | 47.7 (16.8) | <0.0005 | 26.7 (10.7) | <0.0005 |
| Severe OAB | 33.6 (15.6) | <0.0005 | 18.9 (9.5) | <0.0005 |
| Overall | 67.1 (20.4) | | 38.2 (12.8) | |

*ICS* International Continence Society, *LUTS* lower urinary tract symptoms, *OAB* overactive bladder, *OABSS* Overactive Bladder Symptom Score, *PM* post-micturition
[a] data are for both sexes and all three countries combined

Association of lower urinary tract symptoms and OAB severity with quality of life and mental health...

149

**Table 3** Workplace productivity by LUTS and OABSS

| | Number of participants (%) for the overall population | | | | | | |
|---|---|---|---|---|---|---|---|
| | Difficult to get going easily at start of work day[a, b] | Difficult to start on your job as soon as you arrived at work[a, b] | Able to sit, stand, or stay in one position for longer than 15 min while working, without difficulty[a, c] | Able to repeat the same motions over and over again while working, without difficulty[a, c] | Difficult to speak with people in-person, in meetings or on the phone[a, b] | Difficult to handle the workload[a, b] | Difficult to finish work on time[a, b] |
| **LUTS (ICS criteria)** | | | | | | | |
| No LUTS | 60 (3%) | 57 (2%) | 954 (40%) | 967 (40%) | 45 (2%) | 53 (2%) | 66 (3%) |
| PM Only | 13 (8%)[†] | 8 (5%) | 58 (37%) | 64 (42%) | 8 (5%)* | 9 (6%)* | 7 (4%) |
| Storage + PM | 26 (11%)[†] | 23 (10%)[†] | 89 (38%) | 81 (35%) | 16 (7%)[†] | 17 (7%)[†] | 24 (10%)[†] |
| Storage Only | 98 (6%)[†] | 98 (6%)[†] | 566 (38%) | 564 (37%) | 98 (7%)[†] | 94 (6%)[†] | 106 (7%)[†] |
| Voiding + PM | 11 (6%)* | 9 (5%) | 75 (40%) | 74 (39%) | 8 (4%) | 10 (5%)* | 13 (7%)* |
| Voiding + Storage | 183 (22%)[†] | 178 (21%)[†] | 307 (37%) | 293 (35%)* | 166 (20%)[†] | 152 (18%)[†] | 169 (20%)[†] |
| Voiding + Storage + PM | 640 (36%)[†] | 645 (36%)[†] | 590 (33%)[†] | 543 (31%)[†] | 557 (31%)[†] | 511 (29%)[†] | 559 (31%)[†] |
| Voiding Only | 9 (2%) | 10 (3%) | 130 (35%) | 125 (34%)* | 11 (3%) | 14 (4%) | 17 (4%) |
| **OABSS** | | | | | | | |
| No-OAB | 401 (7%) | 365 (6%) | 2150 (38%) | 2142 (37%) | 334 (6%) | 331 (6%) | 374 (7%) |
| Mild-OAB | 114 (20%)[†] | 112 (19%)[†] | 223 (39%) | 212 (37%) | 88 (15%)[†] | 89 (16%)[†] | 97 (17%)[†] |
| Moderate-OAB | 485 (45%)[†] | 506 (47%)[†] | 376 (35%) | 344 (32%)[†] | 446 (41%)[†] | 400 (37%)[†] | 446 (41%)[†] |
| Severe-OAB | 40 (62%)[†] | 45 (69%)[†] | 19 (29%) | 16 (25%)* | 43 (66%)[†] | 39 (60%)[†] | 42 (65%)[†] |
| Overall | 1040 (14%) | 1027 (14%) | 2768 (37%) | 2713 (36%) | 910 (12%) | 859 (12%) | 960 (13%) |

Numbers of individuals are weighted and rounded, therefore category totals may not equal population totals shown in column headings. Percentages are based on the weighted 'n' values

*ICS* International Continence Society, *LUTS* lower urinary tract symptoms, *OAB* overactive bladder, *OABSS* Overactive Bladder Symptom Score, *PM* post-micturition

[a] Because of physical health or emotional problems; excludes those who responded that this did not apply to their job

[b] ≥ ~50% of the time

[c] < ~50% of the time

*$p < 0.05$ vs. No LUTS or No OAB

[†]$p < 0.005$ vs. No LUTS or No OAB

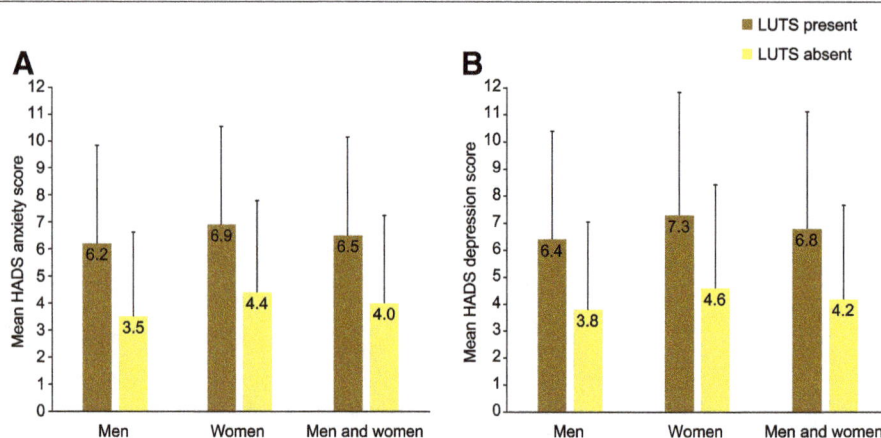

**Fig. 2** HADS by LUTS according to ICS criteria: **a** anxiety and **b** depression. *HADS* Hospital Anxiety and Depression Scale, *ICS* International Continence Society, *LUTS* lower urinary tract symptoms

higher HADS anxiety and depression scores; $p < 0.001$). The associations between HADS scores and OABSS/IPSS severity were evident in both men and women. Statistically significant predictors of high HADS scores ($\geq 8$, indicating clinically relevant levels of anxiety and depression [30]) are shown in Table 5. Urgency with fear of leaking and stress incontinence (different causes) were associated with high depression and anxiety scores in both men and women. Incomplete emptying was a predictor of high scores for anxiety and depression in

**Table 4** HADS by LUTS, IPSS and OABSS

| | Anxiety score[a] | | | Depression score[a] | | |
|---|---|---|---|---|---|---|
| | Men | Women | Men and women | Men | Women | Men and women |
| LUTS (ICS criteria) | | | | | | |
| No LUTS | 3.5 (3.1) | 4.4 (3.4) | 4.0 (3.3) | 3.8 (3.3) | 4.6 (3.9) | 4.2 (3.6) |
| Voiding Only | 4.8 (3.4)[†] | 5.3 (3) | 4.9 (3.3)[†] | 5.5 (4)[†] | 6.3 (4.2)[†] | 5.6 (4)[†] |
| Storage Only | 5.1 (3.4)[†] | 5.7 (3.4)[†] | 5.5 (3.4)[†] | 5.2 (3.8)[†] | 6 (4.1)[†] | 5.7 (4)[†] |
| PM Only | 4.6 (3.1) | 5.8 (3.1)[*] | 5.1 (3.2)[†] | 5 (3.4) | 6.7 (4.4)[†] | 5.7 (3.9)[†] |
| Voiding + Storage | 6.1 (3.5)[†] | 7 (3.6)[†] | 6.5 (3.6)[†] | 6.4 (3.8)[†] | 7.4 (4.3)[†] | 6.9 (4.1)[†] |
| Voiding + PM | 5.1 (3.5)[†] | 6.6 (3.6)[†] | 5.4 (3.5)[†] | 5.8 (3.9)[†] | 7.7 (4.9)[†] | 6.2 (4.2)[†] |
| Storage + PM | 6 (3.4)[†] | 6.7 (3.3)[†] | 6.4 (3.4)[†] | 6.1 (3.8)[†] | 7.3 (4.4)[†] | 6.7 (4.1)[†] |
| Voiding + Storage + PM | 7.5 (3.6)[†] | 8.7 (3.5)[†] | 8.0 (3.6)[†] | 7.5 (3.9)[†] | 9.2 (4.6)[†] | 8.2 (4.3)[†] |
| OABSS | | | | | | |
| No OAB | 4.5 (3.5) | 5.2 (3.5) | 4.9 (3.5) | 4.8 (3.7) | 5.5 (4.2) | 5.1 (4.0) |
| Mild OAB | 6.6 (3.5)[†] | 7.3 (3.2)[†] | 6.9 (3.4)[†] | 7.1 (3.7)[†] | 7.7 (4)[†] | 7.4 (3.9)[†] |
| Moderate OAB | 8.2 (3.4)[†] | 8.7 (3.5)[†] | 8.5 (3.5)[†] | 8.1 (3.8)[†] | 9.3 (4.6)[†] | 8.7 (4.3)[†] |
| Severe OAB | 10.9 (4.3)[†] | 11.9 (4.4)[†] | 11.5 (4.3)[†] | 10.7 (3.6)[†] | 12.1 (5.9)[†] | 11.5 (5.1)[†] |
| IPSS | | | | | | |
| No Symptom | 3 (3.2) | 3.8 (3.5) | 3.4 (3.4) | 3.5 (3.5) | 4.5 (4) | 4 (3.8) |
| Mild | 4.4 (3.3)[†] | 5.2 (3.4)[†] | 4.8 (3.4)[†] | 4.6 (3.5)[†] | 5.3 (4)[†] | 5 (3.8)[†] |
| Moderate | 6.5 (3.4)[†] | 7.5 (3.3)[†] | 6.9 (3.4)[†] | 6.8 (3.8)[†] | 8 (4.4)[†] | 7.3 (4.1)[†] |
| Severe | 9.2 (3.9)[†] | 10 (3.7)[†] | 9.6 (3.9)[†] | 9.1 (4.1)[†] | 10.4 (4.7)[†] | 9.8 (4.4)[†] |
| Overall | 5.2 (3.7) | 5.9 (3.8) | 5.5 (3.8) | 5.4 (3.9) | 6.2 (4.5) | 5.8 (4.2) |

*HADS* Hospital Anxiety and Depression Scale, *ICS* International Continence Society, *IPSS* International Prostate Symptom Score, *LUTS* lower urinary tract symptoms, *OAB* overactive bladder, *OABSS* overactive bladder symptom score, *PM* post-micturition

[*] $p < 0.05$ vs. No LUTS, No OAB or No Symptom

[†] $p < 0.005$ vs. No LUTS, No OAB or No Symptom

[a] mean scores (standard deviation) for all three countries combined

women, while perceived frequency and terminal dribble were predictors of high scores for both parameters in men as well as anxiety in women.

## Discussion

This study provides strong evidence that LUTS are associated with impaired QoL, reduced workplace productivity, and increased tendency towards anxiety and depression. These findings are evident in both men and women from all three countries included in the study. Individuals with all three ICS symptom groups showed greater impairment than those with two ICS symptom groups, and the presence of two ICS symptom groups was associated with greater impairment than one symptom group. Voiding and storage were associated with greater QoL impairment than other pairs of symptom groups. Workplace productivity decreased with increasing severity of OAB, while HADS scores deteriorated with increasing OAB and IPSS severity. Urgency with fear of leaking was a significant predictor of high HADS scores for anxiety and depression in both men and women.

Overall, our results are consistent with data from previous studies assessing the impact of LUTS on QoL and mental health in countries outside Asia. In the EpiLUTS study, conducted in 30,000 adults aged ≥40 years in Sweden, UK and USA, similar methods to the current study were used for assessing LUTS (ICS criteria), HRQoL (SF-12) and mental health (HADS) [9]. As in our study, deteriorations in physical and mental components of the SF-12, as well as anxiety and depression scores, were most pronounced among individuals with all three ICS symptom groups. A study of urinary incontinence in women from France, Germany, UK and USA ($N$ = 1203) showed that the impact of symptoms on HRQoL (measured using the International Consultation on Incontinence Modular Questionnaire Lower Urinary Tract Symptoms Quality of Life [ICIQ-LUTSqol]) increased with increasing symptom severity [6]. Evidence that QoL impairment increases with symptom severity

was also provided by a Mexican study conducted in a population aged ≥70 years ($N$ = 1124): individuals with severe urinary incontinence had worse self-perceived health status and greater disability than those with less severe symptoms [10]. In addition, this study reported increased symptoms of depression among those with severe incontinence. Data from the UREPIK and BACH studies, which were performed in men aged 40–79 years ($N$ = 6486) from five cities (Boxmeer, the Netherlands; Auxerre, France; Birmingham, UK; Seoul, South Korea and Boston, USA), also showed that QoL decreased with increasing severity of LUTS [12]. A 10-point increase in IPSS was associated with a 3.3-point reduction in SF-12 physical health component score, and a 1.4–3.4-point reduction in the mental health component score [12]. A US study reported that storage but not voiding symptoms was significantly associated with anxiety and depression [5]. Our study showed some trends towards greater increases in anxiety and depression scores among individuals with storage versus voiding symptoms, but the differences were small.

Studies conducted in Asian populations also reported similar findings to our study. South Korean women with OAB or stress urinary incontinence (SUI) have been shown to have lower quality of life (i.e. higher scores for all King's Health Questionnaire domains) than controls [15]. The same study reported lower Short Form-36 (SF-36) scores versus controls for four out of eight domains in women with OAB, and for one domain in women with SUI. A door-to-door survey of South Korean men aged ≥40 years showed that generic health status and workplace productivity were impaired among individuals with LUTS compared with those without LUTS [7]. Increased symptoms of major depression were also observed in men with LUTS. A third South Korean study involved 625 men and women with OAB [31]. Increasing severity of incontinence was associated with significantly lower QoL (measured using the Incontinence-Specific

**Table 5** Significant predictors of HADS scores ≥8

|  | Men | Women |
|---|---|---|
| HADS anxiety score | Voiding symptoms: Straining, terminal dribble<br>Storage symptoms: Perceived frequency, nocturia, urgency with fear of leaking, and stress incontinence (in relation to sneezing, exercising, nocturnal enuresis or sexual activity) | Voiding symptoms: Terminal dribble<br>Storage symptoms: Perceived frequency, nocturia, urgency with fear of leaking, and stress incontinence (nocturnal enuresis)<br>Post-micturition symptoms: Incomplete emptying |
| HADS depression score | Voiding symptoms: Terminal dribble<br>Storage symptoms: Perceived frequency, urgency, urgency with fear of leaking, urgency incontinence (how often), and stress incontinence (in relation to coughing or sexual activity) | Storage symptoms: Nocturia, urgency with fear of leaking, and stress incontinence (in relation to laughing or for no reason)<br>Post-micturition symptoms: Incomplete emptying |

*HADS* Hospital Anxiety and Depression Scale

Quality of Life Instrument), increased symptom bother, poorer health-related utility (according to EQ-5D), increased expenditure on incontinence pads, and increased interference with work and regular activities. In the same study, frequency, urgency and nocturia were independently associated with QoL impairment [31]. In Taiwanese women with SUI, significant correlations between the severity of incontinence and incontinence-related QoL have been observed [14]. Another study of Taiwanese women (age range: 35–64 years; $N = 4661$) reported reduced SF-36 scores, including physical and mental components, among individuals with urinary incontinence [8]. This study also showed that urinary incontinence had a greater impact on mental health-related HRQoL than diabetes, hyperlipidaemia, and chronic kidney disease. A third Taiwanese study showed that women with mixed urinary incontinence had lower QoL than those with urge incontinence or stress incontinence [32]. In China, HRQoL was assessed in individuals with LUTS and compared with data for the normal population [33]. Reduced scores were observed among the population with LUTS for the general health and vitality domains and for the physical component, although LUTS was associated with a higher role emotion domain score. HRQoL impairment increased with increased LUTS severity. In another Chinese study, data from >1000 adults showed that increasing episodes of nocturia was an independent predictor of impaired nocturia-related QoL [16].

Our findings also reflect previous Asian mental health data. In Taiwan, the prevalence of depression or anxiety has been found to be twice as high among individuals with LUTS versus matched controls (11.45% vs. 5.72%) [34]. Similarly, the odds ratio of depression in Korean men with versus without LUTS has been reported to be 2.87 [35]. A study performed in Hong Kong reported that the relationship between LUTS and depressive symptoms is robust after adjustment for other factors associated with depression such as divorce, cardiac disease and smoking [36].

Our study suggests considerable scope to reduce the overall burden of LUTS by increasing the percentage of patients who consult healthcare professionals, which will help patients gain access to the most effective available treatment for their condition. A variety of treatments that can be prescribed for LUTS have been shown to improve patients' QoL and/or mental health (e.g. drug treatment such as alpha blockers or antimuscarinics, surgical options such as transobturator tape or transurethral resection, botulinum toxin injections) [37–46].

The survey population is an important strength of our study. Younger individuals were not included because of previous data showing that LUTS are highly prevalent above the age of 40 [2] and numerous other epidemiological studies have focused on populations aged ≥40 years [6, 7, 9, 12, 47]. Additional strengths include the large number of participants and the use of well-established instruments to determine the presence and severity of LUTS and their effects on QoL and mental health. Our survey was conducted in countries with the highest internet penetration rates in Asia (South Korea, 92%; Taiwan, 84% and China 52%) [48]. Use of the internet to conduct a survey encourages full and honest responses to sensitive questions – there can be a tendency for biased answers when questions are asked by an interviewer [49]. On the other hand, we cannot be certain that results among individuals without internet access would be the same as those reported here. Also, when completing a questionnaire online, study participants may potentially interpret questions differently from those asked by a healthcare professional as interviewer. Although our results are similar to other studies around the globe, our study is limited by statistical analyses being undertaken post hoc; ideally these should have been identified a priori. The study was not designed to assess costs associated with LUTS, although impairment of workplace productivity indicates a financial impact and a health economic evaluation may have been useful. Previous investigations have shown that the economic burden of LUTS is significant (e.g. estimated annual costs up to $32 billion in the USA) [50, 51].

## Conclusions

In conclusion, this international study demonstrates the association of both LUTS and increasing OAB severity with impairment of QoL, workplace productivity and mental health in three Asian countries. These results are consistent with previous studies, and highlight the need to ensure that individuals with LUTS consult healthcare professionals to receive appropriate and effective treatment.

**Abbreviations**

ANOVA: Analysis of variance; HADS: Hospital anxiety and depression scale; HRQoL-SF12v2: 12-item short-form health survey for measuring health-related quality of life; ICIQ-LUTSqol: International Consultation on Incontinence Modular Questionnaire Lower Urinary Tract Symptoms Quality of Life; ICS: International Continence Society; IPSS: International Prostate Symptom Score; LUTS: Lower urinary tract symptoms; OABSS: Overactive bladder symptom score; QoL: Quality of life; SD: Standard deviation; WLQ: Work limitations

**Acknowledgements**

The authors would like to thank the participants of the study for their time, Nanjangud Shankar Narasimhamurthy and Koni Raviprakash for statistical analyses and Dr. Ming Liu for intellectual input into the manuscript. Medical writing support was provided by Ken Sutor, BSc and Jackie van Bueren, BSc of Envision Scientific Solutions.

## Funding

This study was designed and funded by Astellas Pharma Singapore Pte. Ltd. Medical writing support was funded by Astellas Pharma Global Development.


## Authors' contributions

K-SL, TKY, LL, JW, Y-CC, S-PL, RC and BS were involved in the study conception and design, analysis and interpretation of data, drafting the manuscript, and critical revision of the manuscript for important intellectual content. BS was additionally involved in acquisition of data and statistical analysis. All authors read and approved the final manuscript.


## Ethics approval and consent to participate

The study was based on a survey, with participants selected via consumer survey panels and as such it was not considered necessary to submit for Institutional Review Board approval. However, principles of the Declaration of Helsinki were followed; the study was performed in compliance with Good Clinical Practice and followed the World Association for Social, Opinion and Market Research (ESOMAR) guidelines that enshrine legal and ethical considerations of panel research, including respondent rights affecting patients/consumers who undertake market research surveys.
Informed consent was obtained from all patients being included in the study.


## Competing interests

K-SL, T-KY, LL, JW, Y-CC, and S-PL: acted as a consultant for Astellas during a meeting to discuss the publications from the study. T-KY also received grants and personal fees from Astellas to act as a consultant. RC: was an employee of Astellas Pharma Singapore Pte Ltd. during the conduct of the study and BS is a current employee of Astellas Pharma Singapore Pte Ltd.

## Author details

[1]Department of Urology, Samsung Medical Center, Sungkyunkwan University School of Medicine, Seoul, Korea. [2]Department of Urology, Nowon Eulji Medical Center, Eulji University School of Medicine, 68, Hangeulbiseok-ro, Nowon-gu, Seoul, Korea. [3]Department of Urology, China Rehabilitation Research Center, Capital Medical University, Beijing, China. [4]Department of Urology, Beijing Hospital, Beijing, China. [5]Department of Urology, Kaohsiung Chang Gung Memorial Hospital, Chang Gung University College of Medicine, Kaohsiung, Taiwan. [6]Department of Urology, National Taiwan University Hospital and College of Medicine, Taipei, Taiwan. [7]Astellas Pharma Singapore Pte. Ltd., Singapore, Singapore. [8]Present address: 5 Pemimpin Drive, #19-03 Seasons View, Singapore, Singapore.

## References

1. Coyne KS, Sexton CC, Thompson CL, Milsom I, Irwin D, Kopp ZS, et al. The prevalence of lower urinary tract symptoms (LUTS) in the USA, the UK and Sweden: results from the epidemiology of LUTS (EpiLUTS) study. BJU Int. 2009;104:352–60.
2. Irwin DE, Milsom I, Hunskaar S, Reilly K, Kopp Z, Herschorn S, et al. Population-based survey of urinary incontinence, overactive bladder, and other lower urinary tract symptoms in five countries: results of the EPIC study. Eur Urol. 2006;50:1306–14.
3. Lee YS, Lee KS, Jung JH, Han DH, Oh SJ, Seo JT, et al. Prevalence of overactive bladder, urinary incontinence, and lower urinary tract symptoms: results of Korean EPIC study. World J Urol. 2011;29:185–90.
4. Wang Y, Hu H, Xu K, Wang X, Na Y, Kang X. Prevalence, risk factors and the bother of lower urinary tract symptoms in China: a population-based survey. Int Urogynecol J. 2015;26:911–9.
5. Martin S, Vincent A, Taylor AW, Atlantis E, Jenkins A, Januszewski A, et al. Lower urinary tract symptoms, depression, anxiety and systemic inflammatory factors in men: a population-based cohort study. PLoS One. 2015;10:e0137903.
6. Abrams P, Smith AP, Cotterill N. The impact of urinary incontinence on health-related quality of life (HRQoL) in a real-world population of women aged 45-60 years: results from a survey in France, Germany, the UK and the USA. BJU Int. 2015;115:143–52.
7. Kim TH, Han DH, Ryu DS, Lee KS. The impact of lower urinary tract symptoms on quality of life, work productivity, depressive symptoms, and sexuality in Korean men aged 40 years and older: a population-based survey. Int Neurourol J. 2015;19:120–9.
8. Horng SS, Huang N, Wu SI, Fang YT, Chou YJ, Chou P. The epidemiology of urinary incontinence and it's influence on quality of life in Taiwanese middle-aged women. Neurourol Urodyn. 2013;32:371–6.
9. Coyne KS, Wein AJ, Tubaro A, Sexton CC, Thompson CL, Kopp ZS, et al. The burden of lower urinary tract symptoms: evaluating the effect of LUTS on health-related quality of life, anxiety and depression: EpiLUTS. BJU Int. 2009;103(Suppl 3):4–11.
10. Aguilar-Navarro S, Navarrete-Reyes AP, Grados-Chavarría BH, Garcia-Lara JM, Amieva H, Avila-Funes JA. The severity of urinary incontinence decreases health-related quality of life among community-dwelling elderly. J Gerontol A Biol Sci Med Sci. 2012;67:1266–71.
11. Currie CJ, McEwan P, Poole CD, Odeyemi IA, Datta SN, Morgan CL. The impact of the overactive bladder on health-related utility and quality of life. BJU Int. 2006;97:1267–72.
12. Robertson C, Link CL, Onel E, Mazzetta C, Keech M, Hobbs R, et al. The impact of lower urinary tract symptoms and comorbidities on quality of life: the BACH and UREPIK studies. BJU Int. 2007;99:347–54.
13. Sexton CC, Coyne KS, Thompson C, Bavendam T, Chen CI, Markland A. Prevalence and effect on health-related quality of life of overactive bladder in older Americans: results from the epidemiology of lower urinary tract symptoms study. J Am Geriatr Soc. 2011;59:1465–70.
14. Huang WC, Yang SH, Yang SY, Yang E, Yang JM. The correlations of incontinence-related quality of life measures with symptom severity and pathophysiology in women with primary stress urinary incontinence. World J Urol. 2010;28:619–23.
15. Oh SJ, Ku JH. Impact of stress urinary incontinence and overactive bladder on micturition patterns and health-related quality of life. Int Urogynecol J Pelvic Floor Dysfunct. 2007;18:65–71.
16. Zhang X, Zhang J, Chen J, Zhang C, Li Q, Xu T, et al. Prevalence and risk factors of nocturia and nocturia-related quality of life in the Chinese population. Urol Int. 2011;86:173–8.
17. Rom M, Schatzl G, Swietek N, Rucklinger E, Kratzik C. Lower urinary tract symptoms and depression. BJU Int. 2012;110:E918–21.
18. Litman HJ, Steers WD, Wei JT, Kupelian V, Link CL, McKinlay JB, et al. Relationship of lifestyle and clinical factors to lower urinary tract symptoms: results from Boston area community health survey. Urology. 2007;70:916–21.
19. Hsieh CH, Kuo TC, Hsu CS, Chang ST, Lee MC. Nocturia among women aged 60 or older in Taiwan. Aust N Z J Obstet Gynaecol. 2008;48:312–6.
20. Norby B, Nordling J, Mortensen S. Lower urinary tract symptoms in the Danish population: a population-based study of symptom prevalence, health-care seeking behavior and prevalence of treatment in elderly males and females. Eur Urol. 2005;47:817–23.
21. Kuritzky L. Role of primary care clinicians in the diagnosis and treatment of LUTS and BPH. Rev Urol. 2004;6(Suppl 9):S53–9.
22. Abrams P, Cardozo L, Fall M, Griffiths D, Rosier P, Ulmsten U, et al. The standardisation of terminology of lower urinary tract function: report from the standardisation sub-committee of the international continence society. Neurourol Urodyn. 2002;21:167–78.
23. Chapple C, Castro-Díaz D, Chuang YC, Lee KS, Liao L, Liu SP, et al. Prevalence of LUTS in China, Taiwan and South Korea: results from a cross-sectional, population-based study. Adv Ther. 2017. doi:10.1007/s12325-017-0577-9 .
24. World Association for Social Opinion and Market Research. ESOMAR guideline for online research. Available at: https://www.esomar.org/uploads/public/knowledge-and-standards/codes-and-guidelines/ESOMAR_Guideline-for-online-research.pdf. Accessed 6 Nov 2017.
25. Barry MJ, Fowler FJ Jr, O'Leary MP, Bruskewitz RC, Holtgrewe HL, Mebust WK, et al. The American urological association symptom index for benign prostatic hyperplasia. The measurement Committee of the American Urological Association. J Urol. 1992;148:1549–57. discussion 64
26. Homma Y, Yoshida M, Seki N, Yokoyama O, Kakizaki H, Gotoh M, et al. Symptom assessment tool for overactive bladder syndrome – overactive bladder symptom score. Urology. 2006;68:318–23.

27. Ware J Jr, Kosinski M, Keller SD. A 12-item short-form health survey: construction of scales and preliminary tests of reliability and validity. Med Care. 1996;34:220–33.

28. Lerner D, Amick BC 3rd, Rogers WH, Malspeis S, Bungay K, Cynn D. The work limitations questionnaire. Med Care. 2001;39:72–85.

29. Zigmond AS, Snaith RP. The hospital anxiety and depression scale. Acta Psychiatr Scand. 1983;67:361–70.

30. Bjelland I, Dahl AA, Haug TT, Neckelmann D. The validity of the hospital anxiety and depression scale. An updated literature review. J Psychosom Res. 2002;52:69–77.

31. Lee KS, Choo MS, Seo JT, Oh SJ, Kim HG, Ng K, et al. Impact of overactive bladder on quality of life and resource use: results from Korean burden of incontinence study (KOBIS). Health Qual Life Outcomes. 2015;13:89.

32. Tsai YC, Liu CH. Urinary incontinence among Taiwanese women: an outpatient study of prevalence, comorbidity, risk factors, and quality of life. Int Urol Nephrol. 2009;41:795–803.

33. Choi EP, Lam CL, Chin WY. The health-related quality of life of Chinese patients with lower urinary tract symptoms in primary care. Qual Life Res. 2014;23:2723–33.

34. Lung-Cheng Huang C, Ho CH, Weng SF, Hsu YW, Wang JJ, Wu MP. The association of healthcare seeking behavior for anxiety and depression among patients with lower urinary tract symptoms: a nationwide population-based study. Psychiatry Res. 2015;226:247–51.

35. Jeong WS, Choi HY, Nam JW, Kim SA, Choi BY, Moon HS, et al. Men with severe lower urinary tract symptoms are at increased risk of depression. Int Neurourol J. 2015;19:286–92.

36. Wong SY, Hong A, Leung J, Kwok T, Leung PC, Woo J. Lower urinary tract symptoms and depressive symptoms in elderly men. J Affect Disord. 2006;96:83–8.

37. Akin Y, Gulmez H, Ucar M, Yucel S. The effect of first dose of tamsulosin on flow rate and its predictive ability on the improvement of LUTS in men with BPH in the mid-term. Int Urol Nephrol. 2013;45:45–51.

38. Cañete P, Ortiz E, Domingo S, Cano A. Transobturator suburethral tape in the treatment of stress urinary incontinence: efficacy and quality of life after 5 year follow up. Maturitas. 2013;74:166–71.

39. Game X, Khan S, Panicker JN, Kalsi V, Dalton C, Elneil S, et al. Comparison of the impact on health-related quality of life of repeated detrusor injections of botulinum toxin in patients with idiopathic or neurogenic detrusor overactivity. BJU Int. 2011;107:1786–92.

40. Hirakawa T, Suzuki S, Kato K, Gotoh M, Yoshikawa Y. Randomized controlled trial of pelvic floor muscle training with or without biofeedback for urinary incontinence. Int Urogynecol J. 2013;24:1347–54.

41. Innerkofler PC, Guenther V, Rehder P, Kopp M, Nguyen-Van-Tam DP, Giesinger JM, et al. Improvement of quality of life, anxiety and depression after surgery in patients with stress urinary incontinence: results of a longitudinal short-term follow-up. Health Qual Life Outcomes. 2008;6:72.

42. Kafri R, Deutscher D, Shames J, Golombp J, Melzer I. Randomized trial of a comparison of rehabilitation or drug therapy for urgency urinary incontinence: 1-year follow-up. Int Urogynecol J. 2013;24:1181–9.

43. Quek KF, Low WY, Razack AH, Loh CS. The psychological effects of treatments for lower urinary tract symptoms. BJU Int. 2000;86:630–3.

44. Quek KF, Razack AH, Chua CB, Low WY, Loh CS. Effect of treating lower urinary tract symptoms on anxiety, depression and psychiatric morbidity: a one-year study. Int J Urol. 2004;11:848–55.

45. Rogers R, Bachmann G, Jumadilova Z, Sun F, Morrow JD, Guan Z, et al. Efficacy of tolterodine on overactive bladder symptoms and sexual and emotional quality of life in sexually active women. Int Urogynecol J Pelvic Floor Dysfunct. 2008;19:1551–7.

46. van Kerrebroeck P, Chapple C, Drogendijk T, Klaver M, Sokol R, Speakman M, et al. Combination therapy with solifenacin and tamsulosin oral controlled absorption system in a single tablet for lower urinary tract symptoms in men: efficacy and safety results from the randomised controlled NEPTUNE trial. Eur Urol. 2013;64:1003–12.

47. Araki I, Tsuchida T, Nomura T, Fukasawa M, Takihana Y, Koyama N, et al. Differential impact of lower urinary tract symptoms on generic and disease-specific quality of life in men and women. Urol Int. 2008;81:60–5.

48. Internet World Stats. Internet usage in Asia. Available at: http://www.internetworldstats.com/. Accessed 6 Nov 2017.

49. Coyne KS, Sexton CC, Kopp ZS, Luks S, Gross A, Irwin D, et al. Rationale for the study methods and design of the epidemiology of lower urinary tract symptoms (EpiLUTS) study. BJU Int. 2009;104:348–51.

50. Levy R, Muller N. Urinary incontinence: economic burden and new choices in pharmaceutical treatment. Adv Ther. 2006;23:556–73.

51. Tapia CI, Khalaf K, Berenson K, Globe D, Chancellor M, Carr LK. Health-related quality of life and economic impact of urinary incontinence due to detrusor overactivity associated with a neurologic condition: a systematic review. Health Qual Life Outcomes. 2013;11:13.

# 24

# Combination therapy only shows short-term superiority over monotherapy on ureteral stent-related symptoms

Qinyu Liu[†], Banghua Liao[†], Ruochen Zhang, Tao Jin, Liang Zhou, Deyi Luo, Jiaming Liu, Hong Li and Kunjie Wang[*]

## Abstract

**Background:** Controversy remains on the superiority of combination therapy over monotherapy on ureteral stent-related symptoms (SRSs). We tend to explore if there is a necessity of combination therapy.

**Methods:** One hundred cases of unilateral upper urinary tract calculi with stent insertion (pre and post flexible ureteroscopy) were randomized into 4 groups, given non-treatment, solifenacin, tamsulosin or combination respectively. Eight times of follow-ups were given after each insertion.

**Results:** SRSs released spontaneously within 4 days after insertion ($p = 0.017$) but then stay with no further improvement. Benefit of solifenacin on flank pain started showing after day4 ($p = 0.002$), which was comparable to that of tamsulosin and combination ($p = 0.914$ vs $0.195$). Combination therapy showed superiority over both monotherapy before day4, but after then solifenacin and tamsulosin showed similar effectiveness with the combination therapy on both bladder pain ($p = 0.229$ vs $0.394$) and urgency ($p = 0.813$ vs $0.974$). No improvement on hematuria or frequency was observed in each group.

**Conclusions:** Combination therapy takes effect faster but shows no supervisory after the first few days compared with monotherapy.

**Keywords:** Stent-related symptoms, Medication therapy management, Muscarinic antagonists, Adrenergic alpha-1 receptor antagonists

## Background

A vast majority of patients with indwelling ureteral stent are suffering from stent-related symptoms (SRSs) with poor quality of life (QoL), and storage symptoms and body pain are the most troublesome [1, 2]. Currently it is hypothesized that bladder discomfort, lower urinary tract symptoms (LUTS) and hematuria are due to mechanical irritation of bladder trigone as well as bladder neck, while flank pain is associated with vesicoureteric reflux and evidences showed antireflux stent can minimize the pain [3]. As a consequence, efforts such as improving stent design and composition and investigating medical therapy have been made to solve this problem [4–6]. So far many researches have shown that α-blockers and anticholinergic agents both can ease these discomforts and ultimately improve the QoL [7] . However, there're still not many researches on comparison between monotherapy and combination. In addition, some most recent published papers made different voices: while former researches with International Prostate Symptom Score (IPSS) found

---
* Correspondence: wangkj@scu.edu.cn
[†]Equal contributors
Department of Urology, Institute of Urology (Laboratory of Reconstructive Urology), West China Hospital, Sichuan University, Chengdu 610041, Sichuan, People's Republic of China

combination therapies provided preferable outcomes, some most current ones declared that monotherapies functioned equally with the combination in Ureteric Stent Symptom Questionnaire (USSQ) assessment [8, 9].

Basing on the background above, we conducted a randomized controlled trial to evaluate the efficacy of solifenacin, tamsulosin and the combination therapy, and meanwhile to explore SRSs' development features with time as secondary outcomes.

## Methods
### Subjects and treatments
An open-label, randomized, controlled study was conducted at West China Hospital of Sichuan University from Feb 2014 to May 2015. Inclusion criteria were as followed: (1) aged 18–60 years with unilateral nephrolithiasis ≤2 cm; (2) 4.7Fr ureteral stent being inserted before and after flexible ureteroscopic lithotripsy. The exclusion criteria included: (1) a history of urinary tract surgery; (2) a history of LUTS related to benign prostatic hyperplasia or infection; (3) concomitant use of other antiadrenergics, anticholinergics, and analgesics; (4) a history of neurogenic bladder, overactive bladder syndrome, neurologic and psychiatric diseases, chronic prostatitis and urinary tract abnormalities; (5) drug allergy; (6) having major complications after the surgery.

4.7Fr ureteral stents (INLAY®, Bard Inc.) of 26 cm were inserted in all cases through cystoscopy 2 weeks before the ureteroscopic surgery. A stent of the same size was inserted after lithotripsy under general anesthesia within the flexible ureteroscopic surgery. X-ray plain films were done after both insertions to make sure the stents were in correct position since inappropriate stent location would worsen LUTS and affect the QoL severely [10, 11]. Patients were told to drink more than 2500 ml water per day and avoid aggravating physical activities after insertion. Patients were discharged on the third day following lithotripsy surgery.

### Randomization, follow-up, assessment of outcomes
Patients were randomized into one of four groups, namely C (control), S (solifenacin 5 mg once daily), T (tamsulosin 0.2 mg once daily), and S + T (solifenacin and tamsulosin combination).

Follow-ups were performed on day 1, 2, 3, 4, 5, 6, 10, and 14 after stent insertion on phone. Questions on urinary symptoms were selected from USSQ to assess bladder irritation, while a visual analogue scale (VAS) and a seven-score QoL scale were adopted for body pain and QoL assessment. Every patient had two series of follow-ups (pre- and post-lithotripsy) as self-control. Data of patients who missed more than twice dose or follow-ups throughout the follow-up duration were excluded in the

final analysis. Also a questionnaire aiming at adverse events was taken on day14 to evaluate the safety.

The primary outcome was the urinary symptom score of the given questionnaire. The secondary outcomes included scores in every single symptom assumed in the current study, the score of quality of life and initial effect time.

### Sample size and statistical analysis
Sample size was calculated with the standard deviation of the urinary symptom domain of 4 as observed in our preliminary test of patients given no treatment and the following assumed post-stent urinary symptom scores: no treatment (14), tamsulosin (11), solifenacin (11) tamsulosin, and solifenacin (10). For $\alpha = 0.05$ and $\beta = 0.1$, the minimal sample size needed for each group was 20. Assuming a 20% withdrawal rate, we decided to have 25 as the least sample size needed for each group and recruit as many as possible during the research period.

SPSS 20.0 was used for statistical analysis. Repeated measures analysis of variance was used to compare variables between groups. Chi-square and ANOVA tests were used to compare ratios and mean values between groups or different follow-up days. Logistic regression was used to reveal relevance between variables. A $p$-value $< 0.05$ indicated statistically significant differences in the current study.

## Results
Finally, a total of 112 cases were recruited. With 12 cases (10.71%) not appropriate for final analysis due to loss of follow-up or poor compliance, the final sample size was 100 (group C 28, S 26, T 22 and S + T 24, Fig. 1). No significant differences showed in age, height, weight or gender among the 4 groups ($p = 0.633$, 0.131, 0.674, 0.337) (Table 1). None of participants were found with a history of urinary tract surgery, LUTS related to benign prostatic hyperplasia or infection, concomitant use of other similar drugs or any other comorbidities that may confuse the assessment of SRSs.

### Characteristics of SRSs in the control group
Outcomes from the group C showed that the total score of all symptoms spontaneously decreased in the first 4 days (from $12.75 \pm 3.52$ to $9.93 \pm 3.64$, $p = 0.017$). However after that, no significant differences showed from day4 to day14 (from $9.93 \pm 3.64$ to $9.18 \pm 3.38$, $p = 0.602$), and a trend of increase was noted after day6 (Fig. 2).

Though the degree of symptoms changed over time, score of quality of life stayed relatively steady throughout the follow-up ($p = 0.674$) and the minimal score was $3.25 \pm 1.08$ (score3 means mostly satisfied while score4 means about equally satisfied and dissatisfied) (Additional file 1: Figure S1).

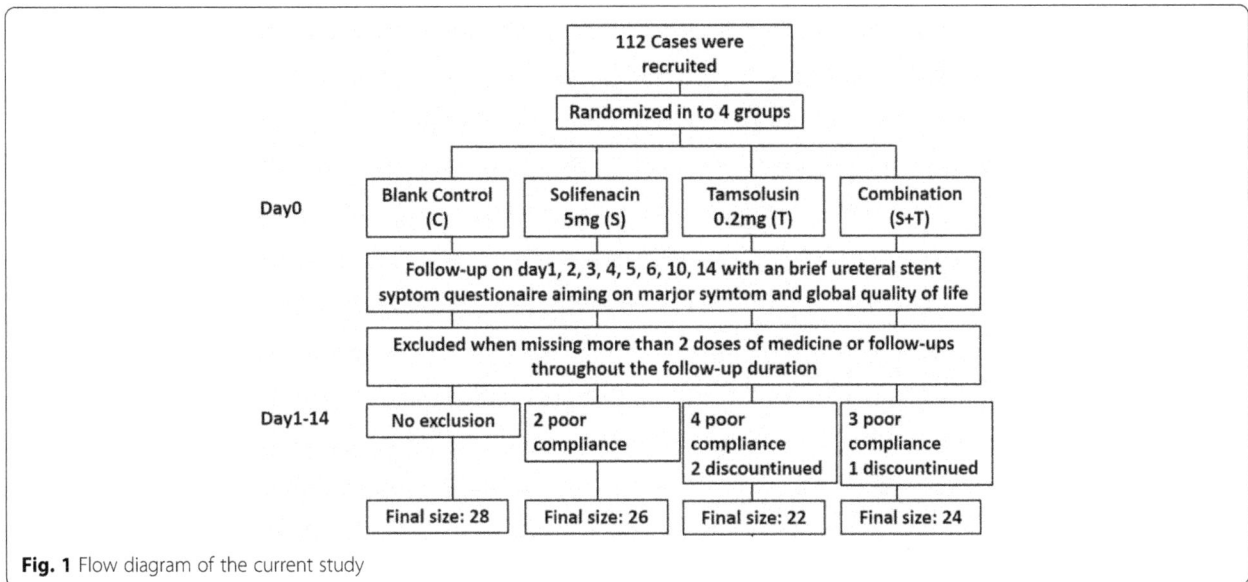

**Fig. 1** Flow diagram of the current study

### Effect of endoscopic procedure on SRSs

Generally no significant differences were found in total scores of symptoms between pre- and post-lithotripsy cases ($p = 0.066$). However, subsection analysis showed that pre-lithotripsy cases had lower scores than those of post-lithotripsy ones before day4 ($p = 0.001$, mean difference = $-1.455$, 95% CI = $-2.334$ to $-0.576$). Subgroup analysis of single symptom suggested that within the first 4 days following insertion, pre-lithotripsy cases had milder bladder area pain ($p = 0.036$, mean difference = $-0.39$, 95% CI = $-0.75$ to $-0.03$), flank pain ($p = 0.005$, mean difference = $-0.60$, 95% CI = $-1.01$ to $-0.19$) and hematuria ($p = 0.001$, mean difference = $-0.065$, 95% CI = $-0.34$ to $-0.09$) comparing to post-lithotripsy cases. Pre- and post-lithotripsy cases had similar level of frequency ($p = 0.232$) and urgency ($p = 0.825$) from the beginning to the end (Additional file 1: Figure S2).

### Efficacy outcomes of medication therapy

Overall, solifenacin, tamsulosin and combination therapy group all had lower levels of SRSs than the control group throughout the follow up ($p = 0.004$ & $0.026$ & $<0.001$).

Before day4, combination therapy provided even lower scores of SRSs than single solifenacin ($p = 0.016$, mean difference = $-1.52$, 95% CI = $-2.76$ to $-0.29$) and tamsulosin ($p = 0.002$, mean difference = $-2.10$, 95% CI = $-3.39$ to $-0.81$), but no significant differences showed up between combination and either single drug group after day5 (solifenacin & tamsulosin, $p = 0.84$ & $0.77$). Solifenacin and tamsulosin showed comparable effect throughout the whole follow up ($p = 0.582$) (Fig. 3).

As for specific symptoms, no statistical differences were found in flank pain scores among all 4 groups before day4 ($p = 0.101$). However, from day5 to the end, a superiority over the control group was noted in solifenacin group ($p = 0.002$, mean difference = $-0.71$, 95% CI = $-1.14$ to $-0.27$), which was comparable with tamsulosin and combination therapy ($p = 0.914$ vs $0.195$). Combination therapy released bladder pain and urgency from the very beginning and remained effective to the end (comparing with the control, bladder pain $p < 0.001$, mean difference = $-1.07$, 95% CI = $-1.43$ to $-0.72$; urgency $p < 0.001$, mean difference = $-0.61$, 95% CI = $-0.91$ to $-0.31$). On the other hand, neither of solifenacin or tamsulosin

**Table 1** Popularity characteristic of the current study

| Variables | Group c | Group s | Group t | Group s+t |
|---|---|---|---|---|
| Number of cases | 28 | 26 | 22 | 24 |
| Gender, n (%) | | | | |
| Male | 20 (71.4) | 20 (76.9) | 12 (54.5) | 18 (75.0) |
| Female | 8 (28.6) | 6 (23.1) | 10 (45.5) | 6 (25.0) |
| Age (year), mean ± SD | 40.00 ± 8.24 | 41.55 ± 10.63 | 43.1 ± 12.10 | 44.00 ± 12.16 |
| Height (cm), mean ± SD | 165.75 ± 7.92 | 167.67 ± 6.05 | 165.30 ± 8.03 | 162.44 ± 5.42 |
| Weight (kg), mean ± SD | 67.08 ± 12.33 | 64.83 ± 10.80 | 67.10 ± 14.71 | 63.00 ± 11.24 |

$P < 0.05$ for age, height, weight and gender among the 4 groups

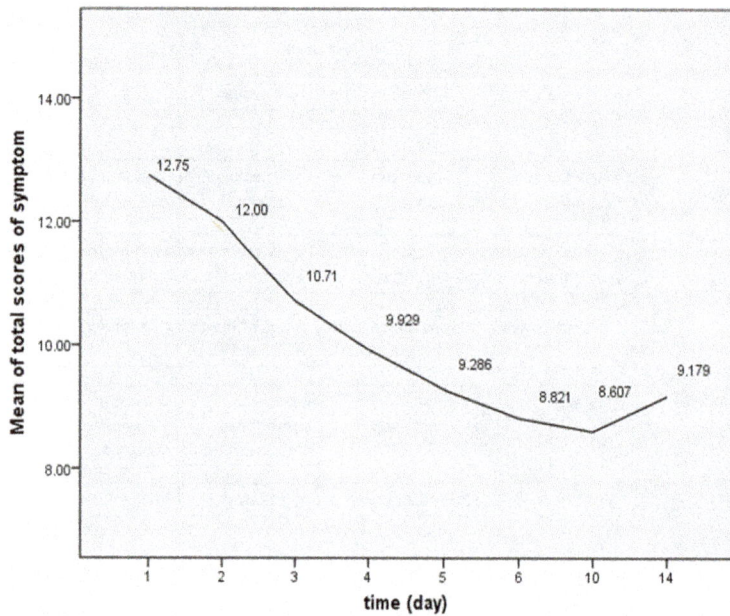

**Fig. 2** Means of total scores of all symptoms in control group on each follow-up day. The means changed statistically over time ($p < 0.001$) and decreased obviously in the first 4 days ($p = 0.017$). However, from then on no significant differences showed from day4 to day14 showed ($p = 0.602$)

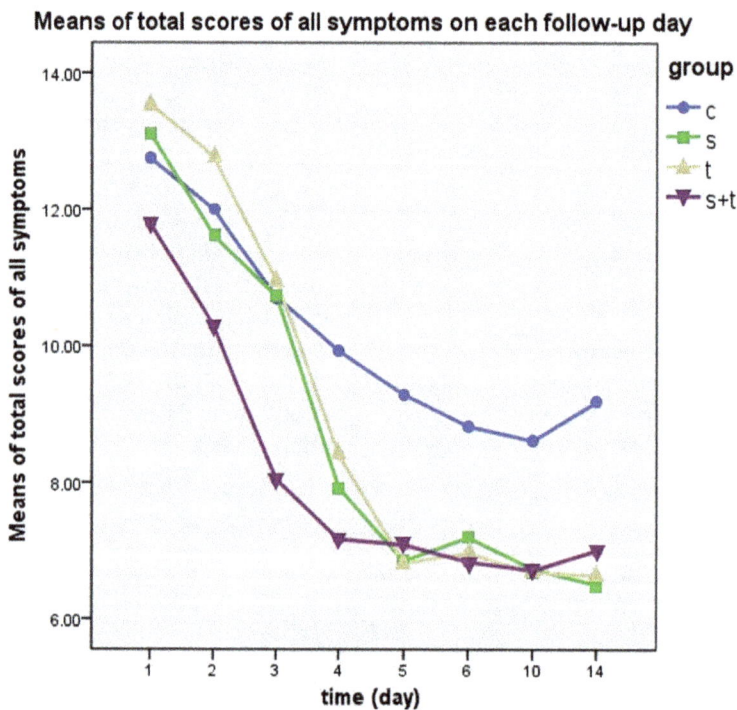

**Fig. 3** Solifenacin, tamsulosin and combination therapy all released SRSs comparing to the control group ($p = 0.004$ vs 0.026 vs <0.001). Combination therapy could release the SRSs much faster than solifenacin ($p = 0.016$) or tamsulosin (0.002) in the first 4 days. No significant differences showed up between combination and solifenacin ($p = 0.842$) or tamsulosin ($p = 0.774$) alone from day5 to day14. Solifenacin and tamsulosin showed comparable effect throughout the whole follow up ($p = 0.582$)

showed significant effects on bladder pain (vs control, $p = 0.589$ & 0.936) or urgency (vs control, $p = 0.806$ & 0.729) before day4. But from the fifth day on, solifenacin and tamsulosin monotherapy both started showing equal benefic effects as the combination therapy on both bladder pain ($p = 0.229$ & 0.394) and urgency ($p = 0.813$ & 0.974) (Fig. 4).

Solifenacin, tamsulosin and combination group all showed no superiority over the control group in hematuria ($p = 0.736$ & 0.924 & 1.000) or frequency ($p = 0.073$ & 0.860

& 0.092) (Additional file 1: Figure S3). Incontinence was observed on only two follow-up days from one single case in solifenacin group.

As for quality of life (QoL), significant difference existed among the 4 groups ($p = 0.046$) but combination therapy wasn't superior to either monotherapy group (solifenacin and tamsulosin, $p = 0.107$ vs 0.670). Medication therapy groups had higher scores than the control at the beginning but finally went down to be lower after day4 (Additional file 1: Figure S4).

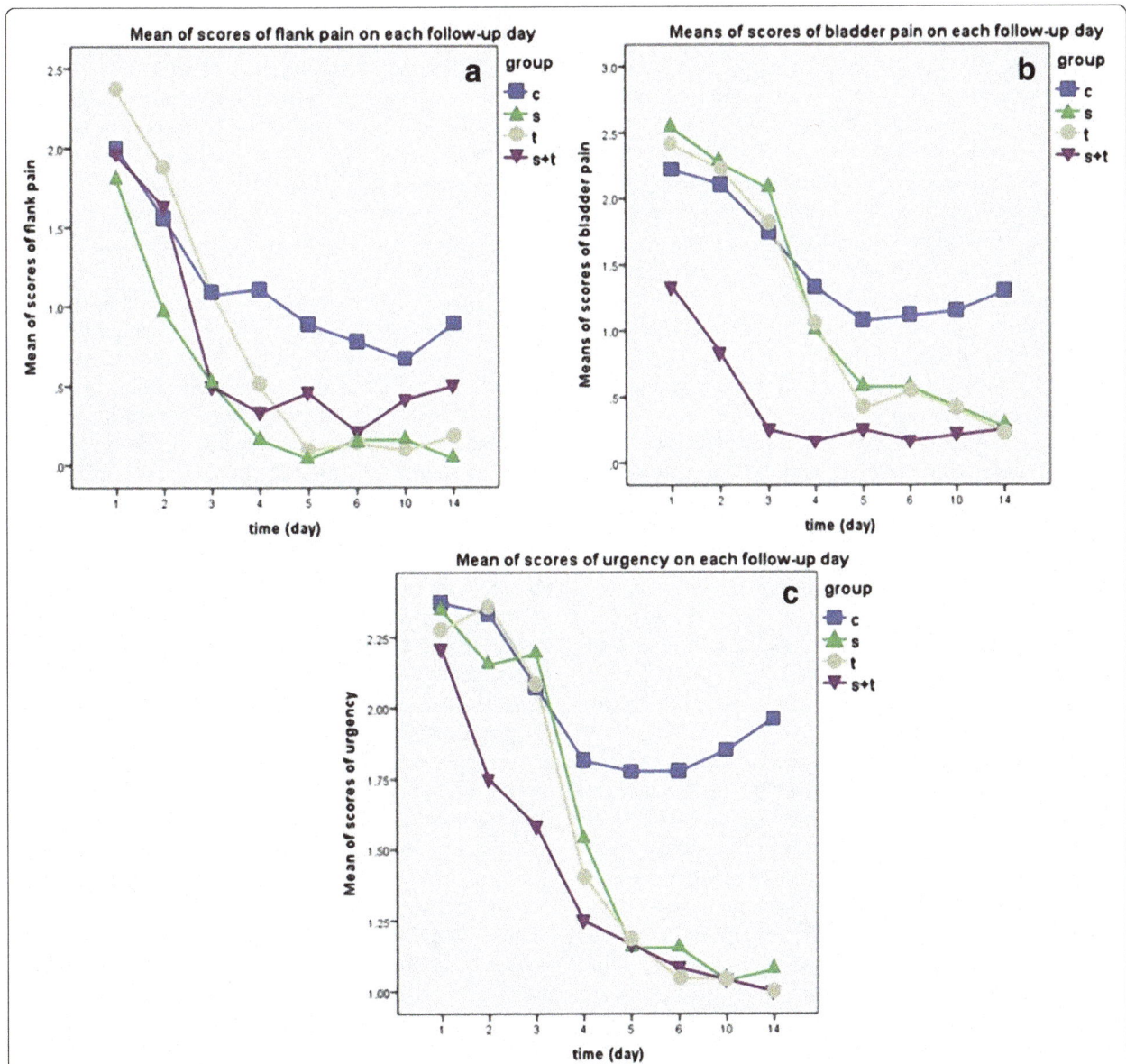

**Fig. 4** Means of scores of flank pain (**a**), bladder pain (**b**) and urgency (**c**). Effect on flank pain started showing up from day5 to the end ($p = 0.006$) and solifenacin is comparable to tamsulosin and combination therapy ($p = 0.914$ vs 0.195) (**a**). Combination therapy released bladder pain and urgency throughout the whole follow-up (comparing with the control, both $p < 0.001$) (**b** and **c**). Before day4, Solifenacin and tamsulosin had no significant effect on bladder pain ($p = 0.589$ vs 0.936) or urgency ($p = 0.806$ vs 0.729) but both showed showed comparable effectiveness as the combination therapy from day5 to day14 (**b** and **c**)

## Adverse events

Main complications of drug therapy groups were as followed: solifenacin group with three patients with dry mouth (3/26, 11.5%); tamsulosin group with two with dizziness (2/22, 9.1%), combination group with three with dry mouth and one with both symptoms in group (4/24, 16.7%). The total incidence rate of adverse events from these three groups and no significant differences ($p = 0.727$). No serious adverse events were reported throughout the study.

## Discussion

In a previous study on SRSs features, J. Irani et al. [12] declared that the general tolerance to SRSs remains unchanged with time while only some symptoms significantly improve, dysuria and hematuria included. And in the current study, we also recorded that though SRSs relieved spontaneously to some degree within a few days after the insertion, it would stay relatively stable after then, and might even relapse or worsen as time went by. The minimal total symptom score was designed as 4, which meant suffering no SRSs, in our questionnaire. But the actual minimal mean of total scores of all symptoms in the control group was 8.607, which again demonstrated that patients would not develop complete tolerance to SRSs within two weeks. We estimate that the symptoms appearing within the very first days after insertion may be also associated with stimulation of transurethral endoscopic procedures, and these parts of symptoms can rapidly improve. The phenomenon that pre- and post-lithotripsy cases suffered differently in the beginning may support this hypothesis to some degree. And since the patients suffer the most in the first few days, we recommend that active managements should be given to patient right after stent-insertion, especially to whom following ureteroscopy surgeries.

Speaking of efficacy, solifenacin and tamsulosin showed comparably promising effect on releasing urgency, bladder discomfort and flank pain. And the long-term effects of both monotherapies were not inferior to the combination therapy in the current study. Meanwhile however, we also noticed that in the first few days a combination therapy would take effect faster than monotherapy, especially on symptoms of bladder pain and urgency. We think that the inhibitors of α- receptor and m-receptor may have synergistic effect on releasing irritative symptoms of bladder. So for patients who have relatively severe SRSs from the beginning or who are urge to release the symptom, a combination therapy is recommended. But after the first few days, an alternation to monotherapy would be a proper choice because the outcome demonstrated that a long-term combination therapy was unnecessary.

Although some transient relieving was observed, no general improvement in hematuria and frequency was found in any medication therapy groups comparing with the control, which disagreed with some previous studies [13–15]. Hematuria is believed to result from mechanical injury on mucosa by stent, so we think it may be more likely to be affected by patients' living habits, exercise habits for example, other than medicine intervention. And for frequency, we believe water-drinking amount also contributes a lot to it apart from stent insertion. In the current study, a daily water intake over 2500 ml resulted in urine volume increasing to about 2000 ml per day. Medication of α-blockers and anticholinergic agents are believed able to release irritating-induced storage symptoms while not affect the normal voiding function of bladder [16, 17], so frequency resulting from increased urine volume wouldn't be improved by solifenacin or tamsulosin. This reminds us that recording daily urine volume may be necessary for an accurate SRSs assessment.

We found it interesting to note that QoL might not improve completely with symptom releasing. On the days just following stent-insertion, patients accepting drug therapies had even poorer score on QoL than the control, although the degrees of their symptoms were about the same or even better. Not satisfied with the slow effect of drug in the first few days may be one of the reasons. Also our advice on water drinking and exercise limitation, which may contribute to the lower incidence of hematuria and flank pain, may also make patients feel bothered. During the follow-up days some patients complained about change in living habits and their QoL scores stayed low even though they have no obvious symptoms.

There are three previous studies adopting the same or similar regimen with the current study. Essam S. et al. found combined therapy of 0.4 mg tamsulosin and 10 mg solifenacin daily significantly alleviated irritative symptoms associated with stent-insertion comparing to either single medication [18]. Lim KT. et al. drew a conclusion of agreement with Essam S. with half the dose [19]. Jinsung P. et al. adopted the same regimen of Lim KT., but resulted in a totally different conclusion. They declared that neither tamsulosin nor solifenacin medications provide beneficial effects for SRSs [8]. In the current study, we conducted a multiple follow-up on several different days to explore SRSs, which can avoid bias of single-day follow-up adopted by the previous studies since SRSs may be affected by aspects like amount of exercise and water-drinking. All the researches mentioned above reached only one agreement that the administration of solifenacin and tamsulosin as well as their combination appeared equally safe and no severe complications were recorded. And so did the current one.

The following limitations should be acknowledged. A major one was that our method inevitably increased the workload of follow-up staffs and participants, so a limitation existed in comprehensiveness of symptom assessment and sample size. However since the size reached our established goal, we still believe our outcomes can make some sense. Another problem was that our center only provided stents with the same size and couldn't adjust the lengths of stents with heights. But while the randomized groups had no significant difference in patients' heights, this limitation would have little influence on the comparison outcomes. Further studies may take more comprehensive symptoms and effects of living habits into account, ending in more accurate assessment of SRSs, so as to bring out a more optimal protocol which can benefit patients the most.

## Conclusion

As our outcomes demonstrated, SRSs would release spontaneously to some degree in the first few days after the insertion, then stay non-improved or even worsen in the following days, which may still be troublesome. Combination of solifenacin and tamsulosin can take effect faster and improve the SRSs better than monotherapy in the first few days. After that, combination and monotherapy relieve the SRSs equally. So for long-term using, patients with SRSs may get comparable benefits from monotherapy and combination. Patients with frequency or hematuria may benefit little from both drugs because these symptoms would be largely affected by living habits. Further studies with lager sample size are expected to collect more detailed data and drawing more accurate conclusions.

## Additional file

**Additional file 1: Figure S1.** Means of total scores of quality of life on each follow-up day. No significant difference existed from day1 to day14 ($p = 0.674$). **Figure S2**. Means of Symptom scores of pre- and post-lithotripsy cases. Generally pre- and post-lithotripsy cases had no significant differences in total scores of all symptoms ($p = 0.066$) but subsection analysis showed significant difference existed before day4 ($p = 0.001$) (a). Subgroup analysis demonstrated difference in scores of bladder area pain ($p = 0.036$), kidney area pain ($p = 0.005$) and hematuria ($p = 0.001$) (b, c, d). No obvious difference showed up on frequency ($p = 0.232$) and urgency ($p = 0.825$) from the beginning to the end. (e, f). **Figure S3**. Solifenacin, tamsulosin and combination group showed no superiority over the control group on hematuria ($p = 0.736$ vs 0.924 vs 1.000) (a). Solifenacin, tamsulosin and combination therapy didn't effectively release the level of frequency ($p = 0.073$ vs 0.860 vs 0.092) (b). **Figure S4**. Mean of scores of quality of life. Significant difference existed among the 4 groups ($p = 0.046$) but combination therapy wasn't superior to either single drug group (solifenacin and tamsulosin, $p = 0.107$ vs 0.670). (DOCX 807 kb)

## Acknowledgements
Not applicable.

## Funding
The current study was supported by the following funds: Technology Support Plan of Science and Technology Department of Sichuan Province (Grant No. 2014SZ0210), Foundation of Sichuan University for Outstanding Youth (Grant No. 2014SCU04B21), Foundation for Academic Leader Fostering of Personnel Department of Sichuan Province (Grant No. JH2014053), Key Project for Applied Research of Organization Department of Sichuan Provincial Party Committee (Grant No. JH2015017) and Natural Science Foundation of China (Grant No. 81470927).

## Authors' contributions
QL and BL contributed equally to this work and share the co-first authors. QL, KW and BL designed the experiments; QL, BL and RZ collected the data. RZ and LZ analyzed while QL, TJ and KW interpreted the data. QL, BL, RZ and LZ wrote the manuscript while DL, TJ, JL and KW provided suggestions for revision. KW and HL obtained the funding. KW and HL did the supervision job throughout this study. All authors read and approved the final manuscript.

## Competing interests
The drug of Solifenacin was provided by Astellas Pharma China Inc. The authors declare that they have no competing interests.

## References
1. Joshi HB, Okeke A, Newns N, et al. Characterization of urinary symptoms in patients with ureteral stents. Urology. 2002;59(4):511–6.
2. Bosio A, Dalmasso E, Destefanis P, et al. How bothersome ureteral stents are after ureteroscopy? A prospective study using a validated questionnaire(USSQ). Eur Urol Suppl. 2005;14(2):e1075.
3. Ritter M, Krombach P, Knoll T, et al. Initial experience with a newly developed antirefluxive ureter stent. Urol Res. 2012;40(4):349–53.
4. Dellis A, Joshi HB, Timoney AG, et al. Relief of stent related symptoms: Review of engineering and pharmacological solutions. J Urol. 2010;184(4):1267–72.
5. Lange D, Bidnur S, Hoag N, et al. Ureteral stent-associated complications - where we are and where we are going. Nat Rev Urol. 2015;12(1):17–25.
6. Walker NAF, Bultitude MF, Brislane K, et al. Management of stent symptoms: what a pain! BJU Int. 2014;114(6):797–8.
7. Zhou L, Cai X, Li H, et al. Effects of α-blockers, antimuscarinics, or combination therapy in relieving ureteral stent-related symptoms: a meta-analysis. J Endourol. 2015;29(6):650–6.
8. Jinsung P, Changhee Y, Deok HH, et al. A critical assessment of the effects of tamsulosin and solifenacin as monotherapies and as a combination therapy for the treatment of ureteral stent- related symptoms: a 2 × 2 factorial randomized trial. World J Urol. 2015;33(11):1833–40.
9. EL-Nahas AR, Tharwat M, Elsaadany M, et al. A randomized controlled trial comparing alpha blocker (tamsulosin) and anticholinergic (solifenacin) in treatment of ureteral stent related symptoms. Eur Urol Suppl. 2015;14(2): e1076–e1076a.
10. Lee SJ, Yoo C, Oh CY, et al. Stent position is more important than α-blockers or anticholinergics for stent-related lower urinary tract symptoms after ureteroscopic ureterolithotomy: a prospective randomized study. Korean J Urol. 2010;51(9):636–41.
11. Giannarini G, Keeley Jr FX, Valent F, et al. Predictors of morbidity in patients with indwelling ureteric stents: results of a prospective study using the validated Ureteric Stent Symptoms Questionnaire. BJU Int. 2011;107(4):648–54.
12. Irani J, Siquier J, Pires C, et al. Symptom characteristics and the development of tolerance with time in patients with indwelling double-pigtail ureteric stents. BJU Int. 1999;84:276–9.
13. Wang CJ, Huang SW, Chang CH. Effects of tamsulosin on lower urinary tract symptoms due to double-J stent: a prospective study. Urol Int. 2009;83(1):66–9.
14. Tehranchi A, Rezaei Y, Khalkhali H, et al. Effects of terazosin and tolterodine on ureteral stent related symptoms: a double-blind placebo-controlled randomized clinical trial. Int Braz J Urol. 2013;39(6):832–40.
15. Beddingfield R, Pedro RN, Hinck B, et al. Alfuzosin to relieve ureteral stent discomfort: a prospective, randomized, placebo controlled study. J Urol. 2009;181:170–6.

16.   Andersson KE. Antimuscarinics for treatment of overactive bladder. Lancet
      Neurol. 2004;3:46–53.
17.   Yamaguchi O. Latest treatment for lower urinary tract dysfunction:
      therapeutic agents and mechanism of action. Int J Urol. 2013;20(1):28–39.
18.   Shalaby E, Ahmed AF, Maarouf A, et al. Randomized controlled trial to
      compare the safety and efficacy of tamsulosin, solifenacin, and combination
      of both in treatment of double-j stent-related lower urinary symptoms. Adv
      Urol. 2013;2013:752382.
19.   Lim KT, Kim YT, Lee TY, et al. Effects of tamsulosin, solifenacin, and
      combination therapy for the treatment of ureteral stent related discomforts.
      Korean J Urol. 2011;52(7):485–8.

# 25

# Adjuvant chemotherapy improves survival of patients with high-risk upper urinary tract urothelial carcinoma

Kazutoshi Fujita[1*], Kei Taneishi[2], Teruo Inamoto[3], Yu Ishizuya[4], Shingo Takada[5], Masao Tsujihata[6], Go Tanigawa[7], Noriko Minato[8], Shigeaki Nakazawa[9], Tsuyoshi Takada[10], Toshichika Iwanishi[11], Motohide Uemura[1], Yasushi Okuno[2], Haruhito Azuma[3] and Nonomura Norio[1]

## Abstract

**Background:** The purposes of this study were to determine whether adjuvant chemotherapy (AC) improved the prognosis of patients with high-risk upper urinary tract urothelial carcinoma (UTUC)and to identify the patients who benefited from AC.

**Methods:** Among a multi-center database of 1014 patients who underwent RNU for UTUC, 344 patients with ≥ pT3 or the presence of lymphovascular invasion (LVI) were included. Cancer-specific survival (CSS) estimates were calculated by the Kaplan-Meier method, and groups were compared by the log-rank test. Each patient's probability of receiving AC depending on the covariates in each group was estimated by logistic regression models. Propensity score matching was used to adjust the confounding factors for selecting patients for AC, and log-rank tests were applied to these propensity score-matched cohorts. Cox proportional hazards regression modeling was used to identify the variables with significant interaction with AC. Variables included age, pT category, LVI, tumor grade, ECOG performance status and low sodium or hemoglobin score, which we reported to be a prognostic factor of UTUC.

**Results:** Of the 344 patients, 241 (70%) had received RNU only and 103 (30%) had received RNU+AC. The median follow-up period was 32 (range 1–184) months. Overall, AC did not improve CSS ($P = 0.12$). After propensity score matching, the 5-year CSS was 69.0% in patients with RNU+AC versus 58.9% in patients with RNU alone ($P = 0.030$). Subgroup analyses of survival were performed to identify the patients who benefitted from AC. Subgroups of patients with low preoperative serum sodium (≤ 140 mEq/ml) or hemoglobin levels below the normal limit benefitted from AC (HR 0.34, 95% CI 0.15–0.61, $P = 0.001$). In the subgroup of patients with normal sodium and normal hemoglobin levels, 5-year CSS was 77.7% in patients with RNU+AC versus 80.2% in patients with RNU alone ($P = 0.84$). In contrast, in the subgroup of patients with low sodium or low hemoglobin levels, 5-year CSS was 71.0% in patients with RNU+AC versus 38.5% in patients with RNU alone ($P < 0.001$).

**Conclusions:** High-risk UTUC patients, especially subgroups of patients with lower sodium and hemoglobin levels, could benefit from AC after RNU.

**Keywords:** Upper urinary tract urothelial carcinoma, Adjuvant chemotherapy, Sodium, Hemoglobin

* Correspondence: kazu.fujita2@gmail.com
[1]Department of Urology, Osaka University Graduate School of Medicine, 2-2 Yamada-oka, Suita, Osaka 565-0871, Japan
Full list of author information is available at the end of the article

## Background

Localized upper urinary tract urothelial carcinoma (UTUC) is treated by radical nephroureterectomy with bladder cuff incision (RNU). However, approximately 30% of patients with localized UTUC suffer disease recurrence and have poor survivals [1]. To improve the prognosis, perioperative chemotherapy before or after surgery was performed. Because of the problem of losing renal function after RNU, neoadjuvant chemotherapy may be better for the patients with high-risk UTUC. However, it is difficult to predict UTUC with adverse pathology preoperatively.

Postoperatively, patients with adverse pathology can be selected for adjuvant chemotherapy (AC), and the overtreatment of the patients with low-risk UTUC can be prevented. In contrast, patients who undergo RNU suffer the loss of renal function resulting in their ineligibility for chemotherapy.

There are limited reports of AC for UTUC patients, but the efficacy of AC for UTUC patients remains controversial [2–7]. No prospective randomized trials have investigated the efficacy of AC for UTUC.

Previously, we reported that lower levels of serum sodium (Na < 141 mEq/L) and hemoglobin (lower than normal range) could predict the prognosis of patients with UTUC who underwent RNU. The subset of patients with high-risk UTUC (≥ pT3, presence of lymphovascular invasion [LVI], or positive lymph nodes) could have a good prognosis and might not benefit from AC to improve survival.

Therefore, the primary purpose of this study was to investigate the effect of AC for high-risk UTUC patients who underwent RNU, and the secondary purpose was to seek effective predictors of AC to select the patients who could benefit from its use.

## Methods

### Patients

We used a database including 1014 patients with UTUC who underwent RNU between 1998 and 2013 at Osaka University Hospital, Osaka Medical College Hospital, and their affiliated hospitals. Among these patients, 359 with localized high-risk UTUC (≥ pT3 or LVI positive and pN negative) were identified. Five patients received neoadjuvant chemotherapy, and 2 patients with incomplete resection were excluded. Eight patients who received only 1 cycle of AC due to side effects were also excluded. Thus, we retrospectively analyzed the remaining 344 patients. RNU was performed laparoscopically in 188 patients (54.7%) and by laparotomy in 156 patients (45.3%). Lymph node dissections were performed in an extended or limited manner, at the surgeon's discretion. The following clinical and pathological data were obtained from the database: age; sex; Eastern Cooperative Oncology Group (ECOG) performance

status (PS); pathological tumor, lymph node, metastasis (TNM) classification; presence of LVI; tumor grade; tumor lesion location; and follow-up data. Serum sodium and hemoglobin levels were measured less than 1 month before RNU. Patients were followed-up every 3 months during 0–2 years after surgery, every 6 months during 2–5 years, and every 6–12 months thereafter. Tumor recurrence was defined as the development of local recurrence, distant metastasis, and/or lymph node metastasis; tumor recurrence did not include intravesical recurrence. Follow-up examinations consisted of routine blood test, urine cytology, cystoscopy, and the chest and abdominal computed tomography scans. This study was approved by the Institutional Review Board of Osaka University Hospital.

### Statistical analysis

Clinical characteristics were analyzed using the Mann-Whitney U test and Fisher's exact test. The association between AC and patient cancer-specific survival (CSS) were tested by Kaplan-Meier survival curve analysis and log-rank tests. Propensity score matching was used to adjust the confounding factors for selecting patients for AC. A logistic regression model, which included age, sex, ECOG PS, pathological findings (pT stage, LVI status, tumor grade), was used to estimate each patient's probability of receiving AC. Patients with RNU only were matched on a one-to-one basis with patients with RNU + AC based on nearest-neighbor matching. To assess the factors affecting CSS, a Cox proportional hazard model was used. Variables included age, pT category, LVI, tumor grade, ECOG PS, and low sodium or hemoglobin score, which we previously reported to be a prognostic factor of UTUC [1, 8]. All of statistical tests were performed with SPSS version 11.0 (SPSS, Chicago, IL, USA) and GraphPad Prism 5 (GraphPad Software, La Jolla, CA, USA). Probability values (P) were two-sided, and statistical significance was defined as a P < 0.05.

## Results

### Analysis in the overall cohort

Among the 344 high-risk patients, 103 (29.9%) patients received AC. A median of 2 cycles (range 2–4 cycles) of platinum-based AC were administered. Patient characteristics are summarized in Table 1. There were several factors that differed significantly between the patients with RNU alone and those with RNU + AC. The median follow-up was 32 months (range 1–184 months), with overall 2- and 5-year CSS of 80.7% (95% CI 75.7–84.7%) and 63.1% (95% CI 56.6–68.8%), respectively. The Kaplan-Meyer curve for the overall cohort showed that no significant differences were found in overall survival between the patients with RNU alone and those with RNU + AC (log-rank test, P = 0.109) (Fig. 1a).

**Table 1** Patient characteristics of overall cohort ($n = 344$)

| | RNU only | RNU plus AC | P value |
|---|---|---|---|
| n (%) | 241 (70) | 103 (30) | |
| Age (years)(median (range)) | 74 (34–91) | 66 (28–82) | < 0.0001 |
| Gender, n (%) | | | 0.20 |
|   Male | 166 (69) | 78 (76) | |
|   Female | 75 (31) | 25 (24) | |
| ECOG performance status | | | 0.40 |
|   0–1 | 199 (83) | 91 (88) | |
|   2–4 | 13 (5) | 3 (3) | |
|   Unknown | 29 (12) | 9 (9) | |
| Pathological T stage, n (%) | | | 0.007 |
|   ≤ T2 | 70 (29) | 18 (17) | |
|   T3 | 158 (66) | 84 (82) | |
|   T4 | 13 (5) | 1 (1) | |
| Tumor grade, n (%) | | | 0.056 |
|   G1 | 13 (5) | 3 (3) | |
|   G2 | 90 (37) | 27 (26) | |
|   G3 | 138 (58) | 73 (71) | |
| LVI, n (%) | | | 0.003 |
|   Absent | 107 (44) | 29 (28) | |
|   Present | 128 (53) | 73 (71) | |
|   Unknown | 6 (3) | 1 (1) | |

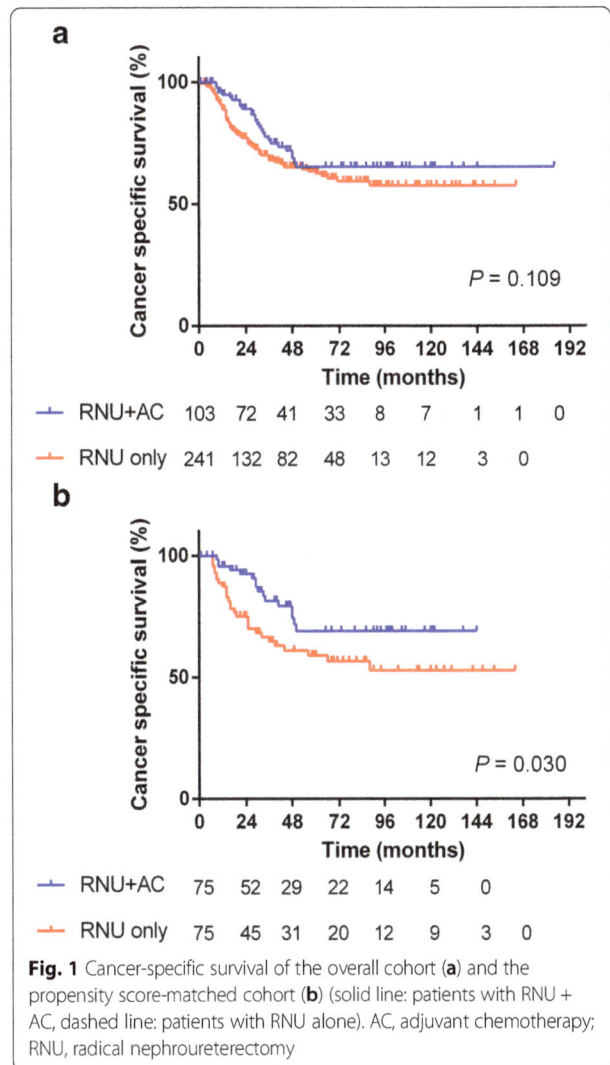

**Fig. 1** Cancer-specific survival of the overall cohort (**a**) and the propensity score-matched cohort (**b**) (solid line: patients with RNU + AC, dashed line: patients with RNU alone). AC, adjuvant chemotherapy; RNU, radical nephroureterectomy

## Propensity score-matched analysis

Because selection bias for AC would exist, we matched the patients using propensity scores for the use of AC, resulting in matched cohorts of 75 patients with RNU only and 75 patients with RNU + AC. The propensity score-matched cohorts are summarized in Table 2. The differences in the variables between the two groups decreased after propensity score matching. In the propensity score-matched cohort, patients with RNU + AC had a better survival rate significantly than the patients with RNU only (Fig. 1b). The 2- and 5-year CSS were 92.6% (95% CI 83.3–96.8%) and 69.0% (95% CI 53.8–80.1%) for patients with RNU + AC compared with 75.0% (95% CI 62.8–83.7%) and 58.9% (95% CI 45.5–70.1%), respectively, for patients with RNU only (HR 0.51, 95% CI 0.28–0.93; $P = 0.030$).

## Subgroup analysis to identify the predictive marker for AC

Subgroup analyses of survival were performed to identify the patients who benefitted from AC to improve CSS. Subgroups of patients with low preoperative serum sodium (≤ 140 mEq/ml) or hemoglobin levels below the normal limit, the presence of LVI, or tumor grade 3 had received benefits from AC (HR 0.34, 95% CI 0.15–0.61, $P = 0.001$; HR 0.51, 95% CI 0.26–0.98, $P = 0.046$; HR 0.41, 95% CI 0.21–0.81, $P = 0.011$, respectively) (Table 3). AC for the patients with these factors resulted in improved survival. In patients with

normal sodium and normal hemoglobin levels, the 5-year CSS was 77.7% in the patients with RNU + AC versus 80.2% in the patients with RNU alone (log rank test, $P = 0.84$). In contrast, in the patients with low sodium or low hemoglobin levels, the 5-year CSS was 71.0% in the patients with RNU + AC versus 38.5% in the patients with RNU alone, resulting in a 32.5% improvement in 5-year CSS (log rank test, $P < 0.001$) (Fig. 2). These results would suggest that the patients with normal sodium and hemoglobin levels would have good prognosis and would not need to receive AC.

## Discussion

UTUC is a rare disease with poor prognosis. More than 40% of patients have advanced-stage cancer at diagnosis, and their prognosis is poor [1]. To improve survival, perioperative chemotherapy is performed. The efficacy of neoadjuvant chemotherapy (NAC) for urinary bladder cancer had been confirmed by randomized study. Immediate AC for patients with advanced urinary bladder cancer did not improved

**Table 2** Patient characteristics of propensity score matched cohort ($n = 150$)

| | RNU only | RNU plus AC | P value |
|---|---|---|---|
| n | 75 | 75 | |
| Age (years)(median (range)) | 66 (34–85) | 68 (28–82) | 0.62 |
| Gender, n (%) | | | 0.28 |
| Male | 50 (67) | 56 (75) | |
| Female | 25 (33) | 19 (25) | |
| ECOG performance status, n (%) | | | 1.0 |
| 0–1 | 72 (96) | 72 (96) | |
| 2–4 | 3 (4) | 3 (4) | |
| Pathological T stage, n (%) | | | 0.51 |
| ≤ T2 | 12 (16) | 15 (20) | |
| T3 | 60 (80) | 59 (79) | |
| T4 | 3 (4) | 1 (1) | |
| Tumor grade, n (%) | | | 0.84 |
| G1 | 2 (2) | 1 (1) | |
| G2 | 23 (31) | 23(31) | |
| G3 | 50(67) | 51 (68) | |
| LVI, n (%) | | | 1.0 |
| Absent | 24 (32) | 23 (31) | |
| Present | 51 (68) | 52 (69) | |

**Table 3** Subgroup analysis to identify the patients who benefit from adjuvant chemotherapy

| | RNU only | RNU + AC | HR | 95% CI | P value |
|---|---|---|---|---|---|
| age | | | | | |
| ≤ 70 | 14/48 | 7/49 | 0.46 | 0.18–1.1 | 0.099 |
| > 70 | 14/27 | 9/26 | 0.56 | 0.24–1.3 | 0.19 |
| pT2 | | | | | |
| ≤ 2 | 4/12 | 4/15 | 0.66 | 0.16–2.6 | 0.56 |
| 3 | 22/60 | 12/59 | 0.51 | 0.25–1.0 | 0.066 |
| 4 | 2/3 | 0/1 | – | – | 1 |
| Na-Hb score | | | | | |
| 0 | 5/30 | 2/19 | 0.84 | 0.16–4.3 | 0.84 |
| 1–2 | 23/45 | 12/54 | 0.30 | 0.15–0.61 | 0.001 |
| ECOG PS | | | | | |
| 0–1 | 27/72 | 16/72 | 0.542 | 0.292–1.01 | 0.053 |
| ≥ 2 | 1/3 | 0/3 | – | – | 1 |
| LVI | | | | | |
| – | 4/24 | 2/23 | 0.483 | 0.088–2.64 | 0.40 |
| + | 24/51 | 14/52 | 0.51 | 0.26–0.98 | 0.046 |
| Grade | | | | | |
| 1–2 | 3/25 | 3/24 | 0.99 | 0.20–4.9 | 0.99 |
| 3 | 25/50 | 13/51 | 0.41 | 0.21–0.81 | 0.011 |

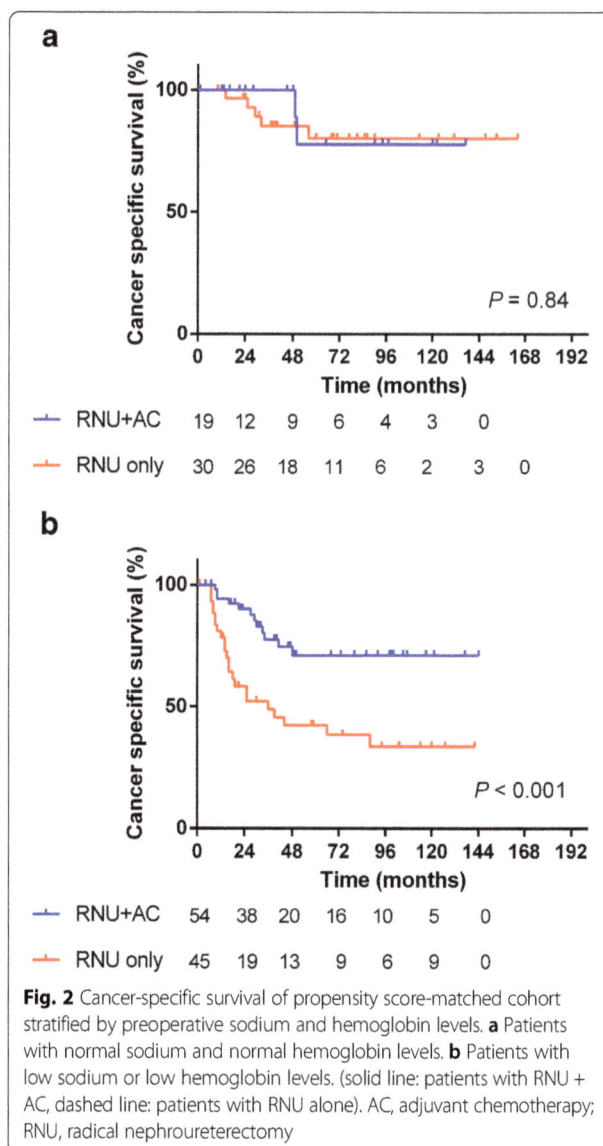

**Fig. 2** Cancer-specific survival of propensity score-matched cohort stratified by preoperative sodium and hemoglobin levels. **a** Patients with normal sodium and normal hemoglobin levels. **b** Patients with low sodium or low hemoglobin levels. (solid line: patients with RNU + AC, dashed line: patients with RNU alone). AC, adjuvant chemotherapy; RNU, radical nephroureterectomy

overall survival over that of patients who underwent deferred chemotherapy, but it might benefit a subgroup of urinary bladder cancer patients, especially pN-positive patients [9]. After RNU, many patients lose nearly 50% of their renal function and can be ineligible to receive chemotherapy [10]. From these points of view, NAC might be preferred for the patients with advanced UTUC. However, the precise preoperative diagnosis of tumor stage or LVI status is difficult, although one study showed the usefulness of magnetic resonance imaging for the prediction of tumor stage [11]. Unlike urinary bladder cancer, for which pathological stage can be accurately diagnosed by transurethral resection of the bladder tumor before radical cystectomy, the accurate staging of UTUC is difficult even with a ureteroscopic biopsy [12].

Because UTUC is a rare malignancy comprising 5% of all urothelial cancer, it is difficult to enroll enough UTUC patients to adequately perform a prospective, randomized study to prove the efficacy of perioperative chemotherapy. For lymph node-positive UTUC patients, the efficacies of adjuvant chemotherapy were reported. Retrospective analysis of 74 lymph node-positive UTUC patients showed the AC improved CSS compared with RNU alone (HR 0.52, 95%CI 0.24–0.82, $P = 0.014$) [2]. Retrospective analysis of 263 lymph node-positive UTUC patients showed that AC did not improve CSS in overall patients (HR 0.89, $P = 0.49$), but improved CSS in the subgroup of patients with pT3–4 N+ (HR 0.67, $P = 0.022$) [13]. Retrospective analysis of 109 locally advanced UTUC patients (pT3–4pN0/xM0) showed that cisplatin-based AC improved recurrence-free survival (HR = 0.41, $P = 0.017$) and CSS (HR 0.33, $P = 0.037$) [14]. Propensity-matched analysis of 1544 UTUC patients with pT2-4 N0 or lymph node-positive showed that AC did not improve overall survival compared with RNU alone (HR 1.14, 95%CI 0.91–1.43, $P = 0.268$). The largest study recently reported used data from the National Cancer Database [5]. This retrospective analysis of the 3253 high-risk UTUC patients showed that AC was statistically associated with an overall survival benefit. A meta-analysis based on this retrospective analysis showed that AC could improve overall survival, CSS, and disease-free survival, but neoadjuvant chemotherapy was more favorable for UTUC than AC in disease-specific survival [3]. The systematic review and meta-analysis of 24 retrospective analysis studied the efficacy of NAC and AC in UTUC [15]. Across 2 retrospective studies about NAC, NAC improved CSS, with a pooled HR of 0.41 (95%CI 0.22–0.76, $P = 0.005$). Across three cisplatin-based studies about AC, the pooled HR for overall survival was 0.43 (95% CI, 0.21–0.89, $P = 0.023$) compared with those who received RNU alone. For disease-free survival, the pooled HR across two studies of AC was 0.49 (95% CI, 0.24–0.99; $p = 0.048$). Benefit was not seen for non- cisplatin–based regimens in AC. Meta-analysis of 31 retrospective studies with 8100 UTUC patients who underwent perioperative treatments also showed that AC improved overall survival (HR 0.71, 95%CI 0.51–0.89), CSS (HR 0.71, 95%CI 0.54–0.89), and recurrence-free survival (HR 0.49, 95%CI 0.23–0.85) [16]. We adopted propensity score-matching analysis, which can reduce the differences between patient characteristics in each group, and the results were consistent with those of this previous study. Furthermore, we identified the patients who benefitted from AC. We previously reported that patients with serum low sodium or hemoglobin levels have a poor prognosis. The supposed mechanism of these markers may be that cells in UTUC with a poor prognosis may secrete inflammatory cytokines such as interleukin-6 that cause anemia and low serum sodium levels. This preoperative prognostic marker may also be useful in the selection of patients to receive AC. AC did not improve the prognosis of patients with normal sodium and hemoglobin levels because these patients already had a better prognosis with or without AC.

There are several limitations in this study. Although we matched the cohorts by propensity scores, this is the retrospective study. A multi-institutional, prospective, randomized study should be performed to prove the efficacy of AC. In this study, a median of 2 cycles of AC were administered, but the optimal number of cycles was not determined. We entered only serum sodium and hemoglobin levels into the Cox proportional analysis, but other prognostic markers might exist to predict the benefit of AC.

## Conclusion
Propensity score-matched analysis showed that AC improved the survival of patients with advanced UTUC. Subgroups of patients with lower sodium and/or hemoglobin levels could benefit from AC after RNU. Further large-scale studies are required to verify these findings.

### Abbreviations
AC: Adjuvant chemotherapy; HR: Hazard ratio; LVI: Lymphovascular invasion; RNU: Radical nephroureterectomy; UTUC: Upper urinary tract urothelial carcinoma

### Acknowledgements
None.

### Funding
None.

### Authors' contributions
KF, TI, MU, HA, NN design this study, and KF wrote this manuscript. KT and YO analyzed the data. YI, ST, MT, GT, NM, SN, TT and TI contributed to the data acquisitions and the interpretation of data. All authors read and approved the final manuscript.

### Competing interests
The authors declare that they have no competing interests.

### Author details
[1]Department of Urology, Osaka University Graduate School of Medicine, 2-2 Yamada-oka, Suita, Osaka 565-0871, Japan. [2]Department of Clinical System Onco-Informatics, Graduate School of Medicine, Kyoto University, Kyoto, Japan. [3]Department of Urology, Osaka Medical College, Takatsuki, Osaka, Japan. [4]Department of Urology, Osaka Medical Center for Cancer and Cardiovascular Diseases, Osaka, Japan. [5]Department of Urology, Osaka General Medical Center, Osaka, Japan. [6]Department of Urology, Osaka Police Hospital, Osaka, Japan. [7]Department of Urology, Sumitomo Hospital, Osaka, Japan. [8]Department of Urology, Osaka Rosai Hospital, Sakai, Osaka, Japan. [9]Department of Urology, Nishinomiya Prefectural Hospital, Nishinomiya, Japan. [10]Department of Urology, Minoh Municipal Hospital, Minoh, Japan. [11]Department of Urology, Higashi Osaka General Medical Center, Higashi-, Osaka, Japan.

### References
1.  Fujita K, Tanigawa G, Imamura R, Nakagawa M, Hayashi T, Kishimoto N, et al. Preoperative serum sodium is associated with cancer-specific survival in

patients with upper urinary tract urothelial carcinoma treated by nephroureterectomy. Int J Urol [Internet]. 2013 [cited 2013 may 10];20:594–601. Available from: http://www.ncbi.nlm.nih.gov/pubmed/23131052.

2.  Fujita K, Inamoto T, Yamamoto Y, Tanigawa G, Nakayama M, Mori N, et al. Role of adjuvant chemotherapy for lymph node-positive upper tract urothelial carcinoma and the prognostic significance of C-reactive protein: a multi-institutional, retrospective study. Int J Urol [Internet]. 2015;22:1006–1012. Available from:. https://doi.org/10.1111/iju.12868.

3.  Yang X, Li P, Deng X, Dong H, Cheng Y, Zhang X, et al. Perioperative treatments for resected upper tract urothelial carcinoma: a network meta-analysis. Oncotarget [Internet]. 2015 [cited 2017 Feb 27];8:3568–3580. Available from: http://www.ncbi.nlm.nih.gov/pubmed/27683040.

4.  Gin GE, Ruel NH, Kardos S V., Sfakianos JP, Uchio E, Lau CS, et al. Utilization of perioperative systemic chemotherapy in upper tract urothelial carcinoma. Urol. Oncol. Semin. Orig. Investig. [Internet]. 2016 [cited 2017 Feb 27]; Available from: http://www.ncbi.nlm.nih.gov/pubmed/28041996.

5.  Seisen T, Krasnow RE, Bellmunt J, Rouprêt M, Leow JJ, Lipsitz SR, et al. Effectiveness of Adjuvant Chemotherapy After Radical Nephroureterectomy for Locally Advanced and/or Positive Regional Lymph Node Upper Tract Urothelial Carcinoma. J Clin Oncol [Internet]. 2017 [cited 2017 Feb 27];JCO2016694141. Available from: http://www.ncbi.nlm.nih.gov/pubmed/28045620.

6.  Hellenthal NJ, Shariat SF, Margulis V, Karakiewicz PI, Roscigno M, Bolenz C, et al. Adjuvant chemotherapy for high risk upper tract urothelial carcinoma : results from the upper tract urothelial carcinoma collaboration. J Urol [internet]. 2009; 182:900–906. Available from. doi: 10.1016/j.juro.2009.05.011.

7.  Kwak C, Lee SE, Jeong IG, Ku JH. Adjuvant systemic chemotherapy in the treatment of patients with invasive transitional cell carcinoma of the upper urinary tract. Urology [Internet]. 2006 [cited 2014 Aug 16];68:53–57. Available from: http://www.ncbi.nlm.nih.gov/pubmed/16806415.

8.  Fujita K, Uemura M, Yamamoto Y, Tanigawa G, Nakata W, Sato M, et al. Preoperative risk stratification for cancer-specific survival of patients with upper urinary tract urothelial carcinoma treated by nephroureterectomy. Int J Clin Oncol [Internet]. 2015 [cited 2014 Apr 21];20. Available from: http://www.ncbi.nlm.nih.gov/pubmed/24740557.

9.  Sternberg CN, Skoneczna I, Kerst JM, Albers P, Fossa SD, Agerbaek M, et al. Immediate versus deferred chemotherapy after radical cystectomy in patients with pT3–pT4 or N+ M0 urothelial carcinoma of the bladder (EORTC 30994): an intergroup, open-label, randomised phase 3 trial. Lancet Oncol. [Internet]. 2015;16:76–86. Available from: http://linkinghub.elsevier.com/retrieve/pii/S147020451471160X

10.  Kaag MG, O'Malley RL, O'Malley P, Godoy G, Chen M, Smaldone MC, et al. Changes in renal function following nephroureterectomy may affect the use of perioperative chemotherapy. Eur Urol [Internet]. 2010 [cited 2012 Oct 1];58: 581–587. Available from: http://www.ncbi.nlm.nih.gov/pubmed/20619530.

11.  Yoshida S, Koga F, Masuda H, Fujii Y, Kihara K. Role of diffusion-weighted magnetic resonance imaging as an imaging biomarker of urothelial carcinoma. Int J Urol [Internet]. 2014 [cited 2017 Apr 12];21:1190–1200. Available from: http://www.ncbi.nlm.nih.gov/pubmed/25074594.

12.  Potretzke AM, Knight BA, Potretzke TA, Larson JA, Bhayani SB. Is Ureteroscopy Needed Prior to Nephroureterectomy? An Evidence-Based Algorithmic Approach. Urology [Internet]. 2016 [cited 2017 Apr 12];88:43–48. Available from: http://www.ncbi.nlm.nih.gov/pubmed/26545850.

13.  Lucca I, Kassouf W, Kapoor A, Fairey A, Rendon RA, Izawa JI, et al. The role of adjuvant chemotherapy for lymph node-positive upper tract urothelial carcinoma following radical nephroureterectomy: a retrospective study. BJU Int. 2015;116:72–8.

14.  Nakagawa T, Komemushi Y, Kawai T, Otsuka M, Miyakawa J, Uemura Y, et al. Efficacy of post-nephroureterectomy cisplatin-based adjuvant chemotherapy for locally advanced upper tract urothelial carcinoma: a multi-institutional retrospective study. World J Urol [Internet]. 2017;35:1569–1575. Available from: http://link.springer.com/10.1007/s00345-017-2032-6

15.  Leow JJ, Martin-Doyle W, Fay AP, Choueiri TK, Chang SL, Bellmunt J. A Systematic Review and Meta-analysis of Adjuvant and Neoadjuvant Chemotherapy for Upper Tract Urothelial Carcinoma. Eur Urol [Internet]. 2014 [cited 2014 Aug 13];66:529–541. Available from: http://www.ncbi.nlm.nih.gov/pubmed/24680361.

16.  Yang X, Li P, Deng X, Dong H, Cheng Y, Zhang X, et al. Perioperative treatments for resected upper tract urothelial carcinoma: a network meta-analysis. Oncotarget [Internet]. 2017;8:3568–3580. Available from: http://www.ncbi.nlm.nih.gov/pubmed/27683040%0Ahttp://www.pubmedcentral.nih.gov/articlerender.fcgi?artid=PMC5356904

# 26

# Female urinary incontinence and wellbeing

Andrew P. Smith

## Abstract

**Background:** Previous research has shown that the severity of symptoms of urinary incontinence impacts on quality of life and wellbeing.
The aim of this article is to investigate the relationship between female urinary incontinence and mental wellbeing. This involved analyses comparing those with UI and those without to determine whether any differences in wellbeing were modified by demographic factors, specific wellbeing domain, or exercise and frequency of sex. Following this, further analyses compared sub-groups of those with UI (based on the impact of the UI) to determine which characteristics were important in influencing wellbeing.

**Methods:** An internet survey of women with UI, aged between 45 and 60 years, has been previously reported and this article reports secondary analyses of that data.
A sample from 4 countries: the UK, France, Germany and the USA.
Two thousand four hundred three women completed the survey, 1203 with UI and 1200 who did not report UI.
The main outcome measures were the scores from the Warwick-Edinburgh Mental Wellbeing Scale (WEMWBS).

**Results:** The results showed that lower wellbeing is observed in UI. This effect is observed in all aspects of wellbeing and most sub-groups of UI sufferers. Lifestyle influences wellbeing and those with UI who exercise less frequently or have sex infrequently are especially likely to report lower wellbeing. Wellbeing decreases as a function of the indirect measures of severity of UI and reductions in HRQol. Again, these changes reflect all aspects of wellbeing measured by WEMWBS.

**Conclusions:** The results show that women with UI, aged 45–60 years, report lower wellbeing. This effect was not modified by demographic factors and was apparent in most of the domains measured by the WEMWBS. The reduced wellbeing was related to the impact of the UI on behaviour, embarrassment associated with it, and frequency of leakage.

**Keywords:** Urinary incontinence, Wellbeing, Female, Quality of life, Exercise, Sex

## Background

The prevalence of urinary incontinence (UI) in adult women has been estimated to be about 18 % [1] and in the elderly this figure can be as high as 55 % [2]. UI can negatively affect many aspects of life, and has been shown to affect overall health-related quality of life (HRQoL) [3–12]. Indeed, a search of PubMed reveals 28 articles that have examined UI and HRQol. A recent survey [13] aimed to develop a clear understanding of the impact of urinary incontinence on the quality of life (Qol) of women of working age. The results showed that the severity of symptoms of UI impacted on quality of life. The results also showed that wellbeing decreased as the symptoms of UI became more severe. The relationship between HRQol and wellbeing was also examined and it was found that UI reduced HRQol which in turn led to reduced wellbeing.

### Wellbeing

Historically, research on wellbeing has mainly been conducted within two traditions: hedonic wellbeing and eudaimonic wellbeing. The hedonic approach to wellbeing measures subjective wellbeing which is comprised

Correspondence: smithap@cardiff.ac.uk
Centre for Occupational and Health Psychology, School of Psychology,
Cardiff University, 63 Park Place, Cardiff CF10 3AS, UK

of life satisfaction, positive affect, and an absence of negative affect. Specifically, focusing on happiness from the perspective of pleasure versus pain including both cognitive evaluation (life satisfaction) and affect (with positive and negative affect comprising separate dimensions). In contrast, the eudaimonic approach to wellbeing is not simply interested in subjective happiness, but in the realisation of human potential. Within this view, wellbeing is linked to a person living in a way which is congruent with their deeply held values: a meaningful life characterised by personal growth, as opposed to a pleasurable life characterised by hedonic enjoyment. There is now international interest in wellbeing and its role in all aspects of life. This interest can be seen at a population level and in specific contexts such as work. In addition, wellbeing is now an outcome of interest in many health-related areas. Wellbeing scales such as the Warwick-Edinburgh Wellbeing Scale (WEMWBS;) [14] measure both hedonic and eudaimonic wellbeing and are correlated with general health, positive and negative affect, life satisfaction and mental ill-health. UI has been shown to negatively impact on these outcomes and it is important to investigate whether wellbeing scores are related to UI as at the moment there is little information on this topic.

### Wellbeing and UI

There have been a number of studies which have investigated associations between incontinence and mental health [15–17]. These generally confirm that UI is associated with an increased risk of depression [15], and show that treatment of the depression associated with UI may be an effective way of reducing the burden of UI [16]. Indeed, interventions aimed at increasing resilience may lessen the impact of depression on those with UI [17].

Two Australian studies have investigated associations between UI and wellbeing [18, 19]. The first study [18] showed that UI was associated with reduced wellbeing but that the relationship between different types of UI and wellbeing was different. The second study [19] investigated associations between UI and wellbeing in young nulligravid women. The results confirmed that women with UI reported lower wellbeing that women without UI. It is now important to replicate and extend these findings using multi-national samples of women of working age and recently developed measures of wellbeing.

### Aims

The primary aim was to conduct secondary analyses of our previous study [13] which focused on UI in women of working age to provide a detailed profile of female UI and wellbeing. This involved comparison of the wellbeing of those with UI with those with no symptoms.

Examination of the individual items of the WEMWBS was carried out to determine whether effects are global or restricted/greatest in specific domains. Further analyses examined whether the associations between UI and wellbeing (and effects on wellbeing of those without UI) varied as a function of demographics and lifestyle (frequency of exercise and sex). Our previous paper from this survey [13] focused on associations between UI severity, HRQoL and WEMBS. UI symptoms were associated with lower HRQoL, which then impacts negatively on wellbeing. In the analyses reported here sub-sets of the UI group (based on indicators of severity - e.g., frequency of wearing pads; interference with activities) were also compared. The general hypothesis being tested was that even relatively mild UI would be associated with reduced wellbeing (compared to those without UI) and that such effects would be global rather than restricted to specific domains or sub-groups. Additionally, the analyses examined whether there was variation within the UI group as a function of the impact of UI on different activities and outcomes. These secondary analyses extend the initial aims of the protocol and address issues that are of practical relevance to women of working age with UI.

### Method

The survey was conducted by Ipsos Market Research and adhered to the Market Research Society code of conduct and was carried out with the informed consent of the participants. The Ipsos samples are representative of the country in terms of demographics and are selected using the recruitment criteria of the specific survey (see below).

### Study population

An internet survey (with the questions in the appropriate language) was conducted in 4 countries (France, Germany, UK and USA) during September 2013. A sample of women aged 45–60 years was recruited by Ipsos Marketing. Their online panels currently consist of approximately 920,000 members in the USA, 535,000 in France, 300,000 in the UK, and 169,000 in Germany. The survey was answered by both women with and without UI and the sampling procedure meant that the UI and non-UI groups did not differ in terms of basic demographics. Informed consent was represented by participation in the survey after the provision of the information about the study. Participants were aware of this procedure when they joined the online panels. The first 300 respondents with UI in each of the four countries were included in the study population, as were the first 300 non-UI respondents. This procedure meant that it was impossible to determine how many would have completed the survey if there was no sample cut-off point nor how many would have refused to participate.

Sample size was based on the need to detect small effect sizes (Cohen's d = 0.2; with power set at 0.9 and $p = 0.05$ a total sample size of 1054 would be needed) in the wellbeing outcomes. Participants were paid for participating in the study and after this the database was anonymised.

## Survey questionnaire

UI categorisation was defined by the answer to the ICIQ-UI Short Form question "how often do you leak urine?; those answering "Never" were classed as without UI while all other answers were classed as having UI. UI severity was based on the response to "How much urine do you usually leak?" [20] with a small amount being classified as "light UI", a moderate amount as "medium UI" and a large amount as "severe UI". Those reporting UI completed questions measuring UI symptoms (ICIQ-UI short form) [21] and UI quality of life (ICIQ-LUTSqol) [20]. Both UI and non-UI participants completed the WEMWBS [14] which has 14 items and a Likert scale of 1–5 giving a maximum score of 70.

Demographic factors (e.g., age; marital status) were recorded as were frequency of exercise and sex. Other questions examined the impact of UI on aspects of life. Outcomes of UI were also recorded (degree of embarrassment; frequency of wearing pads). The complete set of questions are given in supplementary information with our previous publication from the study [13].

## Statistical analysis

The first set of analyses compared those reporting UI with those who did not. Analyses were carried out on the individual items of the wellbeing scale to determine whether any specific domains were more impaired than others. Sub-groups based on demographic factors were also compared. The initial analyses involved a MANOVA to determine whether effects were apparent across all items of the wellbeing scale. Most studies use the WEMWBS total score but analysis of the individual items provided an opportunity to examine the generality of effects. Subsequent analyses examined whether effects were apparent in subgroups of patients (based on demographics, frequency of exercise and sex) and used univariate ANOVAs followed by multiple regression. Factor analyses were carried out to identify categories of outcomes associated with UI. ANOVAs were then carried out to examine changes in wellbeing as a function of the severity of these different types of problem. A similar approach was used to examine the effects of factors leading to leakage on wellbeing. The analyses were carried out using the IBM SPSS Statistics 20 package.

## Results

There was no missing data for the variables considered in the initial analyses comparing those reporting UI with the non-UI group. Those with UI reported significantly lower wellbeing (UI mean: 48.2 s.d. 10.2; Non-UI mean: 50.2 s.d. 8.9; t = 5.3 d.f. 2401 $p < 0.001$) and a multivariate analysis of variance showed this was significant for all items in the scale (Wilks Lambda = 0.97 $p < 0.001$; see Table 1 for means and s.ds.

All of the individual effects remained significant when a Holm-Bonferroni correction for multiple comparisons was applied. Subsequent analyses examined whether the effect varied as a function of country, age and marital status. The results (see Table 2) showed that the effect of UI was observed in the majority of sub-groups groups (the exceptions being the French and those who were widowed). There was no missing data in these analyses.

A multi-variate analysis was then carried out in which UI v non-UI, country, age, marital status, frequency of exercise and frequency of sex were entered into a

**Table 1** Scores for individual wellbeing questions (higher scores = greater wellbeing)

| Question | Group | Mean | SD | Significance |
|---|---|---|---|---|
| Feeling cheerful | UI | 3.39 | 0.91 | $F = 17.0 \; p < 0.001$ |
| | Non-UI | 3.53 | 0.84 | |
| Thinking clearly | UI | 3.71 | 0.95 | $F = 12.2 \; p < 0.001$ |
| | Non-UI | 3.84 | 0.89 | |
| Close to other people | UI | 3.45 | 0.99 | $F = 17.0 \; p < 0.001$ |
| | Non-UI | 3.61 | 0.87 | |
| Feeling confident | UI | 3.35 | 0.97 | $F = 27.0 \; p < 0.001$ |
| | Non-UI | 3.54 | 0.90 | |
| Dealing with problems well | UI | 3.58 | 0.88 | $F = 12.0 \; p < 0.001$ |
| | Non-UI | 3.70 | 0.81 | |
| Energy to spare | UI | 2.79 | 1.05 | $F = 44.8 \; p < 0.001$ |
| | Non-UI | 3.06 | 0.94 | |
| Feeling good about myself | UI | 3.35 | 0.96 | $F = 19.0 \; p < 0.001$ |
| | Non-UI | 3.51 | 0.87 | |
| Interested in new things | UI | 3.46 | 1.00 | $F = 13.4 \; p < 0.001$ |
| | Non-UI | 3.60 | 0.88 | |
| Interested in other people | UI | 3.56 | 0.98 | $F = 9.9 \; p < 0.001$ |
| | Non-UI | 3.68 | 0.87 | |
| Feeling loved | UI | 3.56 | 1.09 | $F = 7.8 \; p < 0.005$ |
| | Non-UI | 3.68 | 1.02 | |
| Feeling optimistic about future | UI | 3.25 | 1.06 | $F = 7.3 \; p < 0.01$ |
| | Non-UI | 3.36 | 0.96 | |
| Able to make up own mind | UI | 4.03 | 0.88 | $F = 12.1 \; p < 0.005$ |
| | Non-UI | 4.15 | 0.79 | |
| Feeling relaxed | UI | 3.21 | 0.95 | $F = 6.7 \; p < 0.01$ |
| | Non-UI | 3.31 | 0.89 | |
| Feeling useful | UI | 3.46 | 0.98 | $F = 25.0 \; p < 0.001$ |
| | Non-Ui | 3.66 | 0.89 | |

**Table 2** Total wellbeing scores in the UI and non-UI groups as a function of country, age and marital status (high scores = greater wellbeing)

| Group | Mean | SD | N |
|---|---|---|---|
| USA UI | 48.2 | 10.9 | 300 |
| USA non-UI | 51.9 | 9.9 | 300 |
| UK UI | 46.1 | 10.2 | 300 |
| UK non-UI | 48.8 | 9.2 | 301 |
| Germany UI | 49.7 | 10.2 | 301 |
| Germany non-UI | 51.6 | 8.6 | 300 |
| France UI | 48.7 | 9.4 | 301 |
| France non-UI | 48.7 | 7.3 | 300 |
| Country x UI group interaction: $F\ (3, 2395) = 3.8\ p < 0.05$ | | | |
| **Age** | | | |
| 45–48 years UI | 47.6 | 9.9 | 262 |
| 45–48 non-UI | 49.4 | 9.2 | 292 |
| 49–53 years UI | 47.4 | 10.3 | 367 |
| 49–53 non-UI | 49.8 | 8.5 | 342 |
| 54–57 years UI | 48.8 | 10.8 | 247 |
| 54–57 non-UI | 51.2 | 8.8 | 233 |
| 58–60 years UI | 49.0 | 10.1 | 327 |
| 58–60 years non-UI | 50.8 | 9.1 | 333 |
| Age x UI group interaction: $F < 1$ | | | |
| **Marital Status** | | | |
| Single UI | 47.0 | 9.5 | 164 |
| Single non-UI | 48.3 | 8.5 | 202 |
| Married/living together UI | 49.0 | 9.9 | 743 |
| Married non-UI | 51.0 | 8.9 | 695 |
| Widowed UI | 47.7 | 8.9 | 51 |
| Widowed non-UI | 46.9 | 10.4 | 49 |
| Divorced/separated UI | 46.6 | 11.8 | 245 |
| Divorced non-UI | 50.3 | 8.7 | 254 |
| Marital status x UI group interaction: $F\ 93,2395) = 2.1\ p > 0.05)$ | | | |

regression with wellbeing as the outcome. All of the effects, except marital status, were significant (see Table 3) confirming the results of the individual analyses.

The next set of analyses examined effects of frequency of exercise (no missing data) and sex (507 participants preferred not to answer this question, with there being

**Table 3** Multi-variate regression with total WEMWBS score as the dependent variable

| Variable | B | Std error | Standardised B | t | Sig |
|---|---|---|---|---|---|
| Age | 1.557 | 0.359 | .086 | 4.334 | <0.001 |
| Exercise | −1.596 | .163 | −.194 | −9.784 | <0.001 |
| Sex | −.684 | .122 | −.111 | −5.588 | <0.001 |
| UI v non-UI | 1.886 | .356 | .105 | 5.302 | <0.001 |

significantly more in this category in the non-UI group) on wellbeing in both groups. Reduced wellbeing in the UI group was greatest in those who did not frequently exercise. Frequency of having sex was associated with greater wellbeing and this was true for both UI and non-UI groups (see Table 4).

The next set of analyses considered the impact of problems associated with UI. Factor analysis showed three categories of problem: Relationships (sex; social life); Work/household/physical activity; and Fatigue/mental health. On the basis of these factor scores the UI sample was split into tertiles in order to provide an initial indication of dose-response. As problems increased, wellbeing decreased (mainly in the last tertile - see Table 5), although the effects were bigger for relationships and fatigue/mental health than the work/household/physical category.

Wellbeing also decreased as a function of the degree of embarrassment associated with UI ($F\ (2,1200) = 68.7$ $p < 0.001$: Never embarrassed: mean = 51.8 s.d. = 9.3; Sometimes embarrassed: mean = 47.6 s.d. = 9.3; Often/All the time: mean = 41.9 s.d. = 11.6). A fourth set of analyses examined when they leaked and the use of pads. Factor analyses ($N = 1177$) showed three categories of leakage: No obvious reason; Cough/sneeze/exercise; and before getting to the toilet. On the basis of these factor scores the UI sample were split into tertiles. An increase in all these types of leakage was associated with reduced wellbeing (see Table 6) as was frequency of wearing pads ($F(3,1199) = 5.1\ p < 0.005$: Never: mean = 50.5 s.d. = 9.2; Sometimes: mean = 48.6 s.d. = 10.2; Often/All the time: mean = 47.1 s.d. = 10.5). Frequency of using pads was associated with more severe UI which in turn was

**Table 4** Frequency of exercise and sex and wellbeing (high scores = greater wellbeing; More exercise = every day or once or twice a week; Less exercise = once or twice a month or never. More frequent sex = once or twice a week or more; Less frequent sex = once or twice a month or I can't remember when)

| Group | Mean | SD | N |
|---|---|---|---|
| UI more exercise | 49.7 | 10.0 | 806 |
| UI less exercise | 45.1 | 10.2 | 397 |
| Non-UI more exercise | 51.1 | 8.7 | 835 |
| Non-UI less exercise | 48.2 | 9.2 | 365 |
| Main effect of exercise: $F(1,2399) = 82.8\ p < 0.001$ | | | |
| Exercise x UI interaction: $F\ (1,2399) = 4.2\ p < 0.05$ | | | |
| UI more sex | 51.4 | 9.6 | 357 |
| UI less sex | 45.9 | 10.4 | 631 |
| Non-UI more sex | 53.1 | 8.0 | 369 |
| Non-UI less sex | 48.0 | 9.4 | 539 |
| Main effect of sex: $F(1,1892) = 145.3\ p < 0.001$ | | | |
| Sex x UI interaction: $F < 1$ | | | |

**Table 5** Wellbeing scores (mean, s.d,) and impact of UI (shown as tertiles, tertile 1 = lowest impact)

| Factor | T1 | T2 | T3 | |
|---|---|---|---|---|
| Relationships | 49.7 9.2 | 51.3 9.5 | 45.5 10.9 | $F_{2,978} = 30.2 \ p < 0.001$ |
| Work/household/physical activities | 49.9 10.1 | 48.9 9.5 | 47.7 10.9 | $F_{2,978} = 4.0 \ p < 0.05$ |
| Mental health | 52.4 9.1 | 49.7 9.7 | 44.4 10.1 | $F_{2,978} = 58.0 \ p < 0.001$ |

associated with lower wellbeing (Light UI: $N$ = mean = 49.4 s.d. = 9.5; Medium UI: mean = 44.6 s.d. = 11.4; Severe UI: mean = 42.2 s.d. = 12.7).

## Discussion

These results showed that reduced wellbeing is observed in UI. This effect is observed in all aspects of wellbeing and most sub-groups of UI sufferers. Factors which reflect greater severity of UI lead to a greater reduction in wellbeing. Lifestyle influences wellbeing and those with UI who exercise less frequently or have sex infrequently are especially likely to report reduced wellbeing. Wellbeing decreases as a function of the severity of UI and reductions in HRQol. Again, these changes reflect all aspects of wellbeing measured by WEMWBS. Previous analyses [13] showed that when both quality of life (ICIQ-LUTSqol) and symptom severity (ICIQ-UI Short Form) were included in the same regression analysis, the only significant effect on mental well-being was ICIQ-LUTSqol. This shows that UI symptoms do not directly affect mental well-being, but that symptoms influence quality of life, which in turn influences well-being.

This is the first multi-national study which has examined the impact of UI on wellbeing. The sample consisted of women aged 45–60 in four developed countries and this population enables assessment of wellbeing in a group with a busy active life which is likely to be more demanding than that of elderly populations who are often studied in UI research. The present sample consisted of women who largely reported light UI and yet the results show a clear reduction in wellbeing in this group. Those with severe incontinence find it extremely difficult to engage in sex and physical exercise but by sampling those with light UI the present study was able to look at how those activities related to wellbeing in both UI and non-UI groups. Improving wellbeing in those with mild UI is clearly very important and shows that clinical management must address this as well as the issue of leakage. UI is often under reported and community education is desirable as those with mild UI

may not see a clinician. It is also important to investigate the extent to which individuals adopt compensatory behaviours which enable them to function and minimize the problems related to UI.

The study has a number of limitations and further research is required to extend the present findings and reduce any potential biases present in this study. The online format of the survey may have excluded certain groups and future research should consider a case-control approach to the comparison of UI and non-UI groups. Type of incontinence (stress, urgency and mixed) is also a factor which can now be assessed using wellbeing outcomes. More specific information about exercise and sexual behaviour is also required, as is information on BMI which may be important in UI and wellbeing. Other psychosocial factors known to influence wellbeing (e.g., personality; stress; social support and coping) should also be measured in order to determine whether the effects of UI and these psychosocial factors have independent, additive or interactive effects on wellbeing. The practical significance of the small difference in wellbeing also needs to be assessed and bench marked against effect sizes seen in other chronic conditions. The WEMWBS was not really designed to determine clinical significance and other measuring instruments should be also used to determine whether any differences are clinically significant.

## Conclusion

In conclusion, the results from the present survey demonstrate that even light UI is associated with lower wellbeing. This appears to be a general problem associated with UI in that it is present in most demographic groups and is observed in all the domains measured by the WEMWBS. Within the UI group the lower wellbeing was related to HRQol and to perceptions of interference with specific activities or the induction of mental health issues. Therapies aimed at increasing wellbeing (e.g., mindfulness; Cognitive Behaviour Therapy) may play a role in the management of UI.

**Table 6** Reason for leakage (shown as tertiles; T1 = not present) and wellbeing (mean, s.d., N)

| Factor | T1 | T2 | T3 | |
|---|---|---|---|---|
| No obvious reason | 50.0 9.0 | 49.0 9.2 | 44.8 11.5 | $F_{2,1174} = 29.9 \ p < 0.001$ |
| Cough/sneeze/exercise | 48.4 10.7 | 48.6 10.3 | 47.0 9.6 | $F_{2,1174} = 2.9 \ p < 0.05$ |
| Before getting to toilet | 48.9 10.5 | 48.8 9.4 | 46.2 10.7 | $F_{2,1174} = 8.7 \ p < 0.001$ |

**Acknowledgements**
N/A.


**Author's contribution**
Professor Smith designed and analysed the wellbeing part of the study. He also wrote the article.


**Funding**
This study was funded by Procter and Gamble Ltd.

**Competing interests**
Professor Smith has received an honorarium from Procter and Gamble Ltd.

**References**

1.  Irwin DE, Milsom I, Hunskaar S, Reilly K, Kopp Z, Herschorn S, Coyne K, Kelleher C, Hampel C, Artibani W, et al. Population-based survey of urinary incontinence, overactive bladder, and other lower urinary tract symptoms in five countries: results of the EPIC study. Euro Urol. 2006;50(6):1306–14. discussion 1314-1305.

2.  Thom D. Variation in estimates of urinary incontinence prevalence in the community: effects of differences in definition, population characteristics, and study type. J Am Geriatr Soc. 1998;46(4):473–80.

3.  Franzen K, Johansson JE, Andersson G, Pettersson N, Nilsson K. Urinary incontinence in women is not exclusively a medical problem: a population-based study on urinary incontinence and general living conditions. Scand J Urol Nephrol. 2009;43(3):226–32.

4.  Fultz NH, Fisher GG, Jenkins KR. Does urinary incontinence affect middle-aged and older women's time use and activity patterns? Obstet Gynecol. 2004;104(6):1327–34.

5.  Coyne KS, Sexton CC, Irwin DE, Kopp ZS, Kelleher CJ, Milsom I. The impact of overactive bladder, incontinence and other lower urinary tract symptoms on quality of life, work productivity, sexuality and emotional well-being in men and women: results from the EPIC study. BJU Int. 2008;101(11):1388–95.

6.  Papanicolaou S, Hunskaar S, Lose G, Sykes D. Assessment of bothersomeness and impact on quality of life of urinary incontinence in women in France, Germany, Spain and the UK. BJU Int. 2005;96(6):831–8.

7.  Broome BA. The impact of urinary incontinence on self-efficacy and quality of life. Health Qual Life Outcomes. 2003;1:35.

8.  Sinclair AJ, Ramsay IN. The psychosocial impact of urinary incontinence in women. Obstet Gynaecol. 2011;13(3):143–8.

9.  Tang DH, Colayco DC, Khalaf KM, Piercy J, Patel V, Globe D, Ginsberg D. Impact of urinary incontinence on healthcare resource utilization, health-related quality of life and productivity in patients with overactive bladder. BJU Int. 2014;113:484–91.

10. Coyne KS, Wein A, Nicholson S, Kvasz M, Chen CI, Milsom I. Comorbidities and personal burden of urgency urinary incontinence: a systematic review. The Int J Clin Pract. 2013;67:1015–33.

11. Osman NI, Chapple CR. The burden of urgency urinary incontinence on health and wellbeing. The Int J Clin Pract. 2013;67:1072–4.

12. Coyne KS, Wein A, Nicholson S, Kvasz M, Chen CI, Milsom I. Economic burden of urgency urinary incontinence in the United States: a systematic review. J Manag Care Pharm. 2014;20:130–40.

13. Abrams P, Smith AP, Cotterill N. The impact of urinary incontinence on quality of life in a real-world population of women aged 45–60 years: results from a survey in France, Germany, the UK and the USA. Br J Urol Int. 2014. doi:10.1111/bju.12852.

14. Tennant R, Hiller L, Fishwick R, Platt S, Joseph S, Weich S, Parkinson J, Secker J, Stewart-Brown S. The Warwick-Edinburgh Mental Well-being Scale (WEMWBS): development and UK validation. Health Qual Life Outcomes. 2007;5:63.

15. Avery J, Braunack-Mayer A, Stocks N, Taylor A, Duggan P. Psychological perspectives in urinary incontinence: a metasynthesis. OA Women's Health. 2013;1:9.

16. Avery J, Stocks N, Duggan P, Braunack-Mayer A, Taylor A, Goldney R, MacLennan A. Identifying the quality of life effects of urinary incontinence with depression in an Australian population. BMC Urol. 2013;13. doi:10.1186/1471-2490-13-11.

17. Avery JC, Braunack-Mayer AJ, Duggan PM, Taylor AW, Stocks NP. 'It's our lot': how resilience influences the experience of depression in women with urinary incontinence. Health Sociol Rev. 2015;24:94–108.

18. Botlero R, Bell RJ, Urquhart DM, Davis SR. Urinary incontinence is associated with lower psychological general well-being in community-dwelling women. Menopause. 2010;17:332–7.

19. O'Halloran T, Bell RJ, Robinson PJ, Davis SR. Urinary incontinence in young nulligravid women. Ann Intern Med. 2012;157:87–93.

20. Avery K, Donovan J, Peters TJ, Shaw C, Gotoh M, Abrams P. ICIQ: a brief and robust measure for evaluating the symptoms and impact of urinary incontinence. Neurourol Urodyn. 2004;23(4):322–30.

21. Bristol Urological Institute. ICIQ-lower urinary tract symptoms quality of life. Available at: http://www.iciq.net/ICIQ.LUTSqolmodule.html. Accessed 20 May 2016.

# 27

# Autoimmune hemolytic anemia associated with renal urothelial cancer

Shuji Isotani[1*], Akira Horiuchi[1], Masayuki Koja[1], Takahiro Noguchi[1], Shouichiro Sugiura[1], Hirofumi Shimoyama[2], Yasuhiro Noma[2], Kousuke Kitamura[2], Toshiyuki China[2], Shino Tokiwa[1], Keisuke Saito[1], Masaki Kimura[1], Shin-ichi Hisasue[2], Hisamitsu Ide[1], Satoru Muto[1], Raizo Yamaguchi[1] and Shigeo Horie[2]

## Abstract

**Background:** Autoimmune hemolytic anemia (AIHA) is hemolytic anemia characterized by autoantibodies directed against red blood cells. AIHA can be induced by hematological neoplasms such as malignant lymphoma, but is rarely observed in the urological field. We report a case of renal urothelial cancer inducing Coombs-positive warm AIHA and severe thrombocytopenia that was responsive to nephroureterectomy.

**Case presentation:** A 52-year-old man presented with a 1-month history of general weakness and dizziness. Hemoglobin level was 4.2 g/dL, and direct and indirect Coombs tests both yielded positive results. Abdominal computed tomography revealed huge left hydronephrosis due to a renal pelvic tumor measuring 4.0 x 4.0 x 3.0 cm, and renal regional lymph-node involvement was also observed and suspected as metastasis. Corticosteroid therapy was administered, and nephroureterectomy was performed. After surgical resection, the hemoglobin level gradually normalized, and direct and indirect Coombs tests yielded negative results. We thus diagnosed warm AIHA associated with renal urothelial cancer.

**Conclusion:** To the best of our knowledge, this represents the first report of AIHA associated with renal urothelial cancer and severe thrombocytopenia responsive to nephroureterectomy. Renal urothelial cancer needs to be included in the differential diagnoses for warm AIHA, and nephroureterectomy represents a treatment option for AIHA.

**Keywords:** Autoimmune hemolytic anemia, Paraneoplastic syndromes, Renal urothelial cancer, Nephroureterectomy

## Background

For over 100 years, paraneoplastic syndromes (PNSs) have been recognized as various symptoms associated with certain cancers but not attributable to direct tumor invasion or compression. These conditions have not been well understood until recently. Currently, PNSs are attributed to tumor secretion of functional peptides and hormones or immune cross-reactivity between tumor and normal host tissues [1]. These syndromes may affect diverse organ systems, including the neurological, hematological, endocrinological, dermatological and rheumatological systems. Medical advances have not only improved our understanding of the pathogenesis of PNSs, but have also enhanced the diagnosis and treatment of these disorders. Treatment of the underlying tumor has been reported to often improve such conditions [1, 2].

## Case presentation

A 52-year-old man without any history of gout presented with a 1-month history of dizziness and weakness, and a 3-month history of mild brown gross macrohematuria. Physical examination showed significant pallor of the skin. Microscopic urine examination confirmed red blood cells by directly examining the centrifuged urinary sediment. Hemoglobin level was 4.2 g/dl (normal, 13.0-16.6 g/dl),

* Correspondence: shujiisotani@gmail.com
[1]Department of Urology, Teikyo University, Kaga 2-11-1, Itabashi-ku, Tokyo, Japan
Full list of author information is available at the end of the article

and mean corpuscular volume (MCV) was 88.2 fl with elevated white blood count ($14.7 \times 10^9$/l) and normal platelet count ($38.0 \times 10^9$/l). Absolute reticulocyte counts were 1.1 thou/µL. Prothrombin time and activated partial thromboplastin time were both within normal ranges. The serum haptoglobin level was 15 mg/dL. Lactate dehydrogenase level was elevated to 325 IU/L (normal, 119–229 IU/L). Serum level of total bilirubin was markedly elevated to 4.85 mg/dL (normal, 0.0-1.1 mg/dL), whereas direct bilirubin level was only slightly elevated (0.5 mg/dL; normal, 0.0-0.4 mg/dL). Iron studies showed that B12 level was markedly elevated to 6030 pg/ml (normal, 249–938 pg/ml), whereas folate level was normal. Serum immunoglobulin (Ig) levels were normal, and electrophoresis revealed no abnormal bands.

A direct Coombs test showed positive results for IgG and negative results for complement C3, while an indirect Coombs test for antiglobulin also yielded positive results. Testing to exclude other autoimmune diseases showed that antinuclear antibodies, antibodies to double-stranded DNA, and antiphospholipid antibodies were all negative. Levels of various tumor markers (prostate-specific antigen, neuron-specific enolase, alpha-fetoprotein, carbohydrate antigen 19–9, carcinoembryonic antigen, squamous cell carcinoma (SCC) antigen were examined and found to be within normal limits. However, serum interleukin (IL)-2 receptor level was elevated to 1503 U/ml (normal, 145–519 U/ml). Urine cytology was negative for cancer. Abdominal computed tomography and magnetic resonance imaging revealed huge left hydronephrosis due to a renal pelvic mass measuring $4.0 \times 4.0 \times 3.0$ cm, and renal regional lymphnode involvement was also observed as a 2-cm mass, which was suspected to represent metastasis of a renal urothelial cancer or malignant lymphoma extension with renal involvement. A diagnosis of IgG-mediated warm autoimmune hemolytic anemia (AIHA) was made on hospital day 3. The patient was transfused with crossmatch-compatible blood. Oral corticosteroid therapy (prednisolone, 60 mg/day) and intravenous Igs 500 mg/day for 3 days were also administered after diagnosis and achieved limited improvement. Surgical treatment was performed on hospital day 7, since tumors that induce AIHA are usually hematological neoplasms such as malignant lymphoma. We planned to eliminate the possibility of malignant lymphoma intraoperatively by intraoperative frozen section diagnosis. If the results of intraoperative biopsy revealed malignant lymphoma of the kidney, initiating chemotherapy as treatment would be considered. Conversely, if some other malignant epithelial tumor was identified, such as renal urothelial cancer or renal cell carcinoma, nephroureterectomy was planned as surgical treatment. The results of intraoperative biopsy indicated reactive hyperplasia of the lymph node, rather than malignant lymphoma. We therefore consecutively performed left nephroureterectomy as a treatment for AIHA. After surgical resection of the left kidney, hemoglobin level and reticulocyte count gradually normalized. Direct and indirect Coombs tests yielded negative results by 7 post-operative weeks. At 10 weeks after surgery, complete blood counts had recovered to within normal ranges and the dose of prednisolone was tapered to 15 mg/day after 10 weeks (Fig. 1).

The diagnosis was confirmed to be warm AIHA associated with renal urothelial cancer. The specimen of the left kidney showed papillary urothelial carcinoma (UC) in the renal pelvis with undifferentiated carcinoma, G2, pT4, INF γ, lt-u0, ew1, ly1, v1, n2), and gradual invasion of the tumor into the renal parenchyma with change to undifferentiated carcinoma. Multiple lung and liver metastases were observed 3 months postoperatively on a CT of the chest and abdomen, so the prednisolone dose was increased to 20 mg/day from 14 weeks to prevent recurrence of AIHA. No symptoms of AIHA or abnormal hemolytic state were observed. Prednisolone was tapered to 5 mg/day and the dosage kept unchanged at 5 mg/day. Although chemotherapy using gemcitabine plus cisplatin for metastases was administered, the patient died 7 months after surgery due to rapid development of metastases and multiple-organ failure (MOF).

## Discussion

Anemia frequently complicates the course of cancer and causes fatigue, representing a very common symptom associated with cancer patients and negatively impacting activities of daily living and quality of life, sometimes becoming life-threating in itself. Some types of anemia associated with cancer involve hematological autoimmune disease, such as AIHA. AIHA is a condition characterized by autoantibodies directed against the red blood cells. Most cases of AIHA are idiopathic, but AIHA can be secondary to some malignancies [3, 4]. These immune-mediated hematological diseases are not usual, but are known as a typical PNS. In the literature, AIHA as a PNS has been demonstrated in patients with a wide variety of tumors, including hematological neoplasms such as malignant lymphoma, squamous cell carcinoma, adenocarcinoma, renal cell carcinoma, oat cell carcinoma and seminoma [4, 5]. However, renal malignancy is rarely associated with hematological PNS, and we have not identified any reports of AIHA associated with renal urothelial cancer.

We examined the literature for AIHA associated with renal tumor, and the results are summarized in Table 1 [1, 3, 5–8]. AIHA secondary to a paraneoplastic process of renal tumor has been reported in association with severe anemia that can lead to significant morbidity and even mortality [7]. From this perspective, correct

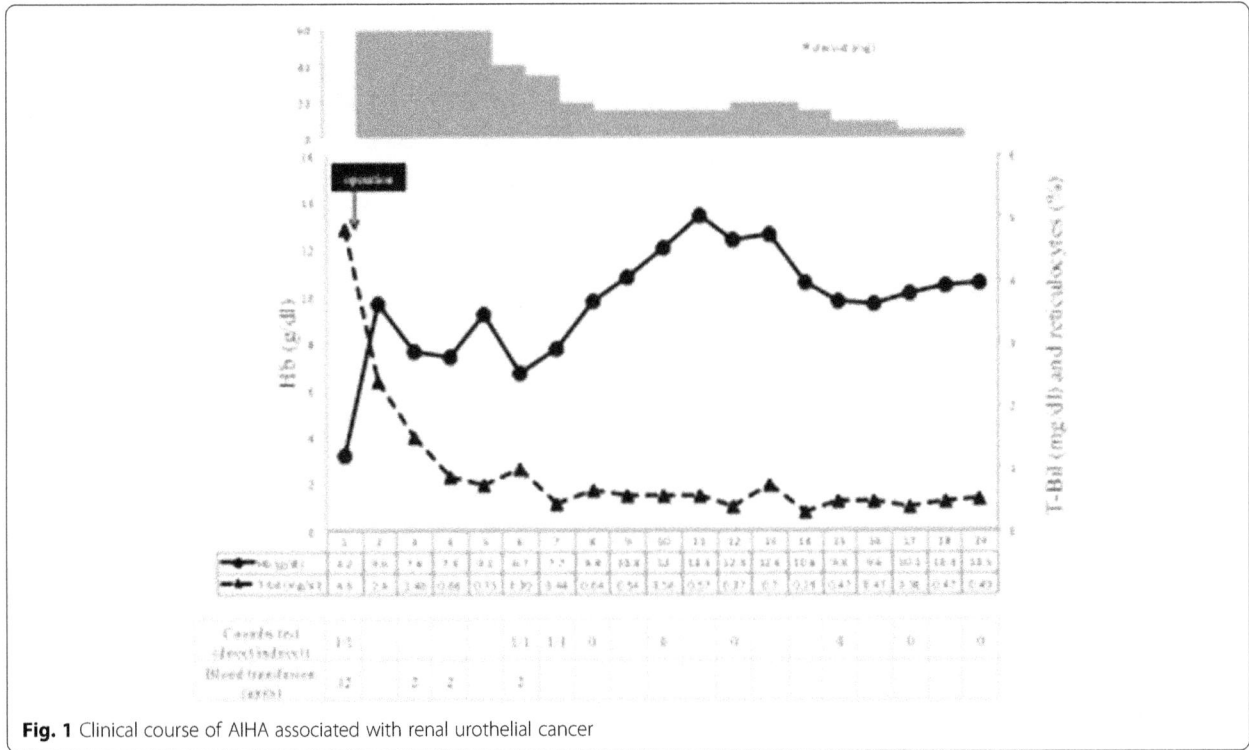

**Fig. 1** Clinical course of AIHA associated with renal urothelial cancer

diagnosis of AIHA as a PNS and start of treatment as soon as possible is very important.

The diagnosis of paraneoplastic AIHA should be made after ruling out metastases, infections, metabolic processes, and vascular alterations. In this case, we diagnosed paraneoplastic AIHA on day 3 of admission and started treatment, performing surgery on day 7. With that clinical decision, given the disadvantage that this case seems to represent the first report of AIHA with renal urothelial cancer, the literature helped us to determine which treatment might be most suitable, even though the pathogenic mechanisms underlying the association between carcinoma and autoimmune hemolytic disease remain poorly understood. The pathogenesis of these PNSs involves the release of substances with endocrine and metabolic activity by tumor cells, or induction of the release of inflammatory mediators, principally cytokines such as interleukin (IL). IL-6 has been identified as being responsible for some inflammatory processes [4]. In this case, such mediators were suggested to be secreted from cancer cells based on blood analysis finding abnormal elevations of the white blood count, B12 level, and serum IL-2 receptor level on admission. These findings also supported our diagnosis of AIHA as a PNS in this case.

Steroids represent the major therapy for idiopathic AIHA. Steroid-resistant cases may require splenectomy, although more recently other immunosuppressants such as azathioprine, mycophenolate, the monoclonal antibody

rituximab, and intravenous immunoglobulins have been successfully applied. Control of the carcinoma through tumor excision or chemotherapy with corticosteroid therapy and/or splenectomy might improve hematological abnormalities [8]. In fact, most reports with renal tumor seem to have described nephrectomy as an effective treatment for AIHA and renal carcinoma [1, 3, 5–8].

In our case, we performed nephroureterectomy to control the AIHA rather than the cancer. Surgical treatment improved the hemolytic state for at least 7 months, even though cancer control failed, with multiple metastases appearing in the liver and lungs within 3 months. We considered increasing the prednisolone dose from 15 mg/day to 20 mg/day to prevent the recurrence of AIHA, because we thought that recurrence of the carcinoma might initiate the hematological abnormalities. If the tumor started to progress, AIHA would thus presumably recur. However, no AIHA symptoms were observed, with negative Coombs reactions observed until the patient died of MOF. This result suggests that once control of AIHA was initiated by surgical intervention, control could be maintained with steroid therapy alone.

## Conclusions

We have reported a case of warm AIHA as a PNS with renal urothelial cancer. Hemolytic anemia as a PNS is diagnosed by excluding other causes such as primary hematological alterations, metastasis, and vascular

**Table 1** Contemporary series of AIHA associated with renal tumor

| References | Age/Sex | Hb | Stage, Pathology | Cooms test (Direct/Indirect) | Treatment | Response to Treatment | Outcome |
|---|---|---|---|---|---|---|---|
| Pirofsky B (1968) | 65/M | Ht:26% | non-metastatic RCC | positive/positive | steroid nephrectomy | CR | NA |
| Spira MA (1979) | 68/F | 8.7 | hypernephroma | positive/positive (IgG) | steroid nephrectomy splenectomy | CR | recurrence-free RCC and AIHA for 5 years |
| Bradley G (1981) | 57/F | 6.8 | non-metastatic clear cell RCC | positive/positive Non-specific (only IgG negative) | steroid nephrectomy | CR | died with lung metastasis after 17 months with AIHA |
| Venzano C (1985) | 71/F | 7.5 | lymph-node metastasis, renal cell carcinoma | positive/positive | steroid | CR | NA |
| Girelli G (1988) | 39/M | 4.0 | T3b clear cell RCC | positive/positive (IgM) | steroid nephrectomy | CR | DAT remained positive, no follow-up data |
| Monga M (1995) | 38/F | | T1N0M0 renal cell cancer | negative/positive | nephrectomy | CR | sustained CR of RCC and AIHA for 2+ years |
| Lands R (1996) | 65/M | 8.1 | T3a adenocarcinoma | positive | steroid nephrectomy | CR | NA |
| Kamra D (2002) | 68/F | 5.6 | T2N0M0 clear cell RCC | negative | steroid globulin therapy nephrectomy | CR | NA |
| Muñoz-Ibarrav EL (2013) | 71/F | 6.7 | T1aN0M0 clear cell RCC | positive | steroid nephrectomy | CR | NA |
| Our case (2015) | 52/M | 3.2 | T4N2M0 UC+RCC | positive/positive (IgG) | steroid globulin therapy nephrectomy | CR | died with multiple metastases after 7 months without AIHA |

processes. The appearance of unusual hematological alterations in patients with renal tumor should be suspected with these hematological paraneoplastic alterations. Our experience suggests that hemolytic anemia as a PNS should be considered in patients with hematological alterations with renal urothelial cancer, and if confirmed, surgical intervention with steroid administration should be considered.

## Consent

Written informed consent was obtained from the patient for publication of this case report and the accompanying images. A copy of the written consent is available for review by the editor of this journal.

**Abbreviations**
AIHA: Autoimmune hemolytic anemia; PNS: Paraneoplastic syndromes; MOF: Multiple-organ failure; UC: Urothelial carcinoma; IL: Interleukin.

**Competing interests**
The authors declare that they have no conflict of interests.

**Authors' contributions**
All authors participated in this case.
All authors read and approved the final manuscript.

**Authors' information**
Qualifications: MD. and Ph.D.
Title: Assistant Professor.
Affiliations: Department of Urology, School of Medicine, Teikyo University, Tokyo, Japan.

**Acknowledgements**
The authors gratefully acknowledge the contribution of Dr. Kazuo Kawasugi and Dr. Naoki Shirafuji of the Department of Hematology. They also thank the staff of the Teikyo Hospital urology unit.

**Financial disclosure**
No financial support was received in relation to this article.

**Author details**
[1]Department of Urology, Teikyo University, Kaga 2-11-1, Itabashi-ku, Tokyo, Japan. [2]Department of Urology, Juntendo University, Graduate School of Medicine, Tokyo, Japan.

**References**
1. Lorraine C, Pelosof MD. Paraneoplastic Syndromes: An Approach to Diagnosis and Treatment. Mayo Clin Proc. 2011;85:838–54.
2. Koike H, Yoshida H, Ito T, Ohyama K, Hashimoto R, Kawagashira Y, et al. Demyelinating neuropathy and autoimmune hemolytic anemia in a patient with pancreatic cancer. Intern Med. 2013;52:1737–40.
3. Krauth M-T, Puthenparambil J, Lechner K. Paraneoplastic autoimmune thrombocytopenia in solid tumors. Crit Rev Oncol Hematol. 2012;81:75–81.
4. Visco C, Barcellini W, Maura F, Neri A, Cortelezzi A, Rodeghiero F. Autoimmune cytopenias in chronic lymphocytic leukemia. Am J Hematol. 2014;89:1055–62.
5. Puthenparambil J, Lechner K, Kornek G. Autoimmunhämolytische Anämie, ein paraneoplastisches Phänomen bei soliden Tumoren: Eine kritische Analyse von 52 publizierten Fällen. Wien Klin Wochenschr. 2010;122:229–36.
6. Kamra D, Boselli J, Sloane BB, Gladstone DE. Renal cell carcinoma induced Coombs negative autoimmune hemolytic anemia and severe thrombocytopenia responsive to nephrectomy. J Urol. 2002;167:1395–5.
7. Lands R, Foust J. Renal cell carcinoma and autoimmune hemolytic anemia. South Med J. 1996;89:444–5.
8. Spira MA, Lynch EC. Autoimmune hemolytic anemia and carcinoma: an unusual association. Am J Med. 1979;67:753–8.

# 28

# Clinical utility of a non-invasive urine test for risk assessing patients with no obvious benign cause of hematuria: a physician-patient real world data analysis

Tony Lough[1], Qingyang Luo[1], Carthika Luxmanan[1,2], Alastair Anderson[1], Jimmy Suttie[1*], Paul O'Sullivan[1,3] and David Darling[1]

## Abstract

**Background:** The non-invasive Cxbladder urine test system has demonstrated clinical utility in ruling out urothelial carcinoma (UC) in patients with asymptomatic microscopic hematuria (AMH), suggesting that the number of invasive diagnostic tests, including cystoscopy, used in this patient population may be reduced by Cxbladder testing prior to conducting a full urological work-up. The aim of this study was to demonstrate the enhanced clinical utility of communicating objective information on diagnostic decisions made by individual physicians on individual patients with AMH.

**Methods:** Three hundred ninety-six physician-patient decisions were generated from twelve participant physicians evaluating real world case notes from the same 33 patients presenting with AMH. Each physician reviewed and recommended diagnostic tests and procedures based on each patient's referral data and then re-evaluated their clinical recommendation following disclosure of the non-invasive Cxbladder urine test result. Changes assessed were the total number of requested diagnostic procedures and the number of invasive procedures, including cystoscopy, following addition of information from Cxbladder in the Triage and Triage and Detect modalities.

**Results:** Physicians made significant changes to their diagnostic behavior for patients with AMH when presented with Cxbladder test results, including a reduction in the number of total and invasive procedures including cystoscopy for individuals identified as having a low probability of UC. The intensity of investigation was targeted and increased, including use of total procedures and cystoscopy, for patients identified by Cxbladder tests as having a high probability of UC: urologists increased the level of investigation for both total procedures and invasive procedures. The outcome resulted in patients with a high risk of UC receiving appropriate guideline-recommended invasive diagnostic tests. Patients who tested negative were offered fewer and significantly less invasive procedures. This change in physician behavior results in an increased clinical and patient utility, lower risk of missed UC and invasive test-related harm incidents.

**Conclusions:** This study demonstrated the potential for increased clinical resolution and significantly enhanced patient management, when physicians consider Cxbladder test results in their clinical evaluation. The change in physician behavior led to more appropriate diagnostic procedure selection and resource allocation to the benefit of both patients and healthcare systems.

**Keywords:** Asymptomatic microscopic hematuria, Biomarker, Clinical parameters, Clinical utility, Cystoscopy, Diagnostic, Hematuria, Molecular diagnostic, Risk assessment, Urothelial carcinoma

* Correspondence: jimmy.suttie@pelnz.com
[1]Pacific Edge Limited, 87 St David Street, Dunedin 9016, New Zealand
Full list of author information is available at the end of the article

## Background

Hematuria, or blood in the urine, is a common occurrence in clinical practice. Asymptomatic microscopic hematuria (AMH; defined as > 3 red blood cells/high-powered field in a properly collected urine sample) is present in up to 24% of the general population [1] and is the primary reason for more than 485,000 referrals to urologists in the US every year [2].

The current American Urological Association (AUA) guidelines recommend a full urological work-up to diagnose or rule out UC in patients with AMH within 180 days [3, 4], however several barriers to referral for a full urological work-up exist. For example, clinical diagnostic algorithms for patients with hematuria are complicated, difficult to follow and enable a degree of latitude in their interpretation [1]. Many physicians are also conscious of the burden of invasive procedures and the potential for harm and there is a lack of compliance by patients when confronted with the prospect of many and varied invasive procedures. Invasive procedures, such as cystoscopy and contrast computed tomography (CT) scans, have the potential to impact their patients in terms of adverse events, financial cost and emotional impact [1, 4–12]. As such, guideline recommendations to administer full urological work-ups to all patients presenting with hematuria may only be selectively adhered to [12, 13].

In particular, as few as 10% of women with hematuria are referred to urologists [14]. Likewise, < 14% of patients with hematuria undergo cystoscopy or radiological investigation within 180 days and a recent Australian study reported delays of up to 1165 days between initial presentation of hematuria and subsequent treatment for UC [15, 16]. This is particularly concerning given that delayed diagnoses are known to negatively influence outcomes for patients with UC with every day increasing the risk of death for a patient with UC by 1% [17].

The high probability of delayed treatment is particularly evident for younger and female patients. Treatment for UC is more likely to be delayed for women than men, and although the incidence of UC is higher for men [18–23], women are less likely to undergo procedures after being referred and have a higher risk of presenting with UC at an advanced stage and have poorer survival outcomes [21, 24]. Therefore, a simple, rigorous and accurate segregation of patients using a non-invasive risk-assessment tool may reduce barriers to referral and focus the intensity and prioritisation of patients for workup.

The need for such a non-invasive UC risk-assessment tool for patients with hematuria contrasts with skepticism regarding the clinical utility of urine biomarkers and molecular diagnostics in diagnosing UC, particularly predictions that routine use of urine biomarker tests will ultimately increase the use of invasive diagnostic procedures [1, 15, 25].

The non-invasive Cxbladder urine test can be used to identify patients with hematuria with a low or high probability of UC in its Triage (sensitivity 0.95; negative predictive value 0.98) and Detect (specificity 0.85; sensitivity 0.82) modalities, respectively [26, 27]. Cxbladder has previously demonstrated population-level clinical utility in reducing the net number of diagnostic tests using real world clinical data in a retrospective evaluation of participating urologist's decisions. [12]. Specifically, invasive procedures, requested by urologists assessing a real-world sample population of patients with AMH [12] led to all patients ultimately diagnosed with UC receiving a cystoscopy and/or CT scan as part of a diagnostic work-up, in line with the AUA guidelines, [4, 12]. There is therefore potential for an increased risk of harm for the one-third of UC-positive cases potentially missed using non-invasive procedures in the baseline case.

Having demonstrated that Cxbladder may decrease the use of invasive tests across a population of patients with AMH, the aim of the present study was to provide greater resolution by investigating the potential change in clinical utility from communicating objective information from Cxbladder tests on the diagnostic decisions made by individual physicians for individual patients with AMH.

## Method

### Participant and patient case details

Full methodological, case and participating physician details were reported in Darling et al. (2017) [12]. Briefly, patients were prospectively recruited and systematically selected to represent a broad patient demographic and clinical spectrum. Three hundred ninety-six physician-patient clinical decisions were evaluated where 12 urologists (participant physicians; Additional file 1: Table S1) with experience in the use and application of Cxbladder in their clinical settings were recruited. Participating physicians were offered honoraria as compensation for the time spent participating in the study. Experience in the use and application of Cxbladder was defined as using Cxbladder more than 10 times in real-world situations. Each participant physician individually evaluated the same 33 case-note clinical referral data from patients presenting with AMH systematically selected from the database of patients enrolled in previous prospective clinical studies of Cxbladder. Patients consented to the anonymous use of their urine sample and clinical information, IRB approval details are presented below.

All patients met the AUA definition of AMH with the possibility of UC requiring a urological work-up, including invasive diagnostic procedures [3]. Each participant physician was asked to review and recommend diagnostic procedures for each case based on the patient's evaluation from normal referral data. Participant physicians were asked to select a set of urological investigation procedures from a list of investigation procedures recommended in the AUA guidelines [3]. For the purposes of this study and to enable the reduction of any systemic bias, participant physicians were instructed to consider all tests and procedures to be fully funded, with no additional cost incurred by the patient. Participant physicians were not informed of the final UC status of each case.

Participant physicians performed further recommended clinical evaluations for each case twice, firstly in the context of the information derived from Cxbladder Triage alone and secondly when both Cxbladder Triage and Detect were presented. The data format was consistent with the commercially available Cxbladder tests, including a report outcome, explanation of the Cxbladder test methodology and guide to interpreting the results [26, 27]. Outcomes were defined as low probability of UC, 'negative', or standard clinical workup, 'physician-directed protocol', for Cxbladder Triage and 'normal', 'elevated' or 'high' gene expression for Cxbladder Detect. Elevated and high results in the Detect modality were presented as 'positive' for UC for the purposes of this study.

### Study endpoints

The co-primary endpoints were changes in the total number of diagnostic procedures used over all patient cases and the number of invasive procedures requested following disclosure of diagnostic information from Cxbladder Triage and Cxbladder Triage and Detect. For the purposes of this study, cystoscopy (flexible or rigid) and CT scans (contrast or non-contrast) were defined as invasive diagnostic procedures whereas ultrasound, urine cytology and UroVysion® fluorescence in situ hybridization were defined as non-invasive procedures and tests.

### Statistical procedures

A random-effect linear mixed model was used for net change analyses for total procedures, invasive procedures and each individual procedure requested, for each physician-patient interaction. Fixed effects were time (baseline, after test) and test results, and random effects were patient and participant physician. The average number of procedures per interaction at baseline was calculated for total procedures, invasive procedures and each individual procedure. 95% confidence intervals (CI) that did not include zero were considered to be statistically significant ($p < 0.05$).

Transition probability analyses were performed for individual invasive procedures. Transition probabilities with a denominator $\geq 10$ and an upper limit of its CI $\geq$ 0.5 were considered to be statistically significant. If the upper and lower limits of the CI were $\geq 0.5$, then the transition probability was considered to be highly statistically significant ($p < 0.01$).

### Heatmap data graphic

Data were graphically presented as heatmap calculations to aid the visualisation of the results at the individual physician-patient interaction level. The heatmaps show the range of variation in decision making and the change in decisions with and without the addition of the Cxbladder result. The baseline heatmaps provide the total count of procedures at each of the 396 physician-patient interactions in the absence of availability of the Cxbladder result. The change, relative to this baseline, made when the Cxbladder result was disclosed reflects the change in physicians decision making. Heatmap columns represent individual physicians and rows represent individual patients with each row and column intersection becoming a physician-patient interaction. Patients (rows) are grouped by Cxbladder result with colour bar linkage, patient ID and test result. The baseline heatmaps include the actual number of procedures per interaction and the associated change heatmap includes the change relative to baseline per interaction. The colour code in the heatmap is used to indicate extent of the change in the number of tests and procedures used in the physician-patient interaction. An increase in the change is represented in shades of red or a decrease in the change is represented in shades of green or no change relative to baseline is in white. The greater the intensity of colour the greater the change in decisions.

### Results

Each participant physician evaluating an individual patient represents an independent physician-patient interaction. Overall, 792 post-baseline decision nodes were generated after 396 baseline physician-patient clinical decisions were made following the provision of firstly Cxbladder Triage followed by Cxbladder Detect data (Fig. 1). At the first decision node, 264/396 clinical decisions (66.7%) tested negative for Cxbladder Triage. No cases where a test was reported as negative for Cxbladder Triage subsequently tested positive using Cxbladder Detect. Of the 132 clinical decisions where a physician-directed protocol was recommended by Cxbladder Triage, 36 (27.3%) carried positive results following Cxbladder Detect.

A total of 688 diagnostic procedures were requested by participating physicians across 278 baseline clinical decisions (Fig. 2a), including 424 invasive procedures in 259 clinical decisions (Fig. 3a). No additional diagnostic procedures were requested in 118 baseline clinical decisions.

### Change in procedure selection following a negative result for Cxbladder triage

Negative Cxbladder Triage results led to a net reduction in procedures in 79/182 (43.4%) clinical decisions where additional diagnostic procedures had been requested based

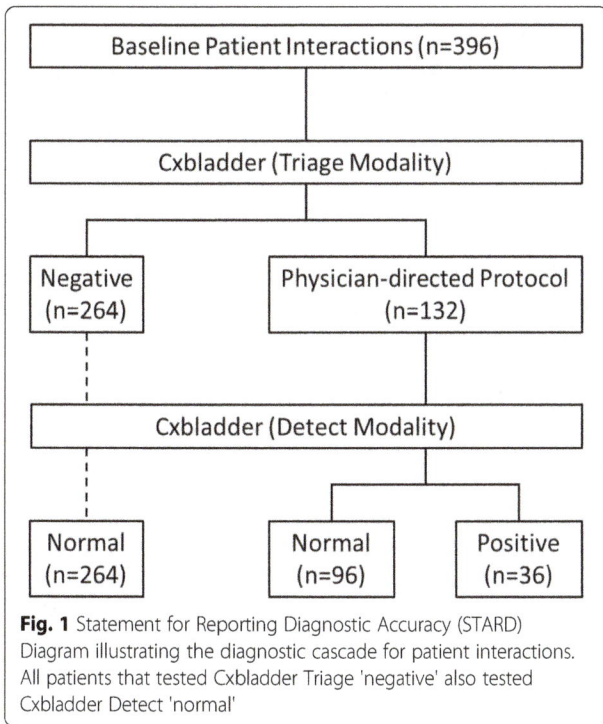

**Fig. 1** Statement for Reporting Diagnostic Accuracy (STARD) Diagram illustrating the diagnostic cascade for patient interactions. All patients that tested Cxbladder Triage 'negative' also tested Cxbladder Detect 'normal'

on baseline data (Fig. 2a+b). This translated into a significant mean reduction in total diagnostic procedures requested per interaction (Table 1). Only one patient with a negative result had a net increase in procedures (Fig. 2b).

Presentation of negative results from Cxbladder Triage resulted in a net removal of invasive procedures in 93/

169 clinical decisions (55.0%) where invasive procedures had been requested at baseline (Fig. 3b). Of the flexible cystoscopies and contrast CT scans requested for this group, 40.4% (67/166) and 46.5% (40/86), respectively, were abandoned (Additional file 2: Figure S1 and Additional file 3: Figure S2).

### Change in procedure selection following a physician-directed protocol from Cxbladder triage and positive result for Cxbladder detect

Following presentation of results from Cxbladder Detect for patients who were guided to a physician-directed protocol by Cxbladder Triage, 19/36 clinical decisions (52.8%), where a patient tested positive, resulted in a net increase in procedures, while three clinical decisions (8.3%) resulted in a net decrease (Fig. 2c). Overall, a positive result for Cxbladder Detect resulted in a significant increase in the total number of procedures per interaction (Table 1).

A net 26 invasive procedures were added across 17 clinical decisions for patients who tested positive using Cxbladder Detect, while three procedures were removed in a further three clinical decisions (Fig. 3c). No net change in the number of clinical decisions involving a request for a flexible cystoscopy occurred in this group (Additional file 2: Figure S1), but 9 additional rigid cystoscopies were requested. Furthermore, a net 13 clinical decisions resulted in the addition of a contrast CT scan (Additional file 3: Figure S2). One extra non-contrast CT scan was also requested.

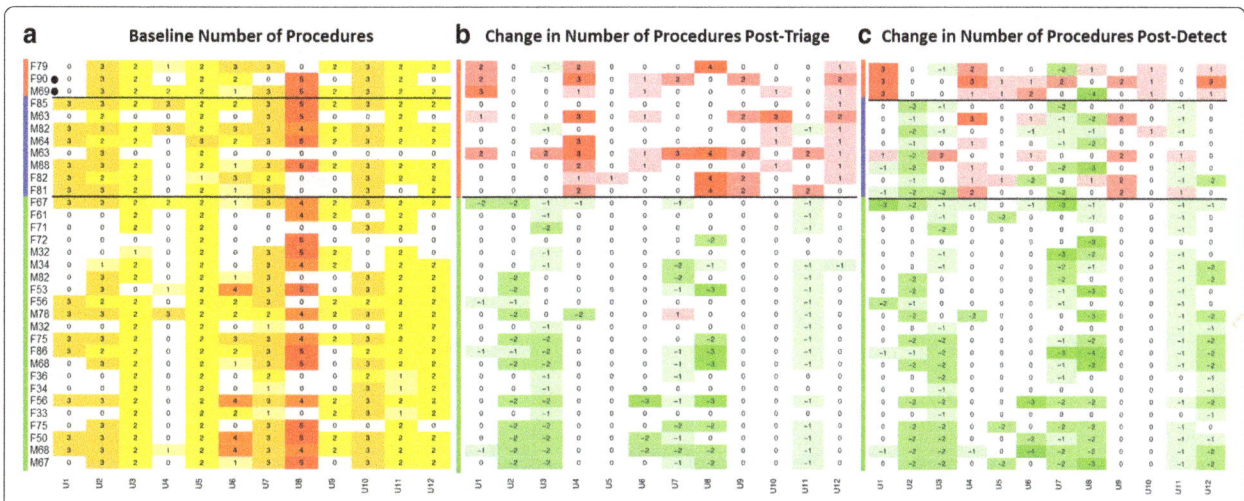

**Fig. 2** Heat maps representing the total number of diagnostic tests. Panel **a**: Baseline number of procedures; Panel **b**: Change from baseline after presenting the results of Cxbladder Triage; Panel **c**: Change from baseline after presenting the results of Cxbladder Triage and Detect. Columns represent participant physicians. Rows represent patients. Each cell represents a patient-physician decision node. Reds represent decisions nodes with added procedures and greens represent decision nodes with removed procedures in panels **b** and **c**. M and F represent male and female gender, respectively, followed by patient age. • denotes a patient who was subsequently diagnosed with urothelial carcinoma of the bladder. Horizontal black lines indicate test result subgroups. The vertical green bar indicates Cxbladder Triage negative and Cxbladder Detect normal results. The vertical blue bar indicates Cxbladder Triage physician directed protocol results. The vertical red bar in panel **b** indicates Cxbladder Triage physician directed protocol results and in panel **c** indicates results that are also Cxbladder Detect positive

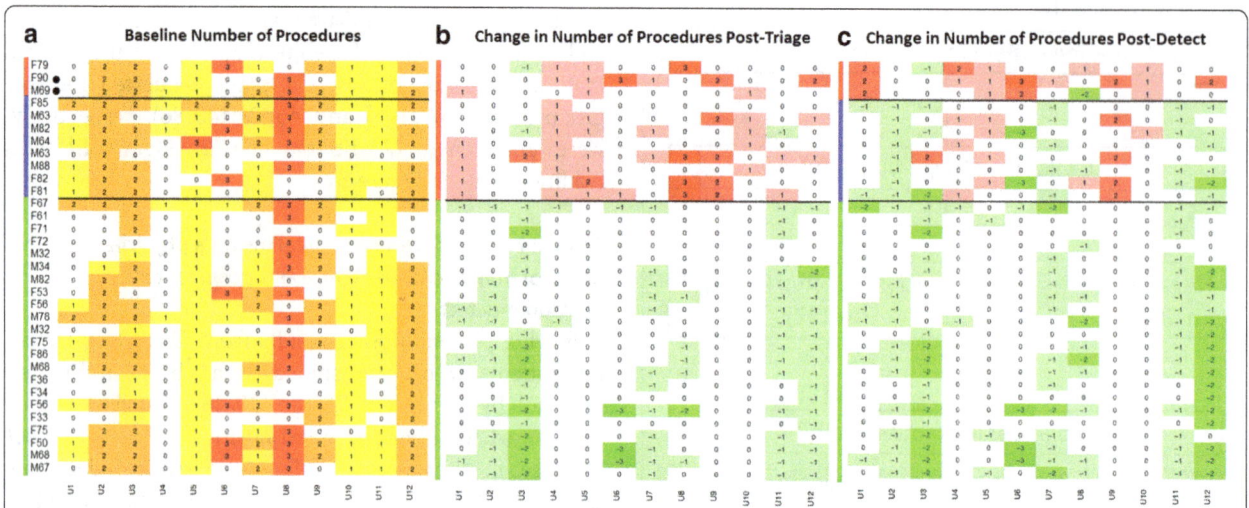

**Fig. 3** Heat maps representing the number of invasive diagnostic tests. Panel **a**: Baseline number of procedures; Panel **b**: Change from baseline after presenting the results of Cxbladder Triage; Panel **c**: Change from baseline after presenting the results of Cxbladder Triage and Detect. Columns represent participant physicians. Rows represent patients. Each cell represents a patient-physician decision node. Reds represent decisions nodes with added procedures and greens represent decision nodes with removed procedures in panels **b** and **c**. M and F represent male and female gender, respectively, followed by patient age. • denotes a patient who was subsequently diagnosed with urothelial carcinoma of the bladder. Horizontal black lines indicate test result subgoups. The vertical green bar indicates Cxbladder Triage negative results and Cxbladder Detect normal results. The vertical blue bar indicates Cxbladder Triage physician directed protocol results. The vertical red bar in panel **b** indicates Cxbladder Triage physician directed protocol results and in panel **c** results that are also Cxbladder Detect positive

### Clinical decisions involving a physician-directed protocol from Cxbladder triage and normal result for Cxbladder detect

Of the 96 clinical decisions resulting in a physician-directed protocol that subsequently tested normal for Cxbladder Detect, 31 had a net increase, and 17 a net decrease in total procedures (Fig. 2c). However, a normal result from Cxbladder Detect was associated with a significant mean reduction in total diagnostic procedures requested per patient interaction versus baseline (Table 1).

A net reduction in invasive procedures compared with baseline occurred in 32/66 (48.5%) clinical decisions following a normal result from Cxbladder Detect, while procedures were added in 14/96 (14.6%) clinical decisions (Fig. 3c). Overall, 28 (42.4%) fewer flexible cystoscopies were requested in this group (Additional file 2: Figure S1), but three rigid cystoscopies were added. Three fewer contrast CT scans (8.1% reduction versus baseline) and one less non-contrast CT scan were requested (Additional file 3: Figure S2).

**Table 1** Mean absolute and proportional change in the use of diagnostic tests per patient

| | Negative | | Physician-directed Protocol /Normal | | Physician-directed Protocol /Positive | |
|---|---|---|---|---|---|---|
| | Δ (95% CI) | Δ% | Δ (95% CI) | Δ% | Δ (95% CI) | Δ% |
| Total | −0.686 (− 0.854, − 0.517)* | −41 | − 0.208 (− 0.488, 0.072) | −11 | 0.722 (0.265, 1.179)* | + 38 |
| Invasive | −0.519 (− 0.639, − 0.399)* | −51 | − 0.198 (− 0.397, 0.001) | −17 | 0.639 (0.314, 0.963)* | + 55 |
| Cystoscopy | | | | | | |
|   Flexible | −0.352 (− 0.422, − 0.283)* | − 56 | 0.187 (− 0.303, − 0.072) | −28 | 0.000 (− 0.188, 0.188) | 0 |
|   Rigid | 0.000 (− 0.021, 0.021) | 0 | 0.031 (− 0.004, 0.067) | + 300 | 0.250 (0.192, 0.308)* | + 900 |
| CT scan | | | | | | |
|   Contrast | −0.155 (− 0.214, − 0.096)* | −48 | −0.031 (− 0.129, 0.067) | −8 | 0.361 (0.201, 0.521)* | + 100 |
|   Non-contrast | −0.011 (− 0.043, 0.020) | −16 | −0.010 (− 0.063, 0.042) | −13 | 0.028 (− 0.058, 0.113) | + 25 |
| Non-invasive tests | | | | | | |
|   Ultrasound | 0.034 (−0.022, 0.090) | + 11 | 0.083 (−0.009, 0.176) | + 26 | − 0.056 (− 0.207, 0.096) | −18 |
|   Urine cytology | − 0.170 (− 0.229, − 0.112) | − 60 | − 0.062 (− 0.159, 0.034) | −18 | 0.167 (0.009, 0.325)* | + 43 |
|   UroVysion® FISH | −0.030 (− 0.051, − 0.009)* | −100 | −0.031 (− 0.066, 0.004) | − 75 | −0.028 (− 0.085, 0.029) | −50 |

*p < 0.05

Abbreviations: *CT* computed tomography, *FISH* fluorescence in situ hybridization

| | Negative | | Physician-directed Protocol / Normal | | Physician-directed Protocol / Positive | | | Negative | Physician-directed Protocol / Normal | Physician-directed Protocol / Positive |
|---|---|---|---|---|---|---|---|---|---|---|
| | Δ (95% CI) | n | Δ (95% CI) | n | Δ (95% CI) | n | | | | |
| Ultrasound → Flexible Cystoscopy | 0.000 (0.000, 0.842) | 40 | 0.000 (0.000, 0.522) | 5 | 0.200 (0.005, 0.716) | 5 | | | | |
| Ultrasound → Contrast CT Scan | 0.000 (0.000, 0.842) | 2 | 0.800 (0.284, 0.995) | 5 | 1.000 (0.478, 1.000) | 5 | | | | |
| Ultrasound → Non-contrast CT Scan | 0.000 (0.000, 0.842) | 2 | 0.000 (0.000, 0.522) | 5 | 0.200 (0.005, 0.716) | 5 | | | | |
| Flexible Cystoscopy → Rigid Cystoscopy | 0.000 (0.000, 0.054) | 67 | 0.143 (0.040, 0.327) | 28 | 0.857 (0.421, 0.996) | 7 | | | | |
| Flexible Cystoscopy → Ultrasound | 0.060 (0.017, 0.146) | 67 | 0.071 (0.009, 0.235) | 28 | 0.143 (0.004, 0.579) | 7 | | | | |
| Contrast CT Scan → Ultrasound | 0.725 (0.561, 0.854) | 40 | 0.769 (0.462, 0.950) | 13 | 0.000 (0.000, 0.842) | 2 | | | | |
| Non-contrast CT Scan → Ultrasound | 1.000 (0.292, 1.000) | 3 | 1.000 (0.158, 1.000) | 2 | 0.000 (0.000, 0.975) | 1 | | | | |

$^{*}p < 0.05$; $^{**}p < 0.01$

**Fig. 4** Transition probabilities for diagnostic tests following disclosure of results from Cxbladder Triage and Detect. $^{*}p < 0.05$; $^{**}p < 0.01$

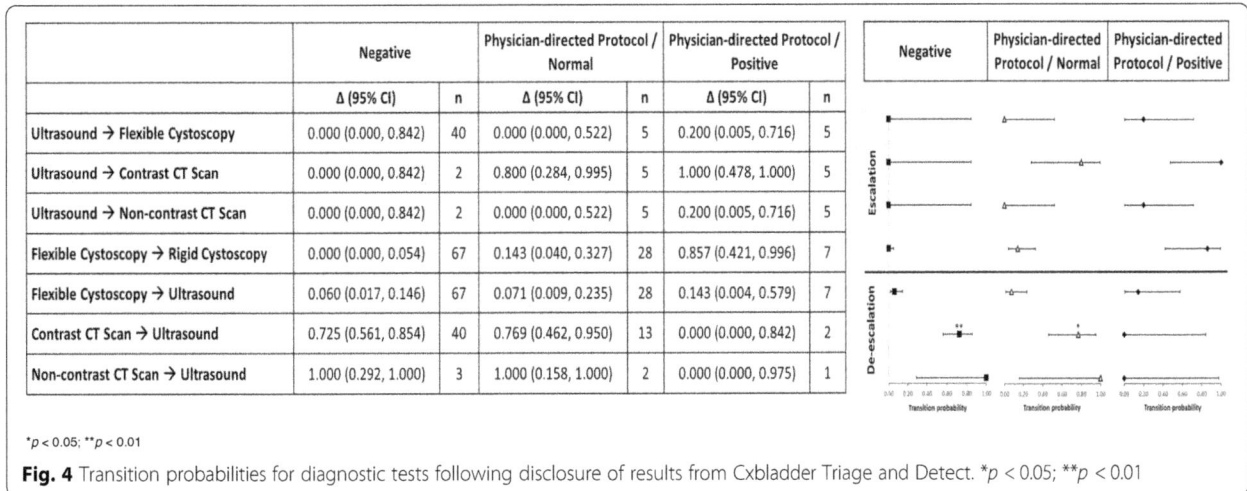

## Transition probability analyses

Transition probability analyses indicate a de-escalation of procedures following a negative result from Cxbladder Triage (Fig. 4). For example, 72.5% (29/40) of patients with negative results who were allocated a contrast CT scan at baseline had this procedure substituted with ultrasound.

Transition analyses also indicate escalation of diagnostic procedures for patients following a physician-directed protocol result (Fig. 4). All five patients with these results who were allocated an ultrasound at baseline had this procedure substituted with a contrast CT scan. Six out of seven (85.7%) patients allocated a flexible cystoscopy at baseline were escalated to rigid cystoscopy.

## Discussion

The assessment process undertaken in this study with participating physicians retrospectively evaluating real world patients extends the previous study [12] by demonstrating that the intensity and focus of the physician recommended workup is influenced by the Cxbladder result without compromising detection of UC. The heatmap data graphic was developed to enhance the visualization of the changes in decisions for the evaluation of these patients, as either an escalation or de-escalation from baseline decisions, after the addition of the Cxbladder test results. This approach provided the opportunity to view changes in decision making and their impact on clinical utility at the level of the individual physician-patient interaction as opposed to the consolidated cohort-wide view of our previous study [12].

The addition of non-invasive Cxbladder urine biomarker test results to the physicians decision making process was shown in this study to provide an overall increase in clinical utility of Cxbladder as an objective risk assessment tool for UC in the work-up of patients presenting with AMH where there are no obvious benign causes. More specifically, presentation of Cxbladder results leads to physicians modifying their diagnostic behavior and resource allocation in a consistent and repeatable manner reflecting the risk of disease for the patient. In addition, 33% (8/24) of the clinical decisions where the patient had UC, would not have been referred for an appropriate work-up that included invasive diagnostics tests in the absence of results from Cxbladder [12].

The addition of Cxbladder test results for decision making was shown to enable patients with a high probability of UC to be identified and prioritized for a full urological work-up in advance of an initial consultation, offering a clear increase in clinical utility. This outcome is expected to be of significant importance in a healthcare system when there are challenges from < 14% of patients with hematuria being referred to a urologist within 180 days [15], and where approximately 20,000 instances of UC are missed annually in the US amongst patients with hematuria who are considered to be moderate-to-high risk [14]. Furthermore, approximately, one-third of patients with hematuria undergo a cystoscopy, providing the potential for approximately 200,000 potentially unnecessary cystoscopies performed on patients who have a low risk of UC every year [14]. Accordingly, Cxbladder has the potential to provide an enhancement to the standard of care for the management and diagnostic workup of patients with hematuria that will provide benefits to the patient and the healthcare system alike from the appropriate targeting and reduction in the total number and invasiveness of tests and procedures used.

The addition of Cxbladder to the decision making by participating physicians evaluating the retrospective patient data showed an increase in the clinical utility from a reduction in the overall diagnostic burden of patients with hematuria. The previous study provided a population-level perspective and demonstrated a reduction in the total number and invasive procedures by 25% and 31%, respectively [12]. The present study extends the analysis at the individual physician-patient level with repeatable outcome results. Specifically the results identified that all participant physicians modified their chosen diagnostic work-ups to reflect the change in risk assessment provided by the addition of Cxbladder test results for each patient, i.e. an escalation or de-escalation of the number and invasiveness of the work-ups appropriately reflecting the change in the probability of UC. Notably, this was often observed as a change in nature or type of the tests and procedures requested, not only the total number. In particular, the prevalence of UC was 3-fold higher in the subset of patients referred for a physician-directed protocol by Cxbladder Triage, providing evidence that the escalation of procedures is appropriate for this subset of patients, while no patients with a negative result had UC, justifying a de-escalation.

Evidence from this study shows that the provision of more objective data on the probability of UC does not result in harm to patients, i.e. a reduced risk of patients who were ultimately diagnosed with UC in the real world not undergoing an appropriate urological work up [12]. On the contrary, more information on the risk of UC is likely to lead to a lowering of the level of variance observed during the diagnostic process to the benefit of patients; high-risk patients may be prioritized, while less invasive diagnostic tests and procedures may be recommended for low-risk patients [12].

The present data provide evidence that the use of a quantitative tool can guide the selection of diagnostic procedures for up to 20% of the general patient population with AMH [14, 15, 18, 20, 25]. Indeed, presenting Cxbladder test results to urologists led to all patients with UC being allocated guideline-recommended procedures compared with 2/3 of patients with baseline referral data alone [12].

Invasive procedures have continued to be relied upon by physicians because, as noted by the US Centers for Medicaid and Medicare [28], studies directly correlating the results of molecular diagnostics with clinical outcomes are lacking. The field of molecular diagnostics has promised to offer superior outcomes compared with invasive options for the patient, healthcare organizations and the wider society, but earlier iterations of non-invasive urine tests remain absent from diagnostic algorithms for patients with hematuria because of their low clinical resolution and lack of demonstrated clinical utility.

Accordingly, routine use of Cxbladder would likely reduce the burden of care for both patients and healthcare systems through the more selective use of invasive procedures, particularly CT scans, without compromising the desire of patients and physicians to achieve direct

visualization and identification of any tumor as part of the diagnostic process [29]. This is consistent with suggestions made by Halpern and colleagues (2017) [2] regarding the cost-effective use of diagnostic procedures in patients with AMH, while also addressing criticism of the clinical implications of advocating for a blanket replacement of CT scans with ultrasound [30]. Furthermore, the utility of Cxbladder as a risk assessment tool is likely to be further enhanced by introduction of the Cxbladder Resolve test as a third step for patients with physician-directed protocol result that identifies patients with a high probability of high-grade UC [31].

### Strengths and weaknesses

In the absence of clear guidance or precedents for assessing the clinical utility of non-invasive diagnostic tests, the investigators considered the study design used here to be the most pragmatic method of evaluating the clinical utility of Cxbladder in a cohort of real-world patients presenting with AMH given the logistical, consistency and ethical challenges in prospectively investigating the selection of diagnostic tests in patients with AMH. Notably, the innovative methodology applied in this study acknowledges and addresses the concerns expressed in the literature by experts in the field regarding the potential risks of using non-invasive urine tests for UC in patients with AMH without risking patient health. Furthermore, the methodology has allowed the challenges in weighing the risk-benefit profile for individual patients using clinical judgement alone to be identified. Accordingly, this methodology has provided hypothesis-generating data to justify further clinical investigation into the use of the new and more sensitive, non-invasive tests such as Cxbladder in increasing clinical resolution of patients being worked up who have presented to the clinic with hematuria.

The design, by requiring each physician to evaluate all patients, takes out 'patient' as a variable, thereby permitting focus on the physician-patient interaction, whose focus is the main aim of the study.

While cases were systematically selected, to provide a broad representation of patients in the prospective studies, data was presented immediately and across a series of patients: the investigators acknowledge that the study may not be reflective of a true clinical scenario. The influence of pre- and intra-study experience influencing decision-making cannot also be ruled out. However, by using the same patients presented to all urologists the study removed any confounding effect caused by different patients for different urologists and accordingly the study measured urologist decision making independent of patient variance. Furthermore, the outcomes of this study have not yet been tested in the real-world where outside influences, such as patient selection, resource availability, costs, alternative diagnostic options and real patient outcomes could influence the translation of these outcomes into clinical practice.

## Conclusion

The non-invasive Cxbladder urine test is being used by physicians to objectively define the risk of UC in patients with AMH with sufficient resolution to guide more efficient diagnostic procedure selection and resource allocation to the benefit of both patients and healthcare systems, particularly underserved groups, such as women, elderly patients and younger patients. The increase in clinical resolution associated with Cxbladder has the potential to significantly improve the identification of patients with UC when compared to the tests and procedures selected in the more conventional or standard work-up without compromising patient safety. Any consequential reduction in total and invasive procedures, coupled with the increased resolution provided by Cxbladder, would minimize the risk of invasive test-related harm and provides an increase in net patient benefit. Translation of the observations reported here into clinical outcomes would simplify the clinical algorithms applied when working up patients with AMH improving outcomes for patients, physicians and healthcare systems.

## Additional files

**Additional file 1: Table S1.** Participating physicians.

**Additional file 2: Figure S1.** Heat maps representing the number of flexible cystoscopies[a,b].

**Additional file 3: Figure S2.** Heat maps representing the number of contrast CT scans[a,b].

## Abbreviations
AMH: Asymptomatic microscopic hematuria; AUA: American Urological Association; CI: Confidence interval; CT: Computed tomography; UC: Urothelial carcinoma

## Acknowledgements
The authors wish to acknowledge the participant physicians who contributed to this study and statistical analysis support provided by Laimonis Kavalieris of Pacific Edge Ltd.

## Funding
This study was funded by Pacific Edge Ltd.

## Availability of data and materials
All authors had full access to all of the data in the study and take responsibility for the integrity of the data and the accuracy of the data analysis. The datasets generated and/or analyzed during the current study are not publicly available due to the proprietary nature of the data set and to protect the privacy of individual participating physicians, but are available from the corresponding author on reasonable request.

## Authors' contributions
Concept and design: DD, CL, POS, JS. Acquisition, analysis, or interpretation of data: All authors. Drafting of the manuscript: All authors. Critical revision of the manuscript for important intellectual content: All authors. Statistical analysis: QL. Study supervision: DD, POS, JS. All authors read and approved the final manuscript.

## Ethics approval and consent to participate
Patients consented to the anonymous use of their urine sample, and clinical information derived from it, in the course of prospective clinical studies of Cxbladder. Ethics approval has been obtained from Human Research Ethics Committee (HREC) of Melbourne Health issued 27th June 2016 (HREC/14/MH/230) for Royal Melbourne Hospital and Royal Brisbane Women's Hospital and also approved by Bellberry HREC under application number 2013-12-684 on 23rd April 2014 for Australian Urology Associates. Separately, approval was obtained from Austin Health HREC (HREC/17/Austin/30) in June 2013 for Northern Hospital.

## Competing interests
All authors are, or were at the time the study was conducted, employees or contractors of Pacific Edge Ltd. Darling, Luxmanan, O'Sullivan and Suttie, also hold shares and/or share options in Pacific Edge Ltd., a public company whose shares trade on the New Zealand Stock Exchange. O'Sullivan and Darling are listed as applicants in a Patent Cooperation Treaty application, and a corresponding US patent application, covering this technology and Suttie has advised on the filing of this application.

## Author details
[1]Pacific Edge Limited, 87 St David Street, Dunedin 9016, New Zealand. [2]University of Otago, Dunedin, New Zealand. [3]Merck, Sharpe & Dohme, Auckland, New Zealand.

## References

1. Schmitz-Dräger BJ, Droller M, Lokeshwar VB, et al. Molecular markers for bladder cancer screening, early diagnosis and surveillance: the WHO/ICUD consensus. Urol Int. 2015;94:1–24.
2. Halpern JA, Chughtai B, Ghomwari H. Cost-effectiveness of common diagnostic approaches for evaluation of asymptomatic microscopic hematuria. JAMA Intern Med. 2017;177:800–7.
3. Davis R, Jones JS, Barocas DA, et al. Diagnosis, evaluation and follow-up of asymptomatic microhematuria (AMH) in adults: AUA guideline. J Urol. 2012; 188(Suppl 6):2473–81.
4. Chang SS, Boorjian SA, Chou R, et al. Diagnosis and treatment of non-muscle invasive bladder cancer: AUA/SUO guideline. J Urol. 2016; 196:1021–9.
5. Burke DM, Shackley DC, O'Reilly PH. The community- based morbidity of flexible cystoscopy. BJU Int. 2002;89:347–9.
6. Stav K, Leibovici D, Goren E, et al. Adverse effects of cystoscopy and its impact on patients' quality of life and sexual performance. Isr Med Assoc J. 2004;6:474–8.
7. Bhatt S, Rajpal N, Rathi V, Avasthi R. Contrast induced nephropathy with intravenous iodinated contrast media in routine diagnostic imaging: an initial experience in a tertiary care hospital. Radiol Res Pract. 2016;2016: 8792984.
8. Herr HW. The risk of urinary tract infection after flexible cystoscopy in bladder tumor patients who did not receive prophylactic antibiotics. J Urol. 2015;193:548–51.
9. Jinzaki M, Kikuchi E, Akita H, Sugiura H, Shinmoto H, Oya M. Role of computed tomography urography in the clinical evaluation of upper tract urothelial carcinoma. Int J Urol. 2016;23:284–98.
10. Schmitz-Dräger BJ, Kuckuck EC, Zuiverloon TCM, et al. Microhematuria assessment an IBCN consensus – based upon a critical review of current guidelines. Urol Oncol. 2016;34:437–51.

11. Blackwell RH, Kirshenbaum EJ, Zapf MAC, et al. Incidence of adverse contrast reaction following nonintravenous urinary tract imaging. Eur Urol Focus. 2017;3:89–93.

12. Darling D, Luxmanan C, O'Sullivan P, Lough T, Suttie J. Clinical utility of Cxbladder for the diagnosis of urothelial carcinoma. Adv Ther. 2017;3: 1087–96.

13. Chamie K, Saigal CS, Lai J, et al. Compliance with guidelines for patients with bladder cancer: variation in the delivery of care. Cancer. 2011;117: 5392–401.

14. David SA, Patil D, Alemozaffar M, Issa MM, Master VA, Filson CP. Urologist use of cystoscopy for patients presenting with hematuria in the United States. Urology. 2017;100:20–6.

15. Friedlander DF, Resnick MJ, You C, et al. Variation in the intensity of hematuria evaluation: a target for primary care quality improvement. Am J Med. 2014;127:633–40.

16. McCombie SP, Bangash H, Kuan M, Thyer I, Lee F, Hayne D. Delays in the diagnosis and initial treatment of bladder cancer in Western Australia. BJU Int. 2017;120(Suppl 3):28-34.

17. Hollenbeck BK, Dunn RL, Ye Z, et al. Delays in diagnosis and bladder cancer mortality. Cancer. 2010;116:5235–42.

18. Lyratzopoulos G, Abel GA, McPhail S, Neal RD, Rubin GP. Gender inequalities in the promptness of diagnosis of bladder and renal cancer after symptomatic presentation: evidence from secondary analysis of an English primary care audit survey. BMJ Open. 2013;3:e002861.

19. Cohn JA, Vekhter B, Lyttle C, Steinberg GD, Large MC. Sex disparities in diagnosis of bladder cancer after initial presentation with hematuria: a nationwide claims-based investigation. Cancer. 2014;120:555–61.

20. Garg T, Pinheiro LC, Atoria CL, Donat SM, Weissman JS, Herr HW, Elkin EB. Gender disparities in hematuria evaluation and bladder cancer diagnosis: a population-based analysis. J Urol. 2014;192:1072–7.

21. Bassett JC, Alvarez J, Koyama T, Resnick M, You C, Ni S, Penson DF, Barocas DA. Gender, race, and variation in the evaluation of microscopic hematuria among Medicare beneficiaries. J Gen Intern Med. 2015;30:440–7.

22. Ngo B, Papa N, Perera M, Bolton D, Sengupta S. Predictors of delay to cystoscopy and adequacy of investigations in patients with haematuria. BJU Int. 2017;119(Suppl 5):19–25.

23. Ark JT, Alvarez JR, Koyama T, Bassett JC, Blot WJ, Mumma MT, Resnick MJ, You C, Penson DF, Barocas DA. Variation in the diagnostic evaluation among persons with hematuria: influence of gender, race, and risk factors for bladder cancer. J Urol. 2017;198:1033-8.

24. Fajkovic H, Halpern JA, Cha EK, et al. Impact of gender on bladder cancer incidence, staging, and prognosis. World J Urol. 2011;29:457–63.

25. Nielsen M, Qaseem A. Hematuria as a marker of occult urinary tract cancer: advice for high-value care from the American College of Physicians. Ann Intern Med. 2016;164:488–97.

26. Kavalieris L, O'Sullivan PJ, Suttie JM, et al. A segregation index combining phenotypic (clinical characteristics) and genotypic (gene expression) biomarkers from a urine sample to triage out patients presenting with hematuria who have a low probability of urothelial carcinoma. BMC Urol. 2015;15:1–12.

27. O'Sullivan P, Sharples K, Dalphin M, Davidson P, Gilling P, Cambridge L, Harvey J, Toro T, Giles N, Luxmanan C, Alves CF, Yoon HS, Hinder V, Masters J, Kennedy-Smith A, Beaven T, Guilford PJ. A multigene urine test for the detection and stratification of bladder cancer in patients presenting with hematuria. J Urol. 2012;188:741–7.

28. Centers for Medicare & Medicaid Services. Technology assessment: Quality, regulation and clinical utility of laboratory-developed molecular tests. https://www.cms.gov/Medicare/Coverage/DeterminationProcess/ Downloads/id72TA.pdf. Accessed 5 May 2017.

29. Jung HS, Park DK, Kim MJ, et al. A comparison of patient acceptance and preferences between CT colonography and conventional colonoscopy in colorectal cancer screening. Korean J Intern Med. 2009;24:43–7.

30. Subak LL, Grady D. Asymptomatic microscopic hematuria – rethinking the diagnostic algorithm. JAMA Intern Med. 2017;177:808–9.

31. Raman JD, Kavalieris L, O'Sullivan P, et al. Prospective evaluation of a clinical tool for segregation of hematuria patients at risk for high-grade urothelial carcinoma. J Urol. 2017;197:e116.

# 29

# Intrathecal administration of TRPA1 antagonists attenuate cyclophosphamide-induced cystitis in rats with hyper-reflexia micturition

Zhipeng Chen[1], Shuqi Du[1,2*], Chuize Kong[2], Zhe Zhang[2] and Al-dhabi Mokhtar[1]

## Abstract

**Background:** The activation of TRPA1 channel is implicated in hyper-reflexic micturition similar to overactive bladder. In this study, we aimed to investigate the effects of blocking TRPA1 via intrathecal administration of antagonists on the afferent pathways of micturition in rats with cystitis.

**Methods:** The cystitis was induced by intraperitoneal cyclophosphamide administration. Cystometry was performed in control and cystitis rats, following the intrathecal injection of the TRPA1 antagonists HC-030031 and A-967079. Real-time PCR, agarose gel electrophoresis, western blotting and immunohistochemistry were used to investigate the levels of TRPA1 mRNA or protein in the bladder mucosa and L6-S1 dorsal root ganglia (DRG).

**Results:** Edema, submucosal hemorrhaging, stiffness and adhesion were noted during removal of the inflamed bladder. The expression of TRPA1 mRNA and protein was higher in the cystitis group in both the mucosa and DRG, but the difference was significant in the DRG ($P < 0.05$). Intrathecal administration of HC-030031 and A-967079 decreased the micturition reflex in the cystitis group. A 50 μg dose of HC-030031 increased the intercontraction interval (ICI) to 183 % of the no-treatment value ($P < 0.05$) and decreased the non-voiding contraction (N-VC) to 60 % of control ($P < 0.01$). Similarly, the treatment with 3 μg A-967079 increased the ICI to 142 % of the control value ($P < 0.05$) and decreased the N-VC to 77 % of control ($P < 0.05$). The effects of both antagonists weakened approximately 2 h after injection.

**Conclusions:** The TRPA1 had a pronounced upregulation in DRG but more slight in mucosa in rat cystitis. The blockade of neuronal activation of TRPA1 by intrathecal administration of antagonists could decrease afferent nerve activities and attenuated detrusor overactivity induced by inflammation.

**Keywords:** TRPA1, Antagonist, Urinary bladder, Cystitis, Rats

## Background

The transient receptor potential (TRP) channel A1 is a non-selective ion channel that can cause an influx of cations into the cell when activated. It is localized predominantly in small-diameter primary sensory neurons of the dorsal root ganglion and trigeminal ganglion [1–3].

The TRPA1 receptor has been shown to play crucial roles in sensory conducting mechanisms in the neural, respiratory, digestive and other systems as a possible mechanosensitive receptor, nociceptor or cold receptor [4–6]. Based on previous studies, TRPA1 has been described as an essential gatekeeper, transducer and amplifier of inflammation and pain [7, 8].

The main syndrome of acute cystitis is urinary frequency, urgency and dysuria in addition to the impairment of patient quality of life. Chemical cystitis is the key adverse effect observed with cyclophosphamide (CY) chemotherapy, and it results from the formation of acrolein, which is a known agonist of TRPA1 [9, 10]. The

\* Correspondence: dushuqi2015@sina.com
[1]China Medical University, No. 77 Puhe Road, Shenyang North New Area 110122, Shenyang, Liaoning Province, People's Republic of China
[2]Department of Urology, The First Affiliated Hospital of China Medical University, No. 155 Nanjing North Street, Heping District 110001, Shenyang, Liaoning Province, People's Republic of China

TRPA1 channel has been suggested to mediate mechanical and nociceptive sensitivity in both physiological and pathological states of the lower urinary tract [11]. In previous studies, we found that intravesical injection of TRPA1 agonists induced hyper-reflexic micturition similar to overactive bladder [12]. Alterations of the TRPA1 channel are known to contribute to mechanical hypersensitivity in primary sensory nerve endings [13]. It is still debated whether the TRPA1 located in neurons become sensitized to nociceptive or mechanical responses in response to visceral inflammation. We hypothesize that the TRPA1 in primary sensory neurons functions as a mechanical or nociceptive receptor and its activation may enhance afferent nerve activities induced by overactive bladder. Therefore the blockade of the TRPA1 channel may be a potential therapeutic target for bladder overactivity.

Thus the present research was conducted to establish the animal model of acute cystitis to assess alterations in the expression and function of TRPA1. We injected intrathecally the highly specific TRPA1 antagonists HC-030031 and A-967079 to evaluate the involvement of TRPA1 in pathological micturition reflex. Two issues were addressed: First, most antagonists have been administered via intravenous or intragastric routes, while the use of intrathecal administration has been rarely reported. The local intrathecal administration could reduce severe gastrointestinal and cardiovascular adverse effects, thus facilitating the identification of potential therapeutic strategies; second, if TRPA1 is involved in the pathological micturition reflex, novel therapeutic drugs could be developed to target this protein.

## Methods
### Animals and ethics statement
Female Sprague–Dawley rats (weight 210 to 245 g) were used. The production, feeding and nursing of the rats were performed by Experimental Animal Center of China Medical University (Certification No.2013002R) and the study was specifically approved by the Animal Ethics Committee of China Medical University. All surgeries were performed under anesthesia, and all efforts were made to minimize suffering. The animals were killed under anesthesia (60 mg/kg sodium pentobarbital) following the recommendations of the US National Institutes of Health.

These rats were housed in standard polypropylene cages, with four animals per cage, at a temperature-controlled, humidity-controlled room and 12–12 light/dark cycle. Cystitis was induced via an intraperitoneal injection of 300 mg/kg CY (Hengrui, China). Sham-treated rats received normal saline (Huaren, China). The expression and function studies were performed 48 h after the injection of CY. For cystometry, the rats were anesthetized via a subcutaneous injection of 1.2 g/kg urethane (Sigma, USA).

### Histopathology
The excised bladder was fixed immediately in 4 % buffered formaldehyde for approximately 24 h, dehydrated in a series of alcohol concentrations, cleared in xylene, embedded in paraffin blocks (Thermo excelsior ES, USA), serially sectioned to a thickness of 5 μm and placed on coated slides. Subsequently, the tissue sections were stained with hematoxylin and eosin (H&E) dehydrated in a graded ethanol series, cleared in xylene, and coverslipped using mounting medium. The slides were examined by light microscopy (Olympus IX71, Japan).

### Quantitative Reverse Transcriptase-Polymerase Chain Reaction and AGE (Agarose Gel Electrophoresis)
The L6-S1 DRG and urinary bladder were harvested ($n = 6$). Under a stereoscopic microscope, the bladder mucosa was separated from the muscular layer. Total RNA was extracted using an RNeasy mini kit and RNase-free DNase kit (Qiagen, Germany). The detail steps were described as before [12]. The 2 % agarose gel (Invitrogen, USA) was resolved in $1 \times$ TBE buffer (Tris, Boric acid, EDTA, pH 7.5). The PCR products supplemented with loading buffer were electrophoresed in a horizontal apparatus (Bio-Rad, USA) at 150 V for 30 min. The bands were imaged using InGenius Imager (Syngene, USA) under UV light.

### Detection of TRPA1 expression by western blotting analysis and localization by immunohistochemistry
The DRG and bladder mucosa were dissolved in RIPA Lysis Buffer (Beyotime, Shanghai, China) containing protease inhibitor ($n = 4$). The protein homogenate was centrifuged at 4 °C and 12,000 rpm for 30 min. The Bio-Rad DC protein assay (model 680; Bio-Rad) was used to detect the concentration via a BSA standard. Equal proteins were separated by 8 % SDS-PAGE and then transferred onto a PVDF membrane. Primary antibodies were incubated on the membranes for TRPA1 (Abcam, ab68848) (1:400) and GAPDH (Santa Cruz) (1:1,000) overnight at 4 °C in TBST and secondary antibodies were incubated at 37 °C for 2 h. The proteins were detected in an ECL detection system (UVP Inc., Cambridge, UK) through enhanced chemiluminescence detection reagents. We used EC3 Imaging System (UVP Inc.) to catch up the specific bands, and relative intensities of all bands were quantified using Image J software. The ratio between the optical density of the TRPA1 and GAPDH protein was calculated as relative content and expressed graphically.

The slides were treated with 3 % hydrogen peroxide to block endogenous peroxidase and with Protein Block Serum-Free to block nonspecific protein binding. The

TRPA1 antibody (Abcam, ab68848) was used as a primary antibody at a dilution of 1:300 for 16 h at 4 °C. After washing, the slides were incubated with the horseradish peroxidase (HRP) conjugated secondary antibody (Maixin, Fuzhou, China) for 30 min at room temperature. Then, DAB was applied for color development. With the use of the Image-Pro plus freeware, the intensity of staining was quantitatively determined in selected areas on digital image of each slice by normalizing with background value.

## Cystometry

Prior to the study, all of the rats had free access to food and water. The rats were fixed to the plate in the prone position. We separated the muscle around the fourth lumbar (L4) spinous process, removed the spinous process and adjacent vertebra, exposed the clearance between L3 and L4 and punctured the yellow ligament gently with a microneedle. Next, a PE-10 catheter's tip was handled by fire in order to avoid neuronal damage; we inserted the catheter parallel to the longitudinal axis through the crevasse and fixed it on the neck of the animal. The rats were carefully turned to the supine position, and another PE-50 catheter was inserted into the bladder through the dome. This catheter was connected through a three-way stopcock to a microinjection pump (Beyond, China) and pressure transducer (RM6240, Chengyi, China) as previously described [12]. We examined the effects of the TRPA1 antagonists via an intrathecal injection of 50 μg HC-030031 and 3 μg A-967079 in normal and cystitis rats [14]. The intravesical pressure was amplified (RM6240, Chengyi) and recorded using a computer (ThinkPad, China). Normal saline (37 °C, pH 7.0 to 7.2) was infused continuously into the bladder at 45 μl/min. The following parameters were calculated as the average of five or six stable successive micturition cycles from the normal ($n = 4$) and cystitis groups ($n = 4$): baseline pressure (BT), pressure threshold (PT), compliance, intercontraction interval (ICI), micturition pressure (MP), and non-voiding contraction (N-VC). N-VC were defined as a rhythmic intravesical pressure increase greater than 5 mmHg from baseline pressure without release of saline from the urethra [12].

## Chemicals

The TRPA1 antagonists HC-030031 and A-967079 were obtained from Sigma-Aldrich. Both antagonists were dissolved in 10 % dimethylsulfoxide (DMSO), 5 % Tween 80 and 85 % sterile saline solution. The durgs or vehicle (sterile saline solution) were injected by intrathecal route contained 0.5 % DMSO. The administration of vehicle did not display any effect.

## Statistical analysis

All of the data were presented as the mean ± standard error (SD). The statistical analysis was performed using Student's $t$-test and one-way analysis of variance, with a significance threshold of $P < 0.05$.

## Results

### Histological analysis

The model of cystitis was induced with CY, which has been used worldwide [15]. Histopathology was conducted 48 h after intraperitoneal injection of saline and CY (Fig. 1). Macroscopically, the inflamed bladder had a much thicker wall and weighed more compared with the normal bladder. Edema, congestion, stiffness and adhesion were noted during removal of the inflamed bladder. In CY-treated group, a thin epithelium, intense edema (Fig. 1a), congestion (Fig. 1b), submucosal hemorrhaging (Fig. 1b), abrasion (Fig. 1c) were markedly increased in large areas. Moreover, the infiltration of large numbers of mononuclear inflammatory cells in the edematous mucosa suggested that CY induced cystitis (Fig. 1d). However, in the control group, microscopic examination of the bladder revealed the gross and histopathological features of the mucosa, urothelium, submucosa and detrusor smooth muscle (Fig. 1e-h).

### Quantification of TRPA1 mRNA level

The levels of TRPA1 mRNA were quantified using the housekeeping gene GAPDH as an internal standard(TRPA1/GAPDH). The values for the normal and cystitis groups were $0.027 \pm 0.01$ and $0.051 \pm 0.02$ in the DRG (Fig. 2a) and $0.007 \pm 0.003$ and $0.008 \pm 0.004$ in the mucosa (Fig. 2b), respectively. The expression of TRPA1 mRNA was higher in the cystitis group in both the mucosa and DRG, but the difference was significant in the DRG ($P = 0.014$). Its expression level for DRG/mucosa was 3 ~ 6:1, demonstrating the more abundant expression in the DRG. We also observed that the TRPA1 had much more expression in the cystitis mucosa than the normal via AGE and the fat tissue did not express TRPA1 mRNA, although they expressed GAPDH mRNA (Fig. 2c).

### Quantification of TRPA1 Protein level

Immunohistochemistry and western blotting analysis of TRPA1 expression in DRG and mucosa of cystitis and normal group. Representative images of the TRPA1 expression in DRG (Fig. 3a) and mucosa (Fig. 3b) with normal group. DRG (Fig. 3c) and mucosa (Fig. 3d) of the cystitis were also be showed. The immunohistochemistry analysis showed that TRPA1 in DRG was markedly upregulated in the cystitis group ($0.224 \pm 0.04$ vs $0.151 \pm 0.02$; Fig. 3g; $P = 0.018$) while the TRPA1 protein level in cystitis mucosa did not have any significant alteration ($0.145 \pm 0.02$ vs $0.127 \pm 0.02$; $P = 0.4$). Accordingly, the western blotting analysis also showed the TRPA1 protein

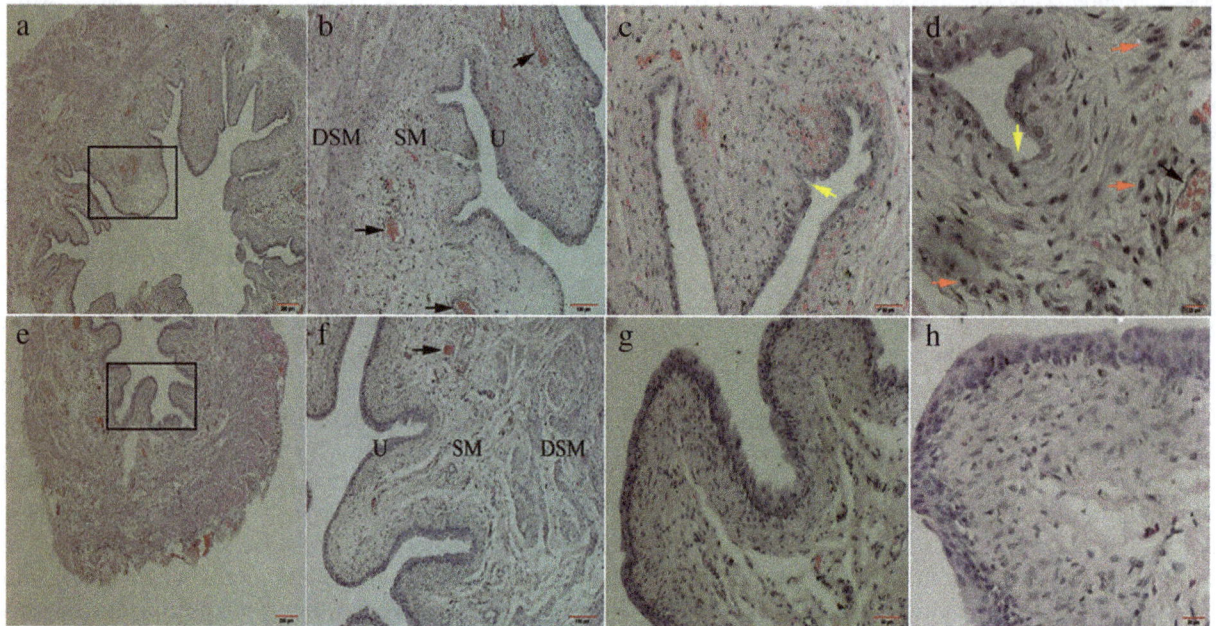

**Fig. 1** Characteristic histological findings in a cross-section of the bladder wall. "**a** to **d**" show the inflamed bladder mucosa consisting of the urothelium (U), submucosa (SM) and detrusor smooth muscle (DSM). Compared with the controls (**e** to **h**), severe submucosal edema (hollow box), hemorrhagia (black arrow), ulceration (yellow arrow), congestion and inflammatory cell infiltrates (red arrow) were observed in CY-treated rats (**a** to **d**). H&E, reduced from 40×, 100×, 200× to 400×

significantly increased in the DRG with cystitis($1.21 \pm 0.12$ vs $0.98 \pm 0.08$; Fig. 3h ,i; $P = 0.018$). Similarly to the data observed in the TRPA1 mRNA levels, there was no significant alteration in the protein expression in mucosa($1.05 \pm 0.07$ vs $0.86 \pm 0.04$; $P = 0.14$).

**Cystometry of rats with cystitis**
In the cystometrograms, the ICI of the cystitis group decreased significantly in comparison with the normal group ($2.55 \pm 0.64$ vs $4.16 \pm 1.02$ min; Fig. 4a; $P < 0.01$). A decrease in bladder compliance with cystitis was observed significantly ($80.83 \pm 21.42$ vs $128.8 \pm 42.07$ μl/mmHg; Fig. 4b; $P = 0.03$). N-VC increased significantly in the cystitis group compared with the normal group ($3.83 \pm 0.75$ vs $0.833 \pm 0.40$; Fig. 4c; $P < 0.01$), while the other parameters such as the baseline pressure, pressure threshold and micturition pressure were not significantly different.

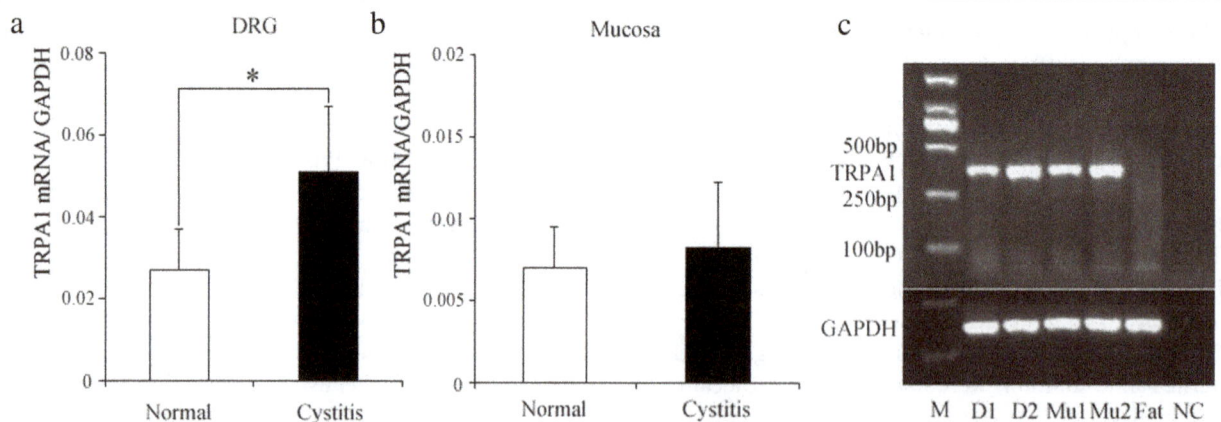

**Fig. 2** The mRNA expression levels of TRPA1 in DRG and bladder mucosa were determined. The TRPA1 mRNA level in DRG (**a**) and mucosa (**b**) during cystitis (filled column, $n = 6$) was 1.89 times and 1.19 times greater than that in the control group (open column, $n = 6$), respectively. The PCR products of the DRG and mucosa (Mu) showed bands of TRPA1 at 358 bp in electrophoresis (**c**). M: marker; Mu1: normal bladder mucosa; Mu2: inflammatory bladder mucosa; D1: normal dorsal root ganglion; D2: inflammatory dorsal root ganglion; NC: no reverse-transcriptase negative control

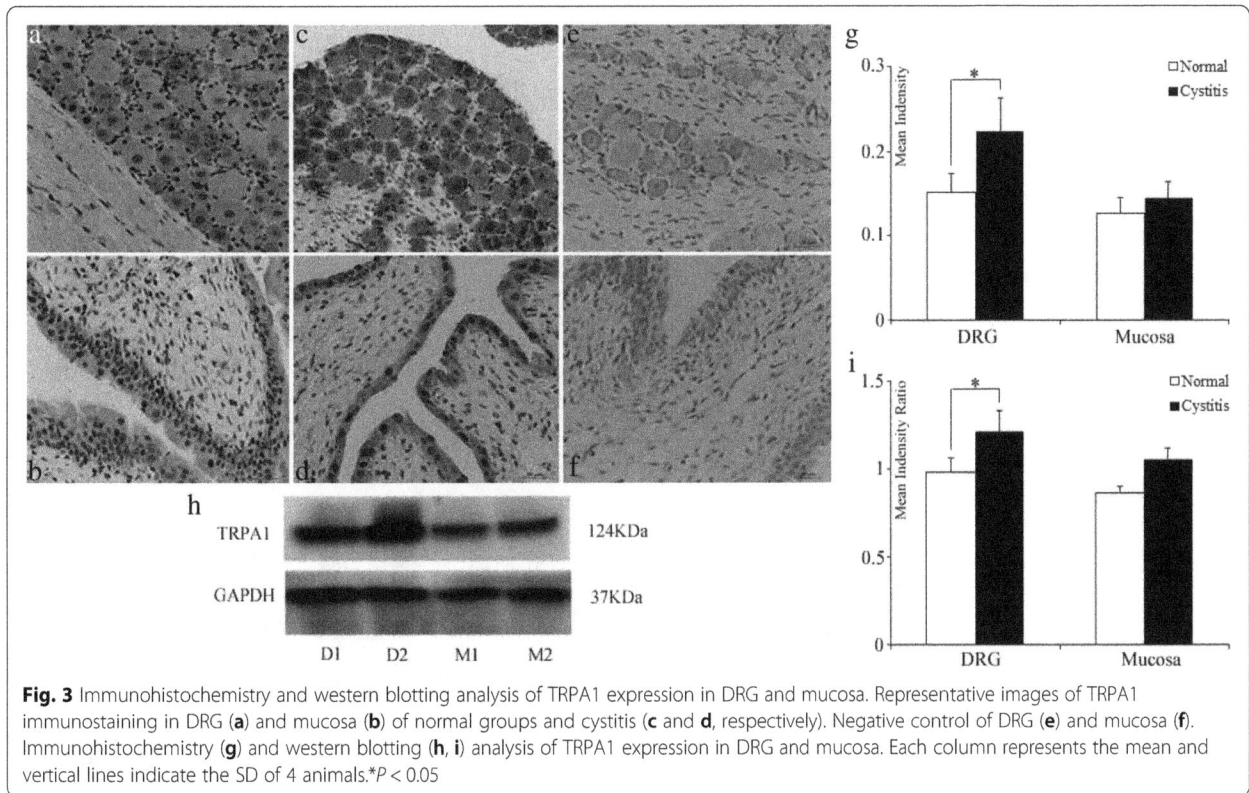

**Fig. 3** Immunohistochemistry and western blotting analysis of TRPA1 expression in DRG and mucosa. Representative images of TRPA1 immunostaining in DRG (**a**) and mucosa (**b**) of normal groups and cystitis (**c** and **d**, respectively). Negative control of DRG (**e**) and mucosa (**f**). Immunohistochemistry (**g**) and western blotting (**h**, **i**) analysis of TRPA1 expression in DRG and mucosa. Each column represents the mean and vertical lines indicate the SD of 4 animals.*$P < 0.05$

## Cystometry of the administered antagonists

Figures 5 and 6 showed the changes of cystometry parameters in cystitis and control group by intrathecal administration of 50 μg HC-030031 and 3 μg A-967079, respectively. In the cystitis group (Fig. 5a ,c), a dose of 50 μg HC-030031 increased the ICI to 183 % of the control value ($P = 0.02$). The reduced effectiveness of the drug resulted in a recovery of the ICI to 140 % of its control value after 2 h ($P = 0.09$). The N-VC decreased to 60 % of the control value ($P < 0.01$) after HC-030031 infusion and then increased to 62 % approximately 2 h later ($P < 0.01$). The baseline pressure, pressure threshold,

micturition pressure and compliance displayed no significant difference before and after intrathecal injection of the drug. The effects of HC-030031 were apparent approximately 30 min after the intrathecal injection, but the recovery was observed after 2 h.

The intrathecal injection of 3 μg A-967079 in the cystitis (Fig. 6a, c) increased the ICI to 142 % of the control value ($P = 0.02$). After approximately 2 h, the ICI recovered to 126 % of the control value due to the decreased drug strength ($P = 0.38$). N-VC decreased to 77 % of the control ($P < 0.01$) after the infusion of A-967079 and increased to 66 % approximately 2 h later. However, a dose

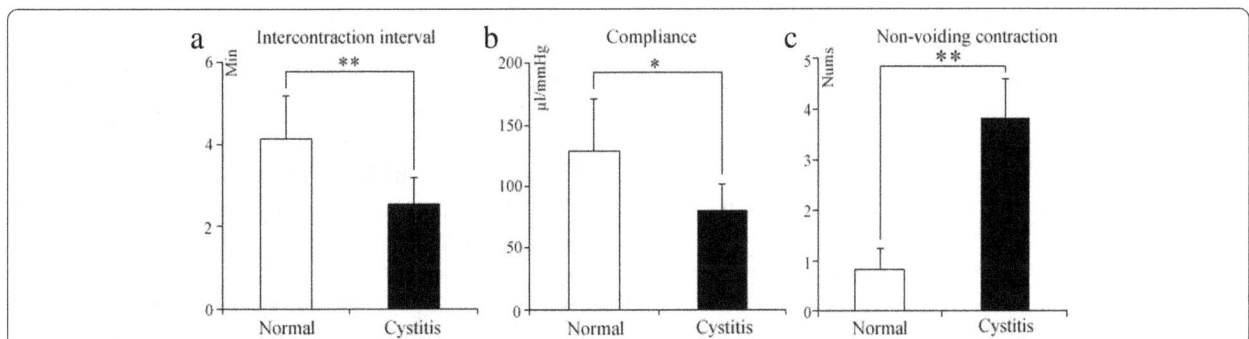

**Fig. 4** Comparison of experimental results between the cystitis and normal group. The cystitis and normal groups were injected with CY and saline, respectively, and cystometry was performed after 48 h. The values of intercontraction interval (**a**), compliance (**b**) and non-voidingcontraction (**c**) were obtained from the cystitis group and the normal group, respectively; Each column represents the mean and vertical lines indicate the SD of 6 animals. *$P < 0.05$, ** $P < 0.01$

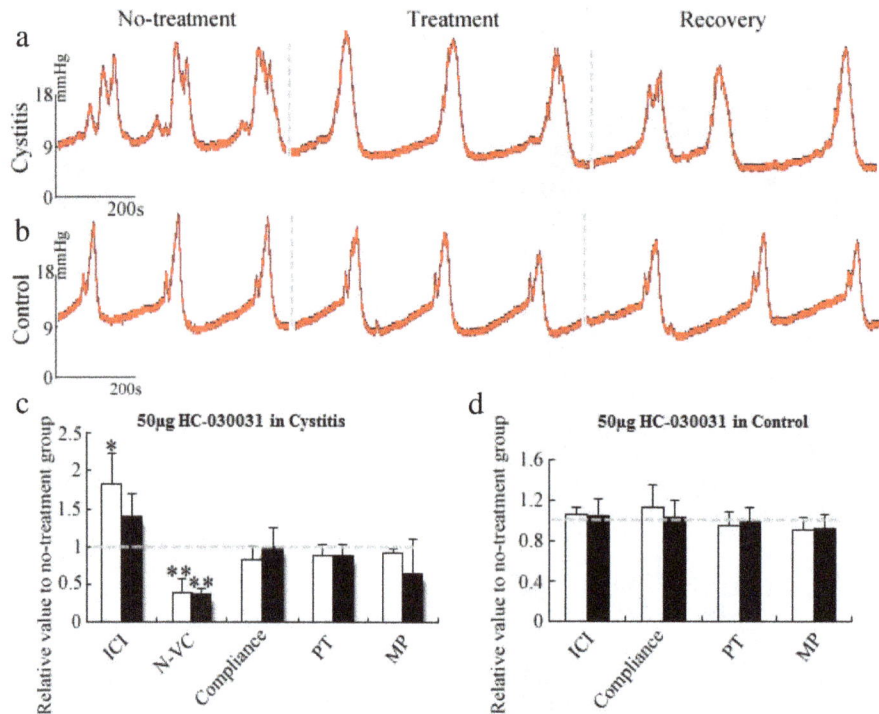

**Fig. 5** Effects of intrathecal injection of TRPA1 antagonist HC-030031. Representative cystometrograms of intrathecal injection in cystitis (**a**) and control (**b**), respectively. Recovery represents 2 h after intrathecal injection of 50 μg HC-030031. The relative value of 50 μg HC-030031(open column) and the recovery (filled column) compared with no-treatment in cystitis (**c**) and control (**d**) on cystometry parameters, respectively. Each column represents the mean and vertical lines indicate the SD of 4 animals. ICI: intercontraction interval, N-VC: non-voiding contraction, PT: pressure threshold, MP: micturition pressure. *$P < 0.05$, ** $P < 0.01$

of 50 μg HC-030031 (Fig. 5b, d) and 3 μg A-967079 (Fig. 6b, d) had no obvious effects on the cystometry parameters in the normal group. The effects of antagonists on micturition were presented in Tables 1 and 2.

## Discussion

The present study demonstrates the TRPA1 was expressed in both bladder and DRG (L6-S1) and had a pronounced upregulation in DRG but more slight in mucosa in rat cystitis. The blockade of TRPA1 via intrathecal administration decreased afferent nerve activities and consequently attenuated detrusor overactivity markly. More recently, Tomonori et al. have shown that TRPA1 channel could improve afferent nerve activities of the rat bladder through both Aδ- and C-fibers pathway [16]. TRPA1 channels have been conducted in multiple-sensation modalities at present including mechanical, nociceptive, and thermal sensation in mammal [17–19].

However, the function of TRPA1 as nociceptor in the DRG innervating bladder is really quite controversial and further research is needed. We suppose the activation of TRPA1 receptors in DRG may lead to hyperalgesia, playing a role in enhanced impulse conduction and detrusor overactivity. We observed hematuria, severe submucosal edema, hemorrhage, ulceration, congestion

and inflammatory cell infiltration following the intraperitoneal injection of CY for 48 h. The symptoms of overactive bladder, a shortened ICI and an increase in unstable contractions, were observed concomitantly. In the present study, the levels of TRPA1 mRNA and protein in DRG were significantly higher in cystitis group than the control group while the TRPA1 in mucosa were slightly higher than the control group without statistical significance, indicating that the TRPA1 in DRG may play a greater role than in mucosa. Similarly, Andrade also found a higher expression of TRPA1 mRNA in DRG neurons in the study investigating bladder overactivity induced by spinal cord injury [20]. It also be demonstrated that the TRPA1 expression level was significantly higher than bladder mucosa [12]. The possible reason may refer to the TRPA1 in mucosa might not function as nociceptive receptor in the case of cyclophosphamide-induced inflammation. The profound results showed that the modulation of intracellular $Ca^{2+}$ could contribute directly to the elevated gene expression of TRPA1 via an influx through voltage-gated channels and/or endoplasmic reticulum [21, 22]. It has also been found that TRPA1 mediates inflammation, hyperalgesia and visceral hypersensitivity in pancreatitis pain as well as in a model of acute gout [23, 24]. The mechanism could be construed as the

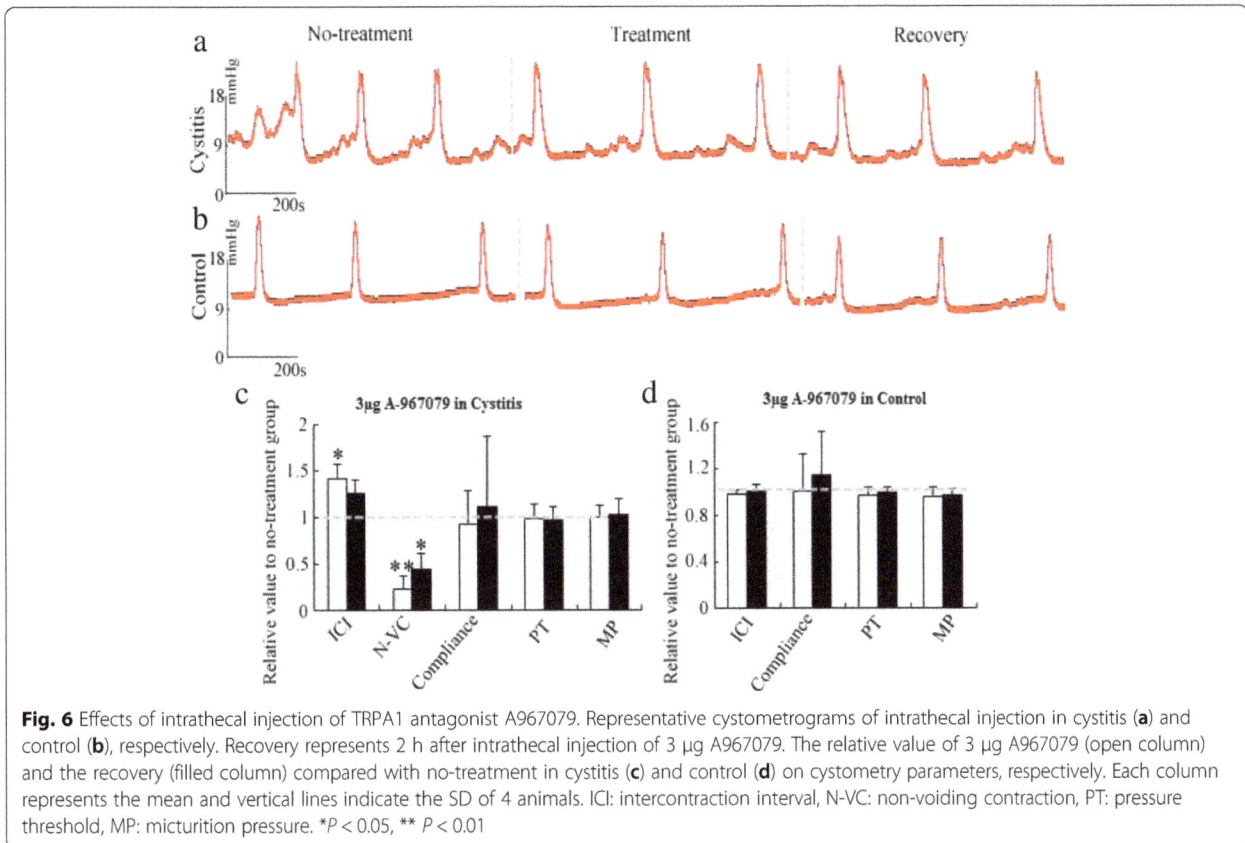

**Fig. 6** Effects of intrathecal injection of TRPA1 antagonist A967079. Representative cystometrograms of intrathecal injection in cystitis (**a**) and control (**b**), respectively. Recovery represents 2 h after intrathecal injection of 3 μg A967079. The relative value of 3 μg A967079 (open column) and the recovery (filled column) compared with no-treatment in cystitis (**c**) and control (**d**) on cystometry parameters, respectively. Each column represents the mean and vertical lines indicate the SD of 4 animals. ICI: intercontraction interval, N-VC: non-voiding contraction, PT: pressure threshold, MP: micturition pressure. *$P < 0.05$, ** $P < 0.01$

TRPA1 in DRG played a crucial role in sensitization of sensory afferent nerves in occurrence of pathological conditions.

Symptoms of overactive bladder such as a shortened ICI and an increase in N-VC were observed in cystitis. We conceive that blocking the TRPA1 in DRG might attenuate the excitability of afferent pathways and thus alleviate detrusor overactivity. Following intrathecal injection of the highly specific TRPA1 antagonists HC-030031 and A-967079,the ICI was extended, and the N-VC was suppressed in cystitis, thereby inhibiting micturition reflex hyperactivity. However, there were no significant changes in BP, PT, MP and compliance in CY-

induced rats before and after the application of each TRPA1 antagonists although the ICI was significantly increased and the number of N-VC was significantly decreased. The probable reason is that the cystometry was performed under anesthetized conditions. Interestingly, neither HC-030031 nor A-967079 had a substantial effect on normal urination, suggesting that TRPA1 might not participate in the physiological micturition reflex. More TRPA1 channels might need to be open under pathological conditions, leading to hyperalgesia in the absence of a physiological pain signal. A study by Perin-Martins A demonstrated the mechanisms that contribute to edema and hyperalgesia induced by TRPA1

**Table 1** The effect of TRPA1 antagonist 50 μg HC-030031 on cystometry parameters of inflammatory rats

|  |  | BP (mmHg) | PT (mmHg) | MP (mmHg) | ICI (min) | Compliance (μl/mmHg) | N-VC (number) |
|---|---|---|---|---|---|---|---|
|  | No-treatment | 13.11 ± 6.14 | 15.86 ± 6.25 | 24.33 ± 8.78 | 3.92 ± 1.41 | 139.10 ± 49.47 | 0.25 ± 0.5 |
| Control | Treatment | 11.24 ± 3.11 | 14.25 ± 3.44 | 21.54 ± 5.34 | 4.08 ± 1.32 | 159.15 ± 76.02 | 0 |
|  | Recovery | 11.17 ± 3.08 | 14.86 ± 3.48 | 21.53 ± 5.14 | 3.90 ± 0.74 | 146.46 ± 65.47 | 0 |
|  | No-treatment | 10.10 ± 5.74 | 11.83 ± 6.16 | 19.11 ± 8.01 | 2.28 ± 0.51 | 124.78 ± 49.52 | 3.25 ± 0.5 |
| Cystitis | Treatment | 7.70 ± 3.29 | 9.83 ± 3.05 | 17.29 ± 6.87 | 4.14 ± 1.05* | 98.12 ± 25.15 | 1.25 ± 0.50** |
|  | Recovery | 7.39 ± 3.75 | 10.05 ± 4.25 | 15.72 ± 7.00 | 3.10 ± 0.31 | 136.80 ± 42.92 | 1.25 ± 0.50** |

Results were expressed as mean ± standard error. The "*" or "**" represented the difference was significant between the treatment or recovery and no-treatment in cystometry parameters. *$P < 0.05$, ** $P < 0.01$

**Table 2** The effect of TRPA1 antagonist 3 μg A-967079 on cystometry parameters of inflammatory rats

|  |  | BP (mmHg) | PT (mmHg) | MP (mmHg) | ICI (min) | Compliance (μl/mmHg) | N-VC (number) |
|---|---|---|---|---|---|---|---|
| Control | No-treatment | 11.83 ± 2.96 | 12.74 ± 3.4 | 21.76 ± 1.63 | 4.80 ± 1.79 | 91.44 ± 18.19 | 0.25 ± 0.5 |
|  | Treatment | 11.66 ± 3.32 | 12.42 ± 3.83 | 20.82 ± 2.84 | 4.76 ± 1.96 | 92.88 ± 43.76 | 0 |
|  | Recovery | 11.71 ± 3.19 | 12.73 ± 3.83 | 21.19 ± 2.22 | 4.68 ± 1.68 | 104.56 ± 40.19 | 0 |
| Cystitis | No-treatment | 10.54 ± 3.23 | 11.94 ± 2.88 | 22.68 ± 4.89 | 3.64 ± 0.78 | 80.07 ± 27.31 | 3.00 ± 0.82 |
|  | Treatment | 10.25 ± 3.99 | 12.00 ± 4.67 | 22.68 ± 5.28 | 5.87 ± 0.93* | 67.40 ± 7.66 | 0.75 ± 0.50** |
|  | Recovery | 9.85 ± 4.37 | 11.46 ± 4.75 | 21.96 ± 5.75 | 4.50 ± 1.59 | 90.86 ± 34.91 | 1.25 ± 0.50* |

Results were expressed as mean ± standard error. The "*" or "**" represented the difference was significant between the treatment or recovery and no-treatment in cystometry parameters. *$P < 0.05$, ** $P < 0.01$

activation [25]. The antagonists prevent and reverse cystitis, suggesting that TRPA1 is pivotal for the maintenance and development of the inflammatory response and hyperalgesia. The effects of both antagonists persist for approximately two hours, which is consistent with previous findings [26]. When the effects of the antagonists disappeared, ICI returned, indicating that continuous activation of the TRPA1 in DRG neurons is crucial to maintain the nociceptor sensitization elicited by inflammatory stimulation. This proposal is further supported by previous findings showing that TRPA1 mediates sustained hyperalgesic responses in different models [14, 27]. Indeed, it has been demonstrated that spinal blockage of the N-type and P/Q-type VGCC (voltage-gated calcium channel) could attenuate inflammatory and nociceptive events associated with cystitis [10]. Consistent to this notion, TRPA1 located on DRG contributes to the transmission of nociceptive information to second-order neurons in the spinal dorsal horn [14, 26].

Studies have showed that HC-030031 and A-967079 were potentially capable of blocking the effect of TRPA1 with a much higher selectivity than other ion channels [28, 29]. Intrathecal administration of antagonists is rarely reported compared with antisense oligonucleotides when blocking the TRPA1 in rats. We use intrathecal injection, which not only can act directly on DRG but can reduce the side effects associated. However, intrathecal administration is a kind of invasive operation which may also accompany related complications such as infection, so its clinical application might be limited. Nevertheless, the intrathecal administration is also a suitable alternative when faced with refractory bladder diseases. Taken together, our results indicate that TRPA1 especially in DRG plays a key role in the occurrence of cystitis, and therefor intrathecal injection of TRPA1 antagonists might be effective in treating detrusor overactivity. It should be noted that this study has examined only the TRPA1 expression and function in the stage of acute inflammation, while a time-dependent change of TRPA1 after cystitis was not involved. Our data also showed the duration of the drug lasted only two hours,

and therefore, further research is needed for possibly clinical applications in future.

## Conclusions
The present findings suggested that TRPA1 might only be involved in pathological rather than physiological micturition reflex. The blockade of neuronal activation of TRPA1 via intrathecal administration could decrease afferent nerve activities and attenuate detrusor overactivity induced by inflammation. Therefore, in multistep sensory pathway, TRPA1 in DRG might be used as a more effective therapeutic target for the treatment of pathological micturition.

### Abbreviations
BP, baseline pressure; CY, cyclophosphamide; DRG, dorsal root ganglia; GAPDH, glyceraldehyde-3-phosphate dehydrogenase; ICI, intercontraction interval; MP, micturition pressure; N-VC, non-voiding contraction; PT, pressure threshold; TRPA1, transient receptor potential channel A1

### Acknowledgements
Not applicable.

### Funding
This research was sponsored by the National Natural Science Foundation of China (No.30801141); the First Affiliated Hospital of China Medical University Foundation for Science and Technology Program (fsfh1305); the Educational Commission of Liaoning Province of China (L2010694) and the Liaoning Provincial Research Foundation for Science and Technology Program (2015020480). The funders had no role in study design, data collection and analysis, decision to publish, or preparation of the manuscript.

### Authors' contributions
SD conceived of the study. SD and ZC designed experiments. ZC and AM performed experiments and prepared manuscript. SD, ZC, CK and ZZ interpreted and analyzed results. SD and ZC prepared figures. SD, ZC, CK, ZZ and AM approved final version of the manuscript. All authors read and approved the final manuscript.

### Competing interests
The authors declare that they have no competing interests.

### References

1. Story GM, Peier AM, Reeve AJ, Eid SR, Mosbacher J, Hricik TR, et al. ANKTM1, a TRP-like channel expressed in nociceptive neurons, is activated by cold temperatures. Cell. 2003;112(6):819–29.
2. Bandell M, Story GM, Hwang SW, Viswanath V, Eid SR, Petrus MJ, et al. Noxious cold ion channel TRPA1 is activated by pungent compounds and bradykinin. Neuron. 2004;41(6):849–57.
3. Jordt SE, Bautista DM, Chuang HH, McKemy DD, Zygmunt PM, Högestätt ED, et al. Mustard oils and cannabinoids excite sensory nerve fibres through the TRP channel ANKTM1. Nature. 2004;427(6971):260–5.
4. Waszkielewicz AM, Gunia A, Szkaradek N, Słoczyńska K, Krupińska S, Marona H. Ion channels as drug targets in central nervous system disorders. Curr Med Chem. 2013;20(10):1241–85.
5. Raemdonck K, de Alba J, Birrell MA, Grace M, Maher SA, Irvin CG, et al. A role for sensory nerves in the late asthmatic response. Thorax. 2012;67(1):19–25.
6. Holzer P. Transient receptor potential (TRP) channels as drug targets for diseases of the digestive system. Pharmacol Ther. 2011;131(1):142–70.
7. Bautista DM, Pellegrino M, Tsunozaki M. TRPA1: a gatekeeper for inflammation. Annu Rev Physiol. 2013;75:181–200.
8. Koivisto A, Chapman H, Jalava N, Korjamo T, Saarnilehto M, Lindstedt K, et al. TRPA1: a transducer and amplifier of pain and inflammation. Basic Clin Pharmacol Toxicol. 2014;114(1):50–5.
9. Nilius B, Appendino G, Owsianik G. The transient receptor potential channel TRPA1: from gene to pathophysiology. Pflugers Arch. 2012;464(5):425–58.
10. Silva RB, Sperotto ND, Andrade EL, Pereira TC, Leite CE, de Souza AH, et al. Spinal blockage of P/Q- or N-type voltage-gated calcium channels modulates functional and symptomatic changes related to haemorrhagic cystitis in mice. Br J Pharmacol. 2015;172(3):924–39.
11. Merrill L, Girard BM, May V, Vizzard MA. Transcriptional and translational plasticity in rodent urinary bladder TRP channels with urinary bladder inflammation, bladder dysfunction, or postnatal maturation. J Mol Neurosci. 2012;48(3):744–56.
12. Du S, Araki I, Yoshiyama M, Nomura T, Takeda M. Transient receptor potential channel A1 involved in sensory transduction of rat urinary bladder through C-fiber pathway. Urology. 2007;70(4):826–31.
13. Nassini R, Materazzi S, Benemei S, Geppetti P. The TRPA1 channel in inflammatory and neuropathic pain and migraine. Rev Physiol Biochem Pharmacol. 2014;167:1–43.
14. Wei H, Koivisto A, Saarnilehto M, Chapman H, Kuokkanen K, Hao B, et al. Spinal transient receptor potential ankyrin 1 channel contributes to central pain hypersensitivity in various pathophysiological conditions in the rat. Pain. 2011;152(3):582–91.
15. Geppetti P, Nassini R, Materazzi S, Benemei S. The concept of neurogenic inflammation. BJU Int. 2008;101 suppl 3:2–6.
16. Minagawa T, Aizawa N, Igawa Y, Wyndaele JJ. The Role of Transient Receptor Potential Ankyrin 1 (TRPA1) Channel in Activation of Single Unit Mechanosensi-tive Bladder Afferent Activities in the Rat. Neurourol Urodyn. 2014;33(5):544–9.
17. Asgar J, Zhang Y, Saloman JL, Wang S, Chung MK, Ro JY. The role of TRPA1 in muscle pain and mechanical hypersensitivity under inflammatory conditions in rats. Neuroscience. 2015;310:206–15.
18. Hatakeyama Y, Takahashi K, Tominaga M, Kimura H, Ohta T. Polysulfide evokes acute pain through the activation of nociceptive TRPA1 in mouse sensory neurons. Mol Pain. 2015;11:24. doi:10.1186/s12990-015-0023-4.
19. Kang K. Exceptionally high thermal sensitivity of rattlesnake TRPA1 correlates with peak current amplitude. Biochim Biophys Acta. 2016;1858(2):318–25.
20. Andrade EL, Forner S, Bento AF, Leite DF, Dias MA, Leal PC, et al. TRPA1 receptor modulation attenuates bladder overactivity induced by spinal cord injury. Am J Physiol Renal Physiol. 2011;300(5):1223–34.
21. DeBerry JJ, Schwartz ES, Davis BM. TRPA1 mediates bladder hyperalgesia in a mouse model of cystitis. Pain. 2014;155(7):1280–7.
22. Fields RD, Eshete F, Dudek S, Ozsarac N, Stevens B. Regulation of gene expression by action potentials:dependence on complexity in cellular information processing. Novartis Found Sym. 2001;239:160–72.
23. Cattaruzza F, Johnson C, Leggit A, Grady E, Schenk AK, Cevikbas F, et al. Transient receptor potential ankyrin 1 mediates chronic pancreatitis pain in mice. Am J Physiol Gastrointest Liver Physiol. 2013;304(11):G1002–12.
24. Trevisan G, Hoffmeister C, Rossato MF, Oliveira SM, Silva MA, Silva CR, et al. TRPA1 receptor stimulation by hydrogen peroxide is critical to trigger hyperalgesia and inflammation in a model of acute gout. Free Radic Biol Med. 2014;72:200–9. doi:10.1016/j.freeradbiomed.
25. Perin-Martins A, Teixeira JM, Tambeli CH, Parada CA, Fischer L. Mechanisms underlying transient receptor potential ankyrin 1 (TRPA1)-mediated hyperalgesia and edema. J Peripher Nerv Syst. 2013;18(1):62–74.
26. da Costa DS, Meotti FC, Andrade EL, Leal PC, Motta EM, Calixto JB. The involvement of the transient receptor potential A1 (TRPA1) in the maintenance of mechanical and cold hyperalgesia in persistent inflammation. Pain. 2010;148(3):431–7.
27. Bonet IJ, Fischer L, Parada CA, Tambeli CH. The role of transient receptor potential A1 (TRPA1) in the development and maintenance of carrageenan-induced hyperalgesia. Neuropharmacology. 2013;65:206–12.
28. Eid SR, Crown ED, Moore EL, Liang HA, Choong KC, Dima S, et al. HC-03003-1, a TRPA1 selective antagonist, attenuates inflammatory- and neuropathy-induced mechanical hypersensitivity. Mol Pain. 2008;4:48.
29. Chen J, Joshi SK, DiDomenico S, Perner RJ, Mikusa JP, Gauvin DM, et al. Selective blocade of TRPA1 channel attenuates pathological pain without altering noxious cold sensation or body temperature regulation. Pain. 2011;152(5):1165–72.

# 30

# High acceptability of a newly developed urological practical skills training program

Anna H. de Vries[1*], Scheltus J. van Luijk[2], Albert J. J. A. Scherpbier[3], Ad J. M. Hendrikx[1], Evert L. Koldewijn[1,3], Cordula Wagner[4,5] and Barbara M. A. Schout[5,6]

## Abstract

**Background:** Benefits of simulation training are widely recognized, but its structural implementation into urological curricula remains challenging. This study aims to gain insight into current and ideal urological practical skills training and presents the outline of a newly developed skills training program, including an assessment of the design characteristics that may increase its acceptability.

**Methods:** A questionnaire was sent to the urology residents (n = 87) and program directors (n = 45) of all Dutch teaching hospitals. Open- and close-ended questions were used to determine the views on current and ideal skills training and the newly developed skills training program. Eight semi-structured interviews were conducted with 39 residents and 15 program directors. All interviews were audiotaped, fully transcribed, and thereafter analyzed.

**Results:** Response was 87.4 % for residents and 86.7 % for program directors. Residents appeared to be still predominantly trained 'by doing'. Structured practical skills training in local hospitals takes place according to 12 % of the residents versus 44 % of the program directors (*p* < 0.001). Ideally, residents prefer to practice certain procedures on simulation models first, especially in endourology. The majority of residents (92 %) and program directors (87 %) approved of implementing the newly developed skills training program (*p* = 0.51). 'Structured scheduling', 'use of peer teaching' and 'high fidelity models' were indicated as design characteristics that increase its acceptability.

**Conclusions:** Current urological residency training consists of patient-related 'learning by doing', although more practice on simulation models is desired. The acceptability of implementing the presented skills-training program is high. Design characteristics that increase its acceptability are structured scheduling, the use of peer teaching and high fidelity models.

## Background

In present time, training outside the patient is widely accepted and several studies have shown that urological skills can be improved by simulation training [1, 2]. The main advantage of training on simulators is that the patient-related learning curve can be shortened without compromising patient safety. In addition to the classical master-apprentice type of training (see one, do one, teach one), new simulation curricula are required due to the evolution of medical technology, the increasing number of minimally invasive procedures that urologists need to master, the decreasing number of patient-related training hours and patient safety issues [3–7].

Several studies have been conducted on how to develop simulation programs. Ahmed et al. concluded that 'proficiency-based curricula with well-structured endpoints and objective tools for validating proficiency are crucial in developing a simulation program' [8]. Sweet et al. emphasized the value of the backward design principle of Wiggins and McTighe [9]. According to this principle, the purpose and learning outcome must be determined first, after which learning objectives are established by working backwards from the desired outcomes.

Within surgery, several practical skills training curricula have been implemented and validated, such as the American College of Surgeons/Association of Program

* Correspondence: a.h.de.vries@hotmail.com
[1]Department of Urology, Catharina Hospital, Eindhoven, The Netherlands
Full list of author information is available at the end of the article

Directors in Surgery surgical skills curriculum and the Fundamentals of Laparoscopic Surgery [10–12]. For urology, only a limited number of urological practical skills training curricula have been developed [13, 14]. Moreover, their structured implementation remains challenging. Possible obstacles in the implementation of a skills curriculum in surgical residency programs are issues like limited personnel, considerable cost and resident working hour restrictions [15].

In the current Dutch urological curriculum, residents are obliged to attend a number of national practical skills courses. However, reports of the Dutch inspection of health services pointed out that residents' knowledge of local medical technology is not optimal [16]. The outline for the Dutch Urology Practical Skills (D-UPS) training program was designed to provide residents and program directors with a structured training program for urological basic skills, including pretest, procedural steps, simulator training, pitfalls and evaluation. One of the first steps in the development and implementation of a new curriculum is the establishment of acceptability [9]. To enhance this aspect, our implementation strategy included the early involvement of residents and program directors in the development of the program, prior to its validation and implementation.

This study presents the outline of the newly developed D-UPS program and aimed to answer the questions: 'How do residents currently and ideally learn their practical urology skills?' and 'Which design characteristics may increase the acceptability of urological practical skills training programs such as D-UPS?'

## Methods
### Development of the Dutch Urology Practical Skills training program
The D-UPS program was designed using the backward design principle of Wiggins and McTighe [17]. The program combines the acquisition and rehearsal of basic theoretical knowledge, based on theory derived from the national courses and expert input, with practical training of basic urological skills and techniques. The first step in developing each specific training session was a Training Needs Analysis (TNA) [18, 19]. In the TNA, procedural steps were identified, potential pitfalls analysed and learning objectives defined [20]. Subsequently, a suitable simulator was selected (Training Media Specification, TMS), with a preference for low fidelity models to limit the costs and simplify logistics.

The D-UPS program was designed by the national project group 'Training in Urology' in collaboration with the Dutch Association of Urologists. In the final development of the program, the opinions of residents and program directors were considered.

### Study design
In this mixed-method research design, we used a questionnaire to collect quantitative data and semi-structured focus group interviews to collect qualitative data.

### Questionnaire
The questionnaire was developed by a multidisciplinary team, consisting of an educationalist (AS) and two experts in urology (BS, AH). The questionnaire contained nine questions or statements rated on a 5-point Likert scale (1 = disagree, 5 = agree), five open-ended questions, one yes/no question and one multiple-choice question. Three questions focused on demographics, three on the participants' opinions on current practical skills training, and ten on the D-UPS program, e.g. positive endpoints and expected difficulties in future implementation. The full version of the questionnaire is added in Additional file 1, including the definitions of various expected positive endpoints.

Between April 2011 and December 2011, the questionnaire was sent to all 87 Dutch urology residents and 45 program directors in the 25 teaching hospitals, using the online program Survey Monkey (http://www.surveymonkey.com).

### Interviews
For the semi-structured focus group interviews, a topic list was developed by a multidisciplinary team, consisting of an educationalist (AS) and two experts in urology (BS, AH). The topic list consisted of three main themes: 1) current way of learning practical skills, 2) ideal way of learning practical skills, and 3) respondents' opinions on the design characteristics of the D-UPS program in relation to its acceptability (Additional file 2).

All residents and program directors in the Netherlands (n = 132) were invited by email (BS) to participate in an interview. Those residents and program directors that responded positively to this electronic invitation were divided into groups based on their geographic distribution. Between March and December 2011 the interviews were conducted in five different teaching hospitals across the Netherlands. The interviews were moderated by an independent expert in medical education (SvL). Besides the moderator, one researcher was present to make field notes (BS or AH). Before the interview, participants received one page of information on the content of the D-UPS program. Interviews continued until no new themes emerged. Needed number of interviews was based on saturation of information.

### Data analysis
Questionnaire data were graphically displayed using frequency figures. Differences in categorical variables

between groups were analysed using the Chi-square test. A p-value <0.05 was considered statistically significant. Analyses were performed using the Statistical Package for Social Sciences version 20.0.

Interviews were audio-recorded and transcribed verbatim by an independent company. Subsequently, transcripts were imported into a software program for qualitative data analysis (Atlas.ti version 7). The transcripts were thematically coded by the principal researcher (BS) using a predefined coding scheme based on the three main themes described earlier. To enhance interobserver reliability, 25 % of transcripts were independently coded by a second researcher (AdV). Discrepancies in initial coding between the two researchers were discussed until consensus was reached, and a final coding scheme was established. Thereafter, all interviews were summarized using the final coding scheme. The responses were categorized into the three themes. Finally, quotes were selected to illustrate findings.

### Ethical aspects

Ethical approval was sought from the Catharina hospital's research and ethics committee. Since patients or patient data were not involved in this study, they ruled that ethical approval was not required according to the Dutch Medical Research (Human Subjects) Act. All included residents and program directors volunteered to participate and anonymity and confidentiality was guaranteed. Informed consent with assurance of anonymity was obtained at the start of each interview.

## Results

### Design characteristics of the D-UPS program

The D-UPS program features mandatory training sessions of one hour per week in the local hospital setting for junior and senior residents. The program starts with the implementation of eight training sessions of basic urological skills that will be yearly repeated, namely: 'ultrasound of kidney and bladder', 'ultrasound of prostate', 'acute penile pathology', 'basic laparoscopy', 'electro surgery', 'mid urethral sling', 'transurethral resection of the prostate', and 'flexible ureterorenoscopy'. After these training sessions have been validated, the next eight sessions will be implemented, consisting of more advanced urological skills (e.g. pyelumplasty).

In preparation for each training hour residents have to study the obligatory theory, based on theory derived from the national courses and expert input, and take a formative online test that consist of approximately ten multiple choice questions. At the start of the training session, the results of this test are discussed, before all procedural steps, pitfalls and non-technical skills of the relevant procedure are trained in a non-patient-related setting under the supervision of an experienced urologist. As residents progress in their specialist training, peer teaching becomes more important, lifting the training sessions to a higher level for senior residents and preparing them for their future role as educators. Each session ends with an evaluation of satisfactory and unsatisfactory aspects of the training. Figure 1 presents the general outline of the training sessions. As an example of the actual content of the training, a summary of the training session

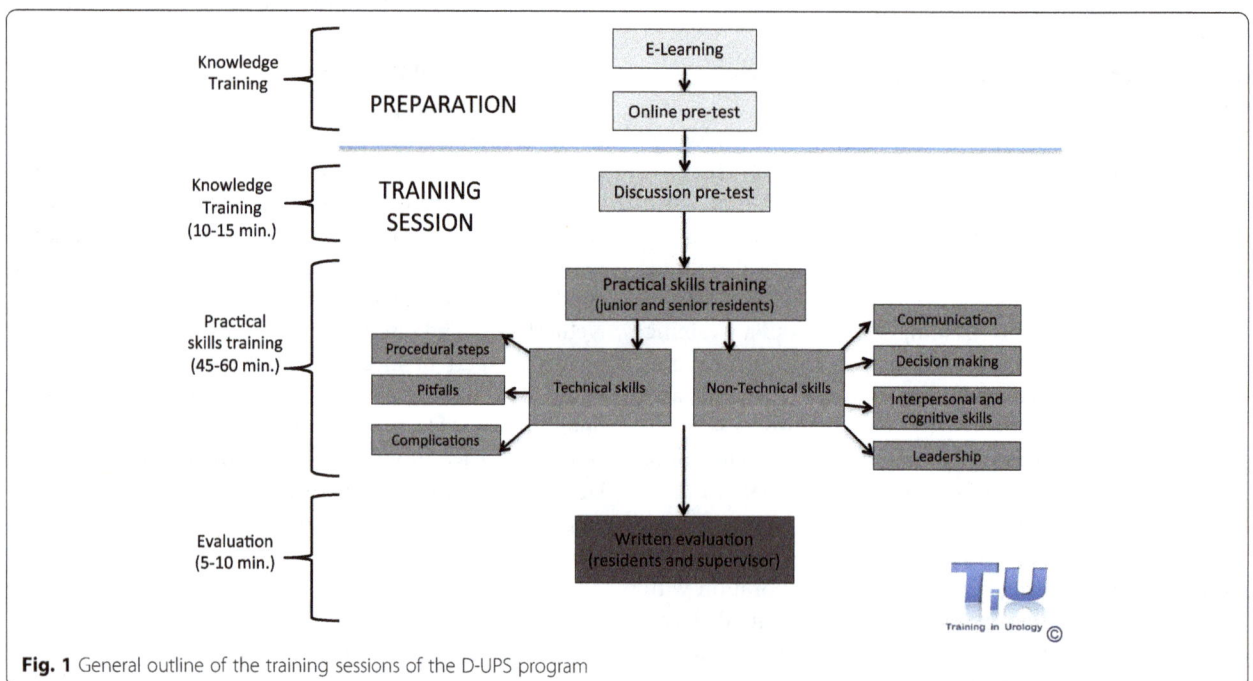

**Fig. 1** General outline of the training sessions of the D-UPS program

'basic laparoscopy' is presented in Additional file 3. The laparoscopic tasks used in this training are derived from the validated European Basic Laparoscopic Urological Skills Exam [21].

## Questionnaire and interviews
The response rate to the questionnaire was 87.4 % for residents and 86.7 % for program directors, representing all the 25 Dutch teaching hospitals. Interviews were conducted with five groups of residents (n = 39) and three groups of program directors (n = 15) from 20 different teaching hospitals. The median number of participants per interview was 6 (range 4–11). Interviews lasted a median of 53 min. (range 39–73).

## Current and ideal practical skills training in general
### Questionnaire-results on general practical skills training
The results of the questionnaire revealed that some form of structured, practical skills training currently takes place in local teaching hospitals according to 12 % of residents versus 44 % of program directors ($p < 0.001$, chi-square test). The frequency of practical skills training sessions varied per hospital, from once a week to once every six months, and training was mostly provided by one of the staff urologists. Residents and program directors who reported to have some form of practical skills training in their hospital mentioned training in laparoscopy as the main practical skills training (80 % and 59 % respectively). Additionally, they mentioned training in sonography, general tips in surgical procedures, vasectomy and circumcision.

### Interview-results on general practical skills training
All the interviewed residents and program directors stated that currently residents learn their practical skills 'by doing'. First they observe and then they do it themselves, step-by-step, with instructions from a supervising urologist. *'See one, do one, teach one. When you feel competent, and the program director feels the same way, they let you go.' (resident).*

The majority confirmed the presence of a skills lab in their teaching hospital. However, only in two hospitals were these skills labs used on a regular basis. Training should be scheduled, since voluntary training does not take place due to residents' busy schedules. Residents stated that materials in the skills lab are often lacking or in bad condition. The majority of residents considered it desirable to practice certain procedures first on a suitable simulation model, especially in endourology and laparoscopy. They would like to practice in a non-patient-related setting more often. *'The question is: would I have preferred to practice on a simulator? The answer is yes, absolutely. But this was not an option.' (resident)* Program directors shared this opinion, provided that adequate simulation models were available for training.

## Quality of the newly developed D-UPS program
### Questionnaire-results on opinions about D-UPS
The majority of residents and program directors considered the D-UPS program to be a useful addition to present education (92 % and 87 % respectively, $p = 0.51$). They expected structured practical skills training to have a positive effect on patient safety, time efficiency in the OR, self-confidence of the residents and uniformity of actions (Fig. 2). There were no significant differences in opinions between residents versus program directors. The main expected difficulties in the implementation of the D-UPS program (Fig. 3) were logistics and lack of

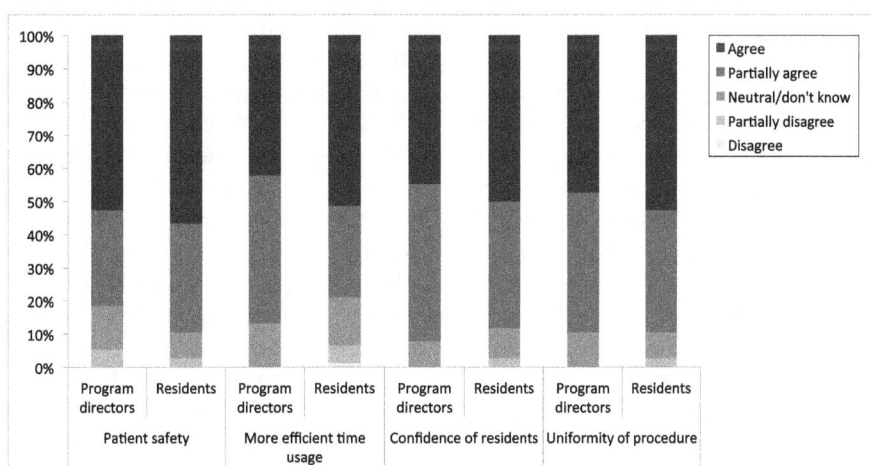

**Fig. 2** Views of residents and program directors on expected positive endpoints in implementation of the D-UPS program. There were no significant differences in opinions of residents versus program directors regarding expected effects on patient safety ($p = 0.35$), time efficiency in the OR ($p = 0.44$), self-confidence of the residents ($p = 0.75$), and uniformity of procedure ($p = 1.0$)

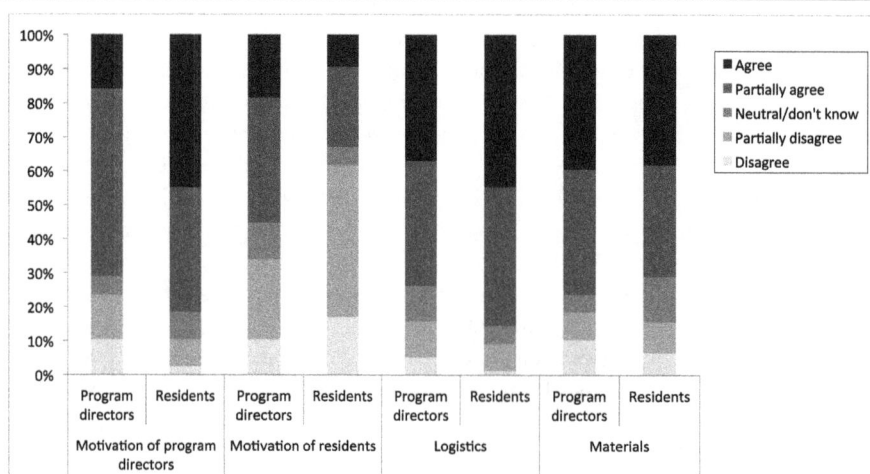

**Fig. 3** Views of residents and program directors on expected difficulties in implementation of the D-UPS program. There were no significant differences in opinions of residents versus program directors regarding expected difficulties in motivation of residents ($p = 0.23$), logistics ($p = 0.13$), and materials ($p = 0.66$). *The majority of residents believed motivation of the program directors would be a difficulty in the implementation of the proposed training program, in contrast to the program directors ($p = 0.02$)

motivation of the program directors. Significantly more residents than program directors expected the motivation of the program director to be a problem ($p = 0.02$).

### Interview-results on opinions about D-UPS

The interviews revealed that residents expected the D-UPS program to provide them with knowledge of instruments and to make them more familiar with procedural steps. They also revealed another challenge, which was adaptation of the training level to senior residents. Moreover, the interviews revealed further details concerning design characteristics in relation to the acceptability of the program. Residents and program directors were enthusiastic about the design of the D-UPS, because it would create a nationwide uniform foundation of basic urology techniques. The use of peer teaching was noted as important for residents' future role as educators and for making the training sessions easily accessible. Some criticism was expressed on the time frame of the training sessions. Various residents and program directors indicated that one hour might not be sufficient for training certain skills, and one afternoon per month was suggested as an alternative. Moreover, residents and program directors stressed structured scheduling of the training sessions as an important condition for successful implementation of the D-UPS program. Residents indicated to be keen on training practical skills on simulation models, particularly in endourology. However, the use of realistic, high fidelity simulation models was emphasized as an important condition for successful implementation. In summary, according to residents and program directors, the design characteristics that could increase the acceptability of urological practical skills training programs

were structured scheduling, the use of peer teaching and high fidelity models.

### Discussion

In this study, we aimed to gain insight into current and ideal Dutch urological skills training and presented the outline of the D-UPS program, including the assessment of design characteristics that may increase its acceptability. The results of this study show that Dutch residents in urology currently learn their practical skills 'by doing', according to the classic master-apprentice model. Ideally, they would prefer to practice certain procedures on simulation models first, especially in endourology. The acceptability of implementing the newly developed D-UPS program is high. Residents and program directors think this program would provide all residents in urology with a nationwide uniform foundation for training urological techniques. Design characteristics that increase acceptability of the D-UPS/related practical skills training programs are discussed in the next paragraphs.

One of the expected difficulties in implementing the skills training program was 'materials'. Residents and program directors expressed the belief that practical skills training is only useful if residents practise on realistic, i.e. high fidelity models. This is contradictory to the present outline of the D-UPS program, in which low fidelity models are preferred. In the decision of which simulator to use for skills training it is of paramount importance that the simulator can serve the goal of training. In the development of the D-UPS program, first the learning objectives for training a certain skill were defined and subsequently a suitable simulator was sought. If possible the choice was for a simulator of low fidelity. This was not only to limit the cost, but also to simplify logistics and because for certain basic skills no high fidelity models are available. In the literature it is confirmed that, especially for training basic skills, low fidelity simulators can be of great value. Matsumoto et al. compared the effectiveness of a strictly didactic training in ureteroscopy with training on a low fidelity model and on a high fidelity model [22]. They showed that training on the low fidelity model had the same degree of benefit as training on the high fidelity model, and both had a significantly higher degree of benefit than the didactic session alone. Since the first eight training sessions focus on basic urological procedures, low fidelity simulators could be suitable. However, when it comes to training more advanced skills sometimes high fidelity simulators, e.g. virtual reality simulation, will be needed. For successful implementation of practical skills training using low fidelity models, it will be of great importance that residents and program directors understand the value of these training models. McDougall et al. designed a 4-year curriculum for urology residency training, with frequent training sessions using mainly low fidelity models [14]. Although this study included only 8 residents so far and evaluation is ongoing, initial results are encouraging. Most participants stated that this 4-year curriculum provided a better learning experience than the curriculum without structured skills training. Furthermore, while residents and program directors in our study expected one-hour training sessions to be insufficient for some parts of practical skills training, McDougall and colleagues found that acceptance of a weekly hour of training was high [14]. In their study, the majority of residents indicated that one hour of training was sufficient and provided new clinical information.

Another important expected obstacle, according to residents and program directors in our study, was the logistic integration of practical skills training into the working week. Structured scheduling was suggested as a condition for successful implementation. The importance of scheduling training sessions and making them obligatory was emphasized by Chang and colleagues, who examined the effectiveness of voluntary training in a simulation laboratory as part of the surgical curriculum [23]. They showed that voluntary use of a surgical simulation laboratory resulted in minimal participation in the curriculum.

Another expected difficulty in implementation was motivation, in particular the motivation of program directors. This concern is in line with the findings of Stefanidis et al., who described the implementation of a proficiency-based laparoscopic skills curriculum in a general surgical residency program and found that this can only be achieved successfully if dedicated faculty

and scheduled training time are ensured [24]. Hence, one of the key success factors for implementation is motivating program directors for their educational role in urology skills training programs.

A remarkable finding was the significant difference in views on the current availability of structured practical skills training in the local teaching hospitals. This was mentioned as current practice by 12 % of residents versus 44 % of program directors. A possible explanation for this difference could be that residents and program directors have different perceptions of the definition of practical skills training, or that some of the residents started their residency only recently, and might not yet have been involved in practical skills training.

To our knowledge, the D-UPS program would be the first curriculum in Europe that provides yearly repetitive practical skills training in the local hospital setting, including the use of the local equipment. The first step in the development and implementation of a new curriculum is the performance of training needs analysis and the establishment of acceptability, which was evaluated in this study. Although the results of this study describe the Dutch situation, which limits generalizability, the outline of the D-UPS program could serve as a blueprint for skills training in other surgical specialties in the Netherlands. Moreover, extrapolation to European countries would be possible, especially those countries with similar residency programs, since up till now there have been limited initiatives for non-patient related skills training curricula.

Where possible, existing validated simulation training is incorporated in the D-UPS program, to avoid duplication and expense. For example, the tasks used in the basic laparoscopy training of the D-UPS program are derived from the validated European Basic Laparoscopic Urological Skills program [21]. Other possibilities should be further explored.

We acknowledge that validation of the curriculum is of paramount importance in the process of innovating educational programs. However, this is a multi-year process and is considered to be the endpoint of the implementation process. In the process towards this validation it is important to inform colleagues in the field of curriculum development regarding the ongoing developments, since they might profit from the outline of this program an our findings on design characteristics that increase the acceptability of implementing practical skills training in a non-patient-related setting.

The use of a questionnaire and interviews is relatively subjective and might have led to socially desirable answers. To counter this effect, the interviews were moderated by an independent educational expert, and anonymity was guaranteed. Furthermore, residents and program directors were interviewed in separate groups to ensure freedom and safety in expressing opinions. As in any qualitative study, investigator objectivity is a limitation [25]. This issue was countered by having 25 % of the transcripts coded by two researchers separately.

## Conclusions

Current urological residency training consists of patient-related 'learning by doing'. Structured, practical skills training takes place in a minority of teaching hospitals. Ideally, residents and program directors would welcome more practice on simulation models. Design characteristics that increase the acceptability of implementing a skills training program are structured scheduling, the use of peer teaching and the use of high-fidelity models. The acceptability of implementing the presented skills training program is high.

## Abbreviations

OR: Operating room; D-UPS program: Dutch Urology Practical Skills program; TNA: Training needs analysis; TMS: Training media specification.

## Competing interests

The authors A.H. de Vries, S.J. van Luijk, A.J.J.A. Scherpbier, A.J.M. Hendrikx, E.L. Koldewijn, C. Wagner and B.M.A. Schout declare that they have no competing interests or financial ties to disclose.

## Authors' contributions

AdV performed statistical and qualitative analysis of the data, contributed to data interpretation and wrote the first draft of the manuscript. SvL made a substantial contribution to the acquisition of data as moderator of the semi-structured focus-group interviews. AS contributed to the conception and design of the study (optimizing questionnaire) and the interpretation of data. AH made a substantial contribution to the conception and design of the study (optimizing questionnaire) and data collection. EK and CW contributed to the interpretation of the data and the second draft of the manuscript. BS designed the study, contributed to data collection, the analysis of qualitative data and interpretation of data. All authors critically revised the manuscript and gave their final approval before submission.

## Acknowledgments

The authors gratefully acknowledge Saskia Houterman for statistical advice, Carolien de Blok for advice in qualitative analyses, Lisette van Hulst for editorial assistance on behalf of 'Text and Training' and all urology residents and program directors for their participation in this study.

## Author details

[1]Department of Urology, Catharina Hospital, Eindhoven, The Netherlands. [2]Academy of Post-graduate Education, Maastricht University Medical Centre, Maastricht, The Netherlands. [3]Faculty of Health, Medicine and Life Sciences, Maastricht University Medical Centre, Maastricht, The Netherlands. [4]Department of Public and Occupational Health, EMGO Institute for Health and Care Research, Amsterdam, The Netherlands. [5]Netherlands Institute for Health Services Research (NIVEL), Utrecht, The Netherlands. [6]Department of Urology, St. Antonius Hospital, Nieuwegein, The Netherlands.

## References

1. Schout BM, Ananias HJ, Bemelmans BL, d'Ancona FC, Muijtjens AM, Dolmans VE, et al. Transfer of cysto-urethroscopy skills from a virtual-reality simulator to the operating room: a randomized controlled trial. BJU Int. 2010;106(2):226–31. discussion 231.
2. Ahmed K, Jawad M, Abboudi M, Gavazzi A, Darzi A, Athanasiou T, et al. Effectiveness of procedural simulation in urology: a systematic review. J Urol. 2011;186(1):26–34.
3. Rodriguez-Paz JM, Kennedy M, Salas E, Wu AW, Sexton JB, Hunt EA, et al. Beyond "see one, do one, teach one": toward a different training paradigm. Postgrad Med J. 2009;85(1003):244–9.
4. Reznick RK, MacRae H. Teaching surgical skills–changes in the wind. N Engl J Med. 2006;355(25):2664–9.
5. Kneebone RL, Scott W, Darzi A, Horrocks M. Simulation and clinical practice: strengthening the relationship. Med Educ. 2004;38(10):1095–102.
6. Rogers DA. Ethical and educational considerations in minimally invasive surgery training for practicing surgeons. Semin Laparosc Surg. 2002;9(4):206–11.
7. Ahmed K, Jawad M, Dasgupta P, Darzi A, Athanasiou T, Khan MS. Assessment and maintenance of competence in urology. Nat Rev Urol. 2010;7(7):403–13.
8. Ahmed K, Amer T, Challacombe B, Jaye P, Dasgupta P, Khan MS. How to develop a simulation programme in urology. BJU Int. 2011;108(11):1698–702.
9. Sweet RM, Hananel D, Lawrenz F. A unified approach to validation, reliability, and education study design for surgical technical skills training. Arch Surg. 2010;145(2):197–201.
10. Henry B, Clark P, Sudan R. Cost and logistics of implementing a tissue-based American College of Surgeons/Association of Program Directors in Surgery surgical skills curriculum for general surgery residents of all clinical years. Am J Surg. 2014;207(2):201–8.
11. Vassiliou MC, Dunkin BJ, Marks JM, Fried GM. FLS and FES: comprehensive models of training and assessment. Surg Clin North Am. 2010;90(3):535–58.
12. Sroka G, Feldman LS, Vassiliou MC, Kaneva PA, Fayez R, Fried GM. Fundamentals of laparoscopic surgery simulator training to proficiency improves laparoscopic performance in the operating room-a randomized controlled trial. Am J Surg. 2010;199(1):115–20.
13. Shamim Khan M, Ahmed K, Gavazzi A, Gohil R, Thomas L, Poulsen J, et al. Development and implementation of centralized simulation training: evaluation of feasibility, acceptability and construct validity. BJU Int. 2013;111(3):518–23.
14. McDougall EM, Watters TJ, Clayman RV. 4-year curriculum for urology residency training. J Urol. 2007;178(6):2540–4.
15. Korndorffer Jr JR, Arora S, Sevdalis N, Paige J, McClusky 3rd DA, Stefanidis D, et al. The American College of Surgeons/Association of Program Directors in Surgery National Skills Curriculum: adoption rate, challenges and strategies for effective implementation into surgical residency programs. Surgery. 2013;154(1):13–20.
16. Stassen LP, Bemelman WA, Meijerink J. Risks of minimally invasive surgery underestimated: a report of the Dutch Health Care Inspectorate. Surg Endosc. 2010;24(3):495–8.
17. Wiggins G, McTighe J. Understanding by Design. NJ: Prentice Hall: Upper Saddle River; 2001.
18. Zevin B, Levy JS, Satava RM, Grantcharov TP. A consensus-based framework for design, validation, and implementation of simulation-based training curricula in surgery. J Am Coll Surg. 2012;215(4):580–586.e3.
19. Schout BM, Hendrikx AJ, Scheele F, Bemelmans BL, Scherpbier AJ. Validation and implementation of surgical simulators: a critical review of present, past, and future. Surg Endosc. 2010;24(3):536–46.
20. Schout BM, Hendrikx AJ, Scherpbier AJ, Bemelmans BL. Update on training models in endourology: a qualitative systematic review of the literature between January 1980 and April 2008. Eur Urol. 2008;54(6):1247–61.
21. Tjiam IM, Persoon MC, Hendrikx AJ, Muijtjens AM, Witjes JA, Scherpbier AJ. Program for laparoscopic urologic skills: a newly developed and validated educational program. Urology. 2012;79(4):815–20.
22. Matsumoto ED, Hamstra SJ, Radomski SB, Cusimano MD. The effect of bench model fidelity on endourological skills: a randomized controlled study. J Urol. 2002;167(3):1243–7.
23. Chang L, Petros J, Hess DT, Rotondi C, Babineau TJ. Integrating simulation into a surgical residency program: is voluntary participation effective? Surg Endosc. 2007;21(3):418–21.

# 31

# Bacteriophages for treating urinary tract infections in patients undergoing transurethral resection of the prostate

Lorenz Leitner[1,2] 🆔, Wilbert Sybesma[1], Nina Chanishvili[3], Marina Goderdzishvili[3], Archil Chkhotua[4], Aleksandre Ujmajuridze[4], Marc P. Schneider[1], Andrea Sartori[1], Ulrich Mehnert[1], Lucas M. Bachmann[5] and Thomas M. Kessler[1]*

## Abstract

**Background:** Urinary tract infections (UTI) are among the most prevalent microbial diseases and their financial burden on society is substantial. The continuing increase of antibiotic resistance worldwide is alarming. Thus, well-tolerated, highly effective therapeutic alternatives are urgently needed. Although there is evidence indicating that bacteriophage therapy may be effective and safe for treating UTIs, the number of investigated patients is low and there is a lack of randomized controlled trials.

**Methods and design:** This study is the first randomized, placebo-controlled, double-blind trial investigating bacteriophages in UTI treatment. Patients planned for transurethral resection of the prostate are screened for UTIs and enrolled if in urine culture eligible microorganisms $\geq 10^4$ colony forming units/mL are found. Patients are randomized in a double-blind fashion to the 3 study treatment arms in a 1:1:1 ratio to receive either: a) bacteriophage (i.e. commercially available Pyo bacteriophage) solution, b) placebo solution, or c) antibiotic treatment according to the antibiotic sensitivity pattern. All treatments are intended for 7 days. No antibiotic prophylaxes will be given to the double-blinded treatment arms a) and b). As common practice, the Pyo bacteriophage cocktail is subjected to periodic adaptation cycles during the study. Urinalysis, urine culture, bladder and pain diary, and IPSS questionnaire will be completed prior to and at the end of treatment (i.e. after 7 days) or at withdrawal/drop out from the study. Patients with persistent UTIs will undergo antibiotic treatment according to antibiotic sensitivity pattern.

**Discussion:** Based on the high lytic activity and the potential of resistance optimization by direct adaptation of bacteriophages, and considering the continuing increase of antibiotic resistance worldwide, bacteriophage therapy is a very promising treatment option for UTIs. Thus, our randomized controlled trial investigating bacteriophages for treating UTIs will provide essential insights into this potentially revolutionizing treatment option.

**Keywords:** Bacteriophages, Antibiotics, Urinary tract infection, Randomized placebo-controlled double-blind trial, Resistance

* Correspondence: tkessler@gmx.ch
[1]Neuro-Urology, Spinal Cord Injury Center & Research, University of Zürich, Balgrist University Hospital, Zürich, Switzerland
Full list of author information is available at the end of the article

## Background

Urinary tract infections (UTI) are highly prevalent and put a substantial financial burden on the health care systems worldwide. In the USA alone, over 7 million physician consultations are due to UTIs [1], resulting in estimated direct and indirect costs of 1.6 billion US dollars [1]. Further, UTIs account for more than 100'000 hospital admissions annually [1], and for at least 40% of all hospital-acquired infections [2]. The increasing threat of antibiotic resistance, mainly due to uncritical use of antibiotics [3, 4], and the subsequent absence of access to effective antimicrobials constitutes a challenge for the future [5]. As UTIs account for approximately 15% of all community-prescribed antibiotics in the USA [6], they play an important role for direct antibiotic selection pressure. Thus, well-tolerated therapeutic alternatives to treat UTIs and to reduce antimicrobial resistances are highly warranted.

In 1917, d'Hérelle proposed the use of bacteriophages to treat bacterial infections. After a colorful episode, the discovery of penicillin by Alexander Fleming declined the interest for bacteriophages in the Western world rapidly [7]. At present, bacteriophage therapy is well accepted and registered in East European and post-Soviet countries like Georgia, Ukraine, Belarus, and Russia. Lately the use of bacteriophages as a target therapy against bacterial pathogens has gained a renewed interest. Reviews about several reports of successfully applied bacteriophage therapies for different medical specializations have been published [7, 8], and the role of bacteriophage as a possible treatment for difficult to treat microorganisms has been encountered [9–11]. A recent in vitro study could show excellent results (i.e. a high lytic activity) of commercially available bacteriophages for the most common bacterial strains found in UTIs [12]. Regarding UTIs, several current clinical studies showed positive effects of the use of bacteriophage therapy [10, 13–15]. Khawaldeh et al. reported on the success of adjunctive bacteriophage therapy after repeated failure of antibiotics alone [10]. An article in Russian language (http://www.bionow.ru/bnows-1020-2.html) describes successful treatments for topically applied (i.e. administrating bacteriophages into the urinary bladder) bacteriophages for several patients. However, well conducted clinical trials, a defined frame for bacteriophage therapy in the current Medicinal Product Regulation, and well-defined, safe bacteriophage preparations are still lacking. In consequence, the use of bacteriophage therapy is still not accepted as an official treatment against infectious diseases in the Western world [16, 17].

In line with recommendations of a multi-disciplinary expert panel on acceptance and re-implementation of bacteriophage therapy [11], we therefore designed a randomized, placebo-controlled, double-blind clinical trial to assess the efficacy and safety of intravesical bacteriophage treatment. We hypothesize that intravesical bacteriophage treatment in patients with UTIs due to *E. coli* and other uropathogens, shows a 40% increase in success rate (normalization of urine culture defined as no evidence of bacteria, i.e. $<10^4$ colony forming units/mL) as compared to placebo treatment within 7 days. This difference is considered to be clinically relevant. We also hypothesize that bacteriophage treatment is non-inferior to antibiotic treatment in terms of treatment success rates, with a non-inferiority margin of 35%.

## Methods and design
### Study design
This study is a randomized, placebo-controlled, double-blind trial investigating bacteriophages in UTI treatment. The study is conducted at the Tzulukidze National Center of Urology (TNCU), Tbilisi, Georgia. Phage preparations (i.e. Pyo bacteriophage solution: commercially available and registered in Georgia) and continuous adaption cycles during the course of the study, to enhance the treatment effect, are done at the Eliava Institute of Bacteriophages, Microbiology, and Virology in Tbilisi (EIBMV), Georgia.

Figure 1 gives an overview of the procedures. Patients planned for transurethral resection of the prostate are screened for UTIs at the TNCU. Urine cultures including antibiotic sensitivity testing are performed in a duplicate manner. If eligible microorganisms which would potentially match with the type of bacteriophage present in Pyo bacteriophage (5 components: Enterococcus spp., *Escherichia coli*, Proteus mirabilis, Pseudomonas aeruginosa, Staphylococcus spp., and Streptococcus spp.) are detected, urine cultures are then sent for bacteriophage sensitivity testing to the EIBMV (Fig. 2) [12]. In case of a positive in-vitro sensitivity testing, concluded within 24 h after receipt of the urine culture, patients will be asked for study participation. After written informed consent, patients are randomized in a double-blind fashion to the study treatment arms in a 1:1:1 ratio to receive either: a) Pyo bacteriophage solution, b) placebo (sterile bacteriology media with identical color as treatment arm a), or c) antibiotic treatment according to the antibiotic sensitivity pattern, respectively. Treatment arms a and b will be double-blind but treatment arm c, i.e. the control arm representing common clinical practice, is open label. All treatments are intended for 7 days starting at the day of surgery (arm c) or one day thereafter (arm a and b). Prior and at the end of treatment (i.e. after 7 days) or at withdrawal / drop out, urinalysis, urine culture, bladder and pain diary [18] and an International Prostate Symptom Score (IPSS) questionnaire [19] will be taken. Patients with persistent bacteriuria will undergo antibiotic treatment according to antibiotic sensitivity.

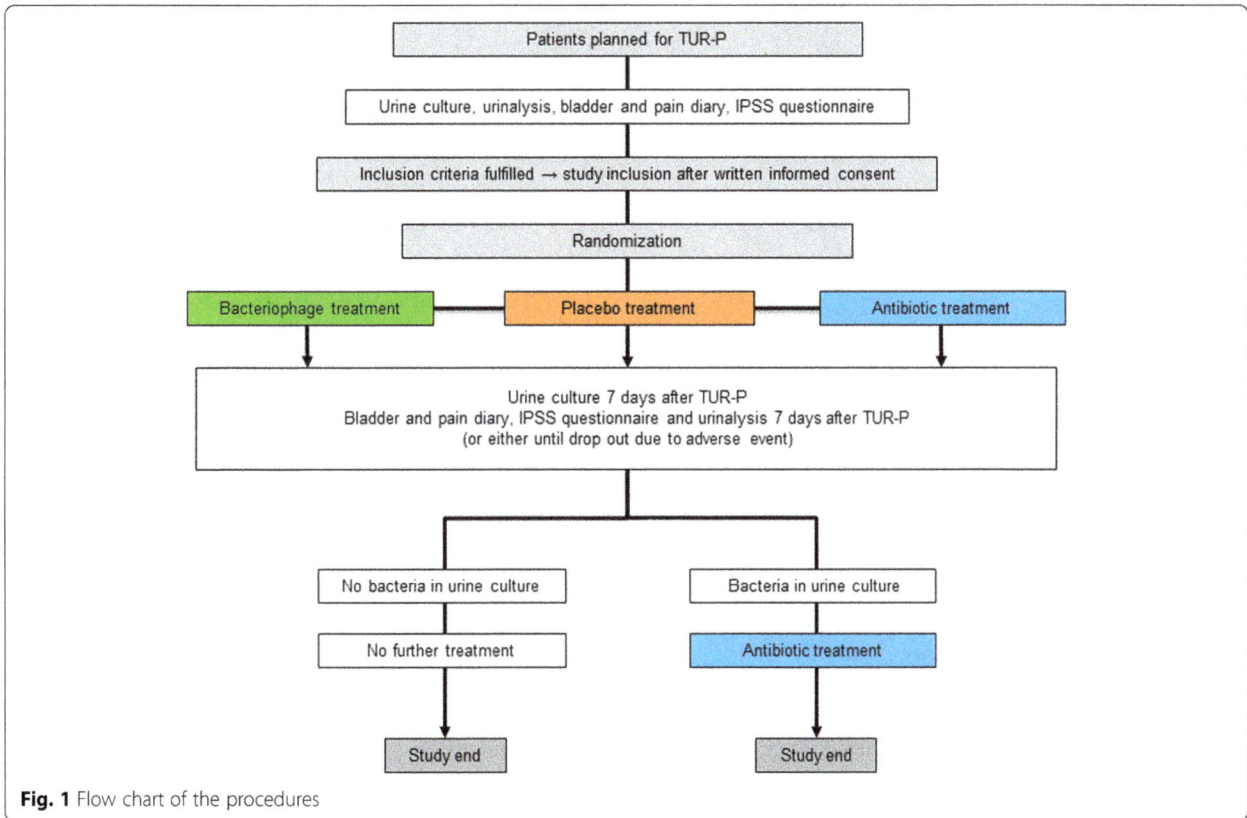

**Fig. 1** Flow chart of the procedures

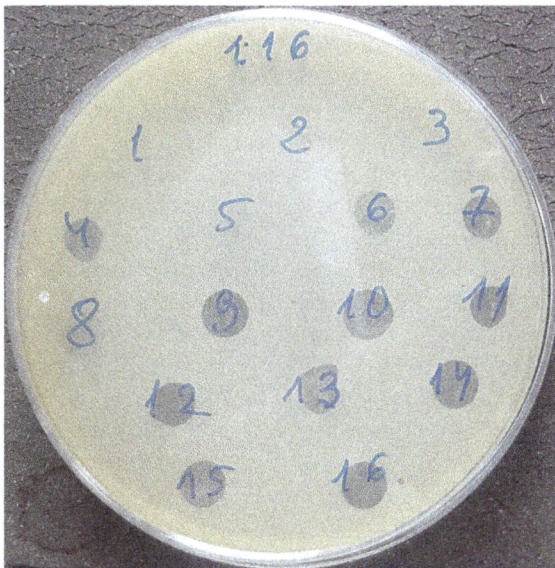

**Fig. 2** Bacteriophage sensitivity testing to *Escherichia coli*: The *Escherichia coli* culture reacts positively to 12 phages out of 16. Confluent (complete) lysis can be seen for phages #9, 14 and 16, overgrown (partial) lysis for phages #4, 6, 7, 8, 10, 11, 12, 13, 15 and 16, respectively

Note: As it is common practice when working with bacteriophage cocktails, the Pyo bacteriophage will be subjected to adaptation cycles during the course of the study.

**Study population and recruitment**

According to the inclusion and exclusion criteria (Table 1), we will investigate patients planned for transurethral resection of the prostate presenting with UTIs (defined as $\geq 10^4$ colony forming units/mL and symptoms such as urgency, frequency, and/or dysuria). The following variables will be considered: age, type of bladder emptying, prostate size, urinalysis, bladder and pain diary, IPSS questionnaire.

**Determination of sample size**

We are planning a study of independent cases and controls with 1 control per case. Superiority of bacteriophage versus placebo treatment: We assume the success rate among controls to be 0.2. If the true success rate for experimental subjects is 0.6, we will need to study 27 experimental and 27 control subjects to be able to reject the null hypothesis that the success rates for experimental and control subjects are equal with probability (power) 0.8. The type I error probability associated with this test of this null hypothesis is 0.05.

Non-inferiority of bacteriophage versus antibiotic treatment: We assume the success rate among subjects

**Table 1** Study inclusion and exclusion criteria

| Inclusion criteria | Exclusion criteria |
|---|---|
| • Age > 18 years<br>• Urine culture (taken by mid-stream urine; or from the existing trans-urethral or suprapubic catheter): ≥10⁴ colony forming units/mL of predefined uropathogens (i.e. Enterococcus spp., Escherichia coli, Proteus mirabilis, Pseudomonas aeruginosa, Staphylococcus spp., and Streptococcus spp.)<br>• Uropathogens sensitive to Pyo bacteriophage<br>• Symptoms: Urgency, frequency, and/or dysuria<br>• Written informed consent | • Fever >38 °C<br>• CRP >100 mg/L<br>• Acute prostatitis<br>• Concomitant fungal urinary tract infection<br>• Current antibiotic treatment or antibiotic treatment within the last 7 days (exceptions: subjects with an active catheter associated urinary tract infection who have received prior antibiotics may be enrolled provided a minimum of 48 h has elapsed between the last dose of the prior antibiotic and the time of obtaining the baseline urine specimen. Subjects receiving current antibiotic prophylaxis for catheter associated urinary tract infection who present signs and symptoms consistent with an active new catheter associated infection may be enrolled provided all other eligibility criteria are met including obtaining a pre-treatment qualifying baseline urine culture)<br>• Any rapidly progressing disease or immediately life-threatening illness including but not limited to: acute hepatic failure, respiratory failure, and septic shock<br>• No informed consent |

receiving bacteriophage treatment to be 0.6 and we accept a non-inferiority margin of 0.35. If the true success rate for experimental subjects is 0.95, we will need to study 27 experimental subjects and 27 control subjects to be able to remain within the non-inferiority margin with a probability (power) 0.8. The type I error probability associated with this test of this alternative hypothesis is 0.05. We will use a continuity-corrected chi-squared statistic or Fisher's exact test to evaluate these hypotheses.

Thus, we will include 27 patients per treatment group, i.e. 81 patients in total. Withdrawn patients will be replaced.

**Study location and partners**

Tzulukidze National Center of Urology, Tbilisi, Georgia: Patient treatment.

Eliava Institute of Bacteriophages, Microbiology, and Virology in Tbilisi, Georgia: Phage preparation and adaptation.

Neuro-Urology, Spinal Cord Injury Center & Research, University of Zürich, Balgrist University Hospital, Zürich, Switzerland: Study design, monitoring and statistical support.

**Investigations**

The patients planned for transurethral resection of the prostate with a positive urine culture (≥10⁴ colony forming units/mL) of predefined uropathogens sensitive to Pyo bacteriophage (i.e. Enterococcus spp., Escherichia coli, Proteus mirabilis, Pseudomonas aeruginosa, Staphylococcus spp., and Streptococcus spp.) and fulfilling the study inclusion criteria will be included into the study after providing written informed consent. The patients will be assessed using bladder and pain diary [18] and an IPSS questionnaire [19]. The Fig. 1 gives an overview of the procedures that patients will undergo during the study.

After inclusion, patients will be randomized in a double-blind fashion to the study treatment arms in a 1:1:1 ratio. Patients of all study arms will undergo monopolar transurethral resection of the prostate and insertion of a suprapubic catheter if not already present. Study arm a) will receive bacteriophage solution (Pyo bacteriophage) and study arm b) placebo solution (sterile bacteriology media). Either solution will consist of 20 mL and will have an identical appearance for both the bacteriophage and the placebo, respectively. An investigator not involved in the assessment of the clinical outcome will deliver the solution and teach the patient / health care provider how to instill the solution into the bladder. The solution will be instilled using the suprapubic catheter, 2 times per 24 h (i.e. 8.00, 20.00) for 7 days, starting the first day after surgery. The patients will be asked to retain the solution in the bladder for approximately 30–60 min. No antibiotic prophylaxes will be given to the study treatment arms a and b.

Study arm c) will receive an antibiotic treatment according to the antibiotic sensitivity pattern and common clinical practice.

At the end of treatment (i.e. after 7 days) or at withdrawal / drop out, urinalysis, urine culture, bladder and pain diary [18] and an IPSS questionnaire [19] will be taken. Patients with persistent UTIs will undergo antibiotic treatment according to antibiotic sensitivity for 7 days.

Drop out criteria for patients in the study arm a and b are fever >38 °C, CRP >100 mg/L, other clinical signs or symptoms for a systemic infection or withdraw from the patients. These patients will undergo antibiotic treatment according to antibiotic sensitivity.

**Safety**

The investigators will inform the patients, the study monitoring board, and the ethics committee if it becomes evident that the disadvantages of participation may be significantly greater than was foreseen in the research proposal. The study will be suspended pending further review by the study monitoring board, except insofar as suspension would jeopardize the patients' health. The investigators will take care that all patients are kept informed.

Adverse events will be assessed and categorized according to the National Cancer Institute Common Terminology Criteria for Adverse Events (CTCAE) version 4 in grade 1 to 5 (http://ctep.cancer.gov/protocolDevelopment/electronic_applications/ctc.htm). All adverse events will be followed until they have abated, or until a stable situation has been reached. Depending on the event, follow-up may require additional tests or medical procedures as indicated, and/or referral to the general physician or a medical specialist.

In the case of withdrawal of consent to participate in the study, all possible efforts will be made to convince the patient to continue to have safety follow-up evaluations.

In the event one of the following situations arises among treated patients during the conduct of the study, the study will be temporarily suspended and a comprehensive safety review conducted evaluating if the study has to be terminated prematurely:

- Any death secondary to rapid unexpected progression of an underlying medical condition.
- Severe clinical or neurological deterioration in more than one subject.
- Any other serious adverse event determined by the study monitoring board to be a reason to suspend the study.

### Study outcome measures

Primary: Success of intravesical treatment, defined as normalization of urine culture (no evidence of bacteria, i.e. $<10^4$ colony forming units/mL) after 7 days of bacteriophage, placebo, or antibiotic treatment.

Secondary: Adverse events, in categorization according to the National Cancer Institute Common Terminology Criteria for Adverse Events (CTCAE) version 4 in grade 1 to 5 (http://ctep.cancer.gov/protocolDevelopment/electronic_applications/ctc.htm) during treatment phase.

Tertiary: a) Changes in bladder and pain diary assessment of number of voids, number of leakages, post void residual, pain assessment using a visual analog scale (0 (no pain) to 10 (strongest possible pain)), b) IPSS items at baseline versus day 7 under intravesical bacteriophage, placebo, or antibiotic treatment.

### Data analysis
#### Statistics
Interval scaled variates will be summarized with means and standard deviations (SD) or medians and interquartile ranges where appropriate. Dichotomous variates will be described as ratios and percentages.

#### Univariate analysis
T-tests will be used to compare means between groups and chi-squared tests to compare dichotomous variables.

#### Multivariate analysis
To adjust for unequal distribution of parameters at baseline, multivariate regression models, linear models in case of an interval scaled outcome and logistic regression in case of a dichotomous outcome will be performed.

## Discussion
UTIs are among the most prevalent microbial diseases and their financial burden on society is substantial. The continuing increase of antibiotic resistance worldwide is alarming; thus, well-tolerated, highly effective therapeutic alternatives are urgently needed. Although there is evidence indicating that bacteriophage therapy may be effective and safe for treating UTIs, the number of investigated patients is low and there is a lack of randomized controlled trials. Thus, well-designed prospective studies are urgently needed to draw definitive conclusions in the ambitious research field of UTIs. We therefore designed this first randomized, placebo-controlled, double-blind clinical trial to assess the efficacy and safety of intravesical bacteriophage for treating UTIs. This trial will significantly influence the future management of UTIs and form a basis for further studies involving bacteriophages for treating different bacterial infections. Moreover, the findings of our research project will provide further stimuli for competent authorities and physicians to use bacteriophages, as additional tools, in the prevention and treatment of otherwise virtually untreatable infections. In addition, the trial is multidisciplinary and will significantly influence all involved disciplines, i.e. urology, microbiology and infectious diseases. It will promote future multidisciplinary, multicenter approaches and collaborations further improving patients' medical care and it will also raise the acceptance to use bacteriophages in western civilizations and accelerate regulations processes.

**Abbreviations**
CTCAE: Common Terminology Criteria for Adverse Events; EIBMV: Eliava Institute of Bacteriophages, Microbiology, and Virology; IPSS: International Prostate Symptom Score; TNCU: Tzulukidze National Center of Urology; UTI: Urinary tract infections

**Acknowledgements**
The authors would like to acknowledge the Swiss National Science Foundation and the Swiss Continence Foundation for financial support.

**Authors' contributors**
WS, NC, AC, AU, UM, LMB and TMK created the study design. LL, WS and TMK drafted the manuscript. NC, NG, AC, AU, MPS, AS, UM and LMB critically reviewed the manuscript. WS, NC, AC, UM and obtained the funding of this study. All the authors read and approved the final manuscript.

## Funding

This study was supported by the Swiss Continence Foundation (www.swisscontinencefoundation.ch), the Swiss National Science Foundation (www.snsf.ch) (Grand application 152,304/Number of the JRP/IP: IZ73Z0_152,304) and the Swiss Agency for Development and Cooperation in the framework of the programme SCOPES (Scientific co-operation between Eastern Europe and Switzerland). The study protocol has been peer-reviewed by the funding bodies.

## Ethics approval and consent to participate

This trial will be performed in accordance with the World Medical Association Declaration of Helsinki [20], the guidelines for Good Clinical Practice [21]. The study protocol has been approved by the The Local Ethic Committee of the National Center of Urology, Tbilisi, Georgia, (TNCU-02/283). The trial has been registered at clinicaltrials.gov (www.clinicaltrials.gov/ct2/show/NCT03140085). The findings of the study will be published in peer-reviewed journals and presented at national and international scientific meetings. Written informed consent will be obtained from all participants.

## Competing interests

The authors declare that they have no competing interests.

## Author details

[1]Neuro-Urology, Spinal Cord Injury Center & Research, University of Zürich, Balgrist University Hospital, Zürich, Switzerland. [2]Department of Urology, University Hospital Basel, Basel, Switzerland. [3]The Eliava Institute of Bacteriophage, Microbiology, and Virology, Tbilisi, Georgia. [4]Tsulukidze National Center of Urology, Tbilisi, Georgia. [5]Medignition Inc., Research Consultants, Zürich, Switzerland.

## References

1. Foxman B. Epidemiology of urinary tract infections: incidence, morbidity, and economic costs. Am J Med. 2002;113(Suppl 1A):5S–13S.
2. Ruden H, Gastmeier P, Daschner FD, Schumacher M. Nosocomial and community-acquired infections in Germany. Summary of the results of the First National Prevalence Study (NIDEP). Infection. 1997;25(4):199–202.
3. Carlet J, Collignon P, Goldmann D, Goossens H, Gyssens IC, Harbarth S, Jarlier V, Levy SB, N'Doye B, Pittet D, et al. Society's failure to protect a precious resource: antibiotics. Lancet. 2011;378(9788):369–71.
4. Verbeken G, Huys I, Pirnay JP, Jennes S, Chanishvili N, Scheres J, Gorski A, De Vos D, Ceulemans C. Taking bacteriophage therapy seriously: a moral argument. Biomed Res Int. 2014;2014:621316.
5. Holmes AH, Moore LS, Sundsfjord A, Steinbakk M, Regmi S, Karkey A, Guerin PJ, Piddock LJ. Understanding the mechanisms and drivers of antimicrobial resistance. Lancet. 2016;387(10014):176–87.
6. Mazzulli T. Resistance trends in urinary tract pathogens and impact on management. J Urol. 2002;168(4 Pt 2):1720–2.
7. Abedon ST, Kuhl SJ, Blasdel BG, Kutter EM. Phage treatment of human infections. Bacteriophage. 2011;1(2):66–85.
8. Chanishvili N. A Literature Review of the Practical Application of Bacteriophage Research. Nova Science Publishers. 2012;
9. Merabishvili M, Vervaet C, Pirnay JP, De Vos D, Verbeken G, Mast J, Chanishvili N, Vaneechoutte M. Stability of Staphylococcus aureus phage ISP after freeze-drying (lyophilization). PLoS One. 2013;8(7):e68797.
10. Khawaldeh A, Morales S, Dillon B, Alavidze Z, Ginn AN, Thomas L, Chapman SJ, Dublanchet A, Smithyman A, Iredell JR. Bacteriophage therapy for refractory Pseudomonas aeruginosa urinary tract infection. J Med Microbiol. 2011;60(Pt 11):1697–700.
11. Expert round table on a, re-implementation of bacteriophage t: Silk route to the acceptance and re-implementation of bacteriophage therapy. *Biotechnol J* 2016, 11(5):595–600.
12. Sybesma W, Zbinden R, Chanishvili N, Kutateladze M, Chkhotua A, Ujmajuridze A, Mehnert U, Kessler TM. Bacteriophages as Potential Treatment for Urinary Tract Infections. Front Microbiol. 2016;7:465.
13. Perepanova T, Debreeva O, Koliatarova G, Kondratieva E, Aitskaia I, Malysheva V, al. e: The efficacy of bacteriophages preparations in treatment of inflammatory urogenital diseases. Urology & Nephrology 1957;5:14–17.
14. Kolomintsev N, Goroeinko I, Shakmatov V, Brazhnik P. Treatment of urological infections with different antibiotics and specific coli-proteus bacteriophages. Strategy and tactics of antibiotic therapy Krasnodar. 1966:172–4.
15. Danilova T. Phage therapy of the inflammatory urogenital infections in women. Proceedings of Dermatology and Venerology. 1996;
16. Merabishvili M, Pirnay JP, Verbeken G, Chanishvili N, Tediashvili M, Lashkhi N, Glonti T, Krylov V, Mast J, Van Parys L, et al. Quality-controlled small-scale production of a well-defined bacteriophage cocktail for use in human clinical trials. PLoS One. 2009;4(3):e4944.
17. Pirnay JP, De Vos D, Verbeken G, Merabishvili M, Chanishvili N, Vaneechoutte M, Zizi M, Laire G, Lavigne R, Huys I, et al. The phage therapy paradigm: pret-a-porter or sur-mesure? Pharm Res. 2011;28(4):934–7.
18. Abrams P, Cardozo L, Fall M, Griffiths D, Rosier P, Ulmsten U, van Kerrebroeck P, Victor A, Wein A. Standardisation Sub-committee of the International Continence S: The standardisation of terminology of lower urinary tract function: report from the Standardisation Sub-committee of the International Continence Society. Neurourol Urodyn. 2002;21(2):167–78.
19. Barry MJ, Fowler FJ Jr, O'Leary MP, Bruskewitz RC, Holtgrewe HL, Mebust WK, Cockett AT. The American Urological Association symptom index for benign prostatic hyperplasia. The Measurement Committee of the American Urological Association. J Urol. 1992;148(5):1549–57. discussion 1564
20. Declaration of Helsinki - Ethical principles for medical research involving human subjects. [https://www.wma.net/policies-post/wma-declaration-of-helsinki-ethical-principles-for-medical-research-involving-human-subjects].
21. Good clinical practice guideline [http://www.ich.org/products/guidelines/efficacy/article/efficacy-guidelines.html].

# 32

# Eviprostat has an identical effect compared to pollen extract (Cernilton) in patients with chronic prostatitis/chronic pelvic pain syndrome

Hiromichi Iwamura, Takuya Koie[*], Osamu Soma, Teppei Matsumoto, Atsushi Imai, Shingo Hatakeyama, Takahiro Yoneyama, Yasuhiro Hashimoto and Chikara Ohyama

## Abstract

**Background:** Previously reported results of a prospective, randomized placebo-controlled study showed that the pollen extract (Cernilton) significantly improved total symptoms, pain, and quality of life in patients with inflammatory prostatitis/chronic pelvic pain syndrome (CP/CPPS) without severe side effects. A phytotherapeutic agent, Eviprostat, is reportedly effective in a rat model of nonbacterial prostatitis. The aim of the present study was to compare the efficacy and safety of Eviprostat to that of the pollen extract in the management of CP/CPPS.

**Methods:** The patients with category III CP/CPPS were randomized to receive either oral capsules of Eviprostat (two capsules, q 8 h) or the pollen extract (two capsules, q 8 h) for 8 weeks. The primary endpoint of the study was symptomatic improvement in the NIH Chronic Prostatitis Symptom Index (NIH-CPSI). Participants were evaluated using the NIH-CPSI and the International Prostate Symptom Score (IPSS) at baseline and after 4 and 8 weeks.

**Results:** In the intention-to-treat analysis, 100 men were randomly allocated to Eviprostat ($n = 50$) or the pollen extract ($n = 50$). Response (defined as a decrease in the NIH-CPSI total score by at least 25 %) in the Eviprostat group and the pollen extract group was 88.2 and 78.1 %, respectively. There was no significant difference in the total, pain, urinary, and quality of life (QOL) scores of the NIH-CPSI between the two groups at 8 weeks. This was also the case with the total, voiding, and storage symptoms of the IPSS. There were no severe adverse events observed in any patients in this study.

**Conclusion:** Both the pollen extract and Eviprostat significantly reduced the symptoms of category III CP/CPPS without any adverse events. Eviprostat may have an identical effect on category III CP/CPPS compared the pollen extract.

**Keywords:** Chronic prostatitis/chronic pelvic pain syndrome, Eviprostat, Pollen extract

* Correspondence: goodwin@cc.hirosaki-u.ac.jp
Department of Urology, Hirosaki University Graduate School of Medicine, 5 Zaifucho, Hirosaki, Aomori 036-8562, Japan

## Background

Prostatitis is a relatively common urological disease that occurs in adult men [1]. The U.S. National Institutes of Health (NIH) Advisory Committees divided prostatitis into four categories [2, 3]. Of these, the incidence of category III disease, chronic prostatitis/chronic pelvic pain syndrome (CP/CPPS) is believed to be very high [1]. Category III prostatitis is subdivided into the inflammatory type (IIIA; similar to nonbacterial CP) and non-inflammatory type (IIIB; similar to prostatodynia) based on the presence (IIIA) or absence (IIIB) of leukocytes in prostatic secretions or seminal plasma [2, 3].

While the cause of CP/CPPS is presently unknown, it is a disease that has many clinical issues because it is often resistant to various treatments [4–6]. To date, CP/CPPS has been treated using alpha-blockers, antibacterial agents, anti-inflammatory agents, and phytotherapeutic agents with varying outcomes [4–12]. Phytotherapeutic agents that have been used include pollen extract, quercetin, and saw palmetto. Several years ago, Wagenlehner FM et al. announced the results of a prospective, randomized placebo-controlled study, which indicated that the pollen extract (Cernilton) significantly improved the total symptoms, pain, and quality of life in patients with inflammatory prostatitis/chronic pelvic pain syndrome (CP/CPPS) without any severe adverse effects [6].

Eviprostat is a phytotherapeutic agent widely used in the treatment of prostatic hypertrophy and has been used in Japan and Germany for more than 40 years [13–15]. Eviprostat consists of five components: four are extracted from the umbellate wintergreen Chimaphila umbellata, the aspen Populus tremula, the small pasque flower Pulsatilla pratensis, and the field horsetail Equisetum arvense, and the fifth is germ oil from wheat (Tritium aestivum) [13–15].

Oka et al. administered Eviprostat treatment in a rat model of nonbacterial prostatitis and reported that oxidative stress and proinflammatory cytokines in the enlarged prostate were considerably suppressed, and that Eviprostat may be useful in the clinical treatment of CP/CPPS [13–15]. Here we conducted a randomized prospective study to determine the effectiveness and safety of Eviprostat to treat CP/CPPS in comparison with pollen extract.

## Methods

### Study design

This double-blind, prospective, randomized and multi-centre clinical phase 3 study was conducted in 8 Japan urologic centers to ascertain the safety and efficacy of 8-weeks Eviprostat in men diagnosed with inflammatory CP/CPPS.

The design of the study was in accordance with the guidelines for clinical trials in CP/CPPS described by the NIH Chronic Prostatitis Collaborative Research Network [16].

Inclusion criteria were [1] men between 20 and 80 year of age with symptoms of pelvic pain for 3 months or more before study [2]. Patients with a total National Institutes of Health Chronic Prostatitis Symptom Index (NIH-CPSI) score ≥15 point [3]. Patients diagnosed with NIH category IIIA and IIIB using the PPMT (pre- and post-massage test) . Category IIIA refers to the presence of white blood cells (WBC) after a prostate massage urine specimen (VB3) (WBC in VB3 > 10/hps). Category IIIB refers to patients with pelvic pain with no evidence of inflammation on VB3.

Exclusion criteria were [1] documented urinary tract infection (midstream urine culture with at least 100,000 colony-forming units per milliliter), [2] history of urethritis, epididymitis or sexually transmitted disease (STD) [3] history of prostate surgery [4] history of urogenital cancer [5] treatment with phytotherapeutic agents, a-blocker agents, or antimicrobials. [6] residual urine volume >50 ml resulting from bladder outlet obstruction (BOO).

The study protocol was approved by the ethical committee of Hirosaki University School of Medicine, Aomori, Japan. Written informed consent was obtained from all patients to participation in this study. This study was registered with the Hirosaki University Hospital Clinical Trials Registry in Japan (2009-013) on 24 May 2009 and was registered with the University Hospital Medical Information Network Clinical Trials Registry in Japan (UMIN000019618) on 3 November 2015.

### Study procedure

We included in our study patients with urinary symptoms who met our inclusion criteria from among patients who had been diagnosed with clinically chronic prostatitis in medical interviews. The significance, objectives, and methods of this clinical study were fully explained to the patients, and their voluntary written informed consent was obtained. The patients' subjective symptoms were evaluated using NIH-CPSI (Japanese version) and International Prostate Symptom Score (IPSS) (Japanese version) [17, 18].

We checked patients 1 week after initiating drug therapy to ascertain whether they met the inclusion criteria. Patients were then allocated to receive either Eviprostat [two capsules q8h, with the active substance consisting of the umbellate wintergreen Chimaphila umbellate extract 0.5 mg, the aspen Populus tremula extract 0.5 mg, the small pasque flower Pulsatilla pratensis extract 0.5 mg, the field horsetail Equisetum arvense extract 1.5 mg and germ oil from wheat (Tritium aestivum) 15.0 mg.] or pollen extract (two capsules q8h, with the active substance consisting of 60 mg Cernitin T60 and 3 mg Cernitin GBX) The allocation

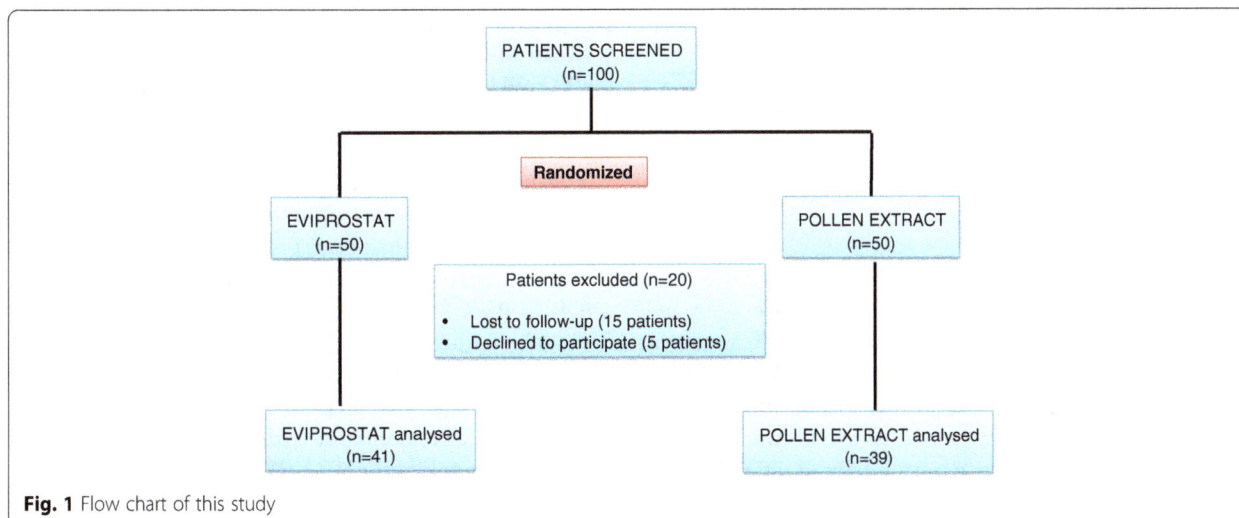

**Fig. 1** Flow chart of this study

manager randomly determined which of the 2 drugs would be administered to each patient. Cards detailing the drug to be used were sealed in numbered envelopes and distributed to patients from the smallest number to the largest. The drug to be used was decided on the basis of the card.

### Statistical analysis

We used the SPSS 21.0 software package (SPSS, Chicago, IL) for statistical analyses. Intergroup differences were analyzed by the Student's $t$-test. Intragroup differences were analyzed by a paired $t$-test. A value of $P < 0.05$ was considered statistically significant.

### Results

We randomized 100 patients diagnosed Category III A/III B prostatitis. 80 patients completed 12 weeks of follow-up and had primary and secondary outcomes ascertained. Flow chart of this study was presented in Fig. 1. In Eviprostat group, 7 patients were lost to follow-up and 2 patients declined to participate the study. In pollen extract group, 8 patients were lost to follow up and 3 patients declined to participate the study.

In Eviprostat group, there were 26 category IIIA patients and 15 category IIIB patients. In pollen extract group, there were 20 category IIIA patients and 19 category IIIB patients. There were no differences from baseline in the number of leukocytes in the prostatic secretion between the two groups.

The baseline characteristics of each study group are presented in Table 1. In the Quality of Life (QOL) domain of NIH-CPSI, there were significant differences between two groups. ($p = 0.014$) Except for QOL domain, there were no significant differences between the two groups at the start of this study.

Response (defined as a decrease in the NIH-CPSI total score by at least 25 %) in the Eviprostat group and the pollen extract group at 4 week was 68.3 and 61.5 %, respectively. Response in the Eviprostat group and the pollen extract group was 88.2 and 78.1 %, respectively. There were no severe adverse events observed in any patients in this study (Table 2). There was no significant difference in the total, pain, urinary, and the QOL scores of the NIH-CPSI between the two groups at 4 weeks and 8 weeks (Fig. 2). There were no significant differences about the total, voiding, and storage symptoms of the IPSS between two groups (Fig. 3). There were no severe adverse events observed in any patients in this study.

### Discussion

Antibiotics administration is the standard treatment for chronic bacterial prostatitis [19], however, the standard treatment for CP/CPPS has not yet been established [20].

**Table 1** Patients background

|  | Eviprostat | Pollen extract | p value |
|---|---|---|---|
| Number | 41 | 39 | n.s. |
| Age | $50.1 \pm 13.7$ | $53.0 \pm 14.6$ | n.s. |
| CategoryIIIA/IIIB | 26/15 | 20/19 | n.s. |
| Duration of current symptoms (months) | $8.2 \pm 10.6$ | $9.5 \pm 11.2$ | n.s. |
| IPSS | $10.8 \pm 7.5$ | $11.6 \pm 7.3$ | n.s. |
| NIH-CPSI |  |  |  |
| Total score | $22.3 \pm 4.7$ | $20.3 \pm 5.8$ | n.s. |
| Pain domain | $9.4 \pm 4.2$ | $9.2 \pm 4.0$ | n.s. |
| Urinary domain | $4.6 \pm 2.8$ | $3.8 \pm 2.7$ | n.s. |
| QoL domain | $8.3 \pm 1.6$ | $7.3 \pm 2.0$ | 0.014 |

**Table 2** 25% response rates for NIH-CPSI

|  | Eviprostat | | Pollen extract | |
|---|---|---|---|---|
|  | 4 weeks | 8 weeks | 4 weeks | 8 weeks |
| Total variation | -8.9 | -11.1 | -7.8 | -10.5 |
| Adverse event (%) | 1.7 | 2.3 | 2.3 | 4.7 |
| 25 % response rates (%) | 68.3 | 88.2 | 61.5 | 78.1 |

To date, various treatments for CP/CPPS have been reported, including α-blockers, antibiotics, anti-inflammatory agents, phytotherapeutics, and various other modalities [4–12]. However it is believed that these treatments have little effect on major symptoms, such as pain and urinary disturbance, experienced in CP/CPPS that reduce the QOL [21].

In general, patients with CP/CPPS undergo long-term treatment, and therefore, phytotherapeutics such as pollen extract, quercetin, Saw palmetto, or terpenes may be useful because they have few side effects [5]. However, there is no scientific evidence supporting these agents, and only few prospective controlled clinical trials have been conducted.

Since a long time, Cernilton has been used for the treatment of prostatitis [6]. Wagenlehner et al. conducted a prospective, randomized, double-blind, placebo-controlled study to study the effect of Cernilton in patients with CP/CPPS (NIH IIIA). They reported that compared with a placebo, Certilton improved total symptom, pain, and QOL without any side effects [6].

Eviprostat is a phytotherapeutic agent commonly used to treat prostatic hypertrophy in Japan [13–15]. An experiment using nonbacterial prostatitis model suggested that Evoprostat is potentially effective for the treatment of CP/CPPS. Oka et al previously reported that by using a model of non-bacterial prostatitis (NBP) induced in castrated aging rats by the injection of 17b-estradiol, they showed that the increased production of oxidative-stress marker malondialdehyde (MDA) and the proinflammatory cytokines TNF-a, IL-6, and IL-8 in prostate tissue homogenates from NBP rats. Eviprostat treatment significantly suppressed oxidative stress and proinflammatory cytokines in the NBP rats [13]. Sugimoto et al reported that chemokines, including CCL2/MCP-1 and CXCL1/CINC-1, were elevated in the prostate and urine of NBP rats, and Eviprostat potently suppressed the increases in CCL2/MCP-1 and CXCL1/CINC-1 [14].

The aim of the present study was to compare the efficacy and safety of Eviprostat to that of the pollen extract in the management of CP/CPPS.

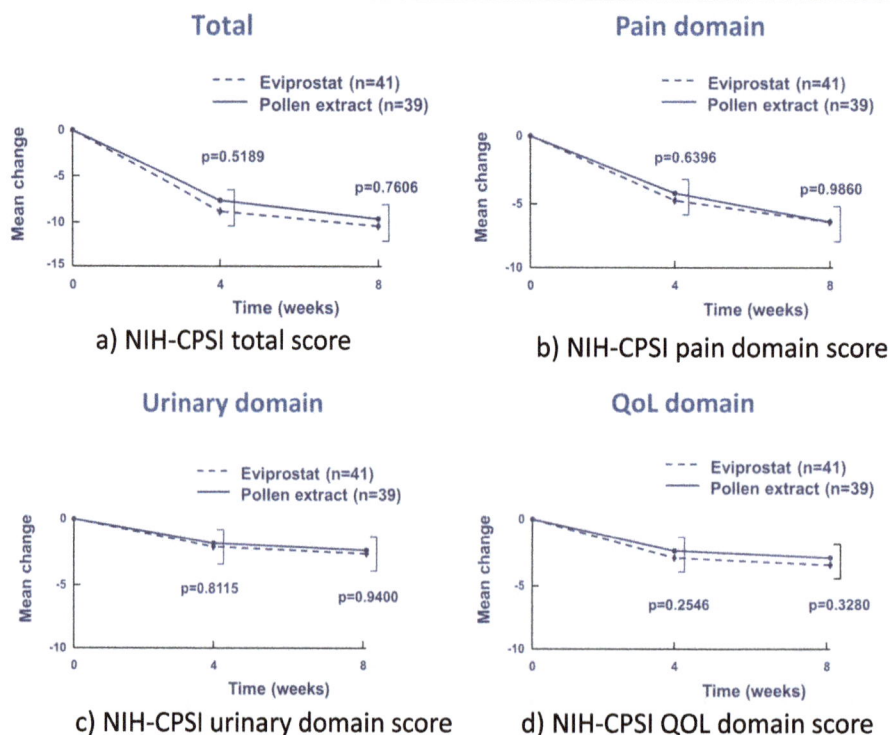

**Fig. 2** Mean change from baseline in the NIH-CPSI total score and in the sub-score after 4 and 8 week of treatment with Cernilton group or Eviprostat group. **a** NIH-CPSI total score. **b** NIH-CPSI pain domain score. **c** NIH-CPSI urinary domain score. **d** NIH-CPSI QOL domain score

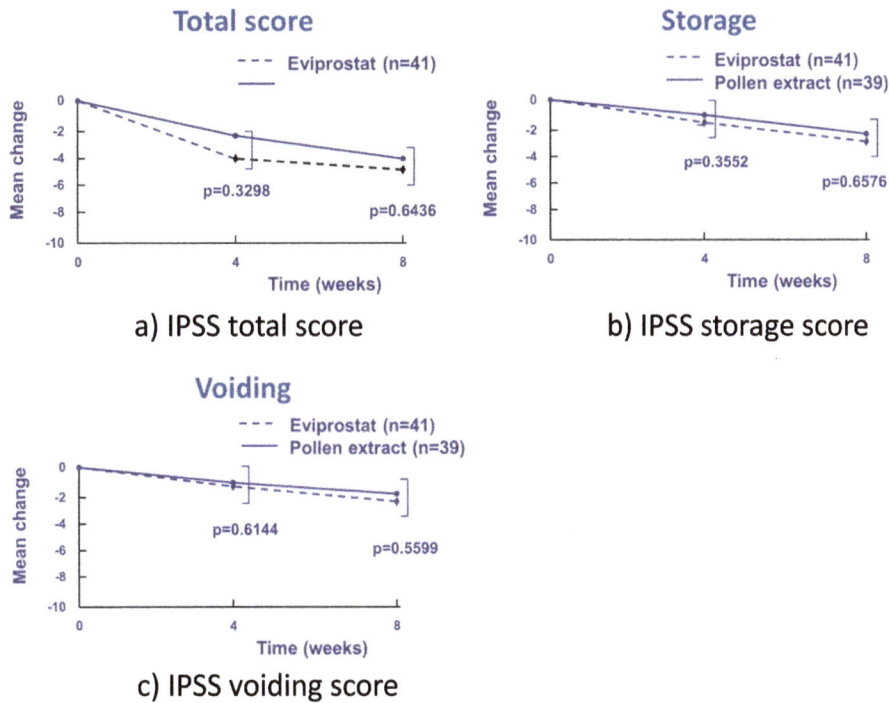

**Fig. 3** Mean change from baseline in the IPSS total score and in the sub-score after 4 and 8 week of treatment with Cernilton group or Eviprostat group. **a** IPSS total score. **b** IPSS storage score. **c** IPSS voiding score

In the intention-to-treat analysis, 100 Category III CP/CPPS patients were randomly allocated to Eviprostat ($n = 50$) or the pollen extract ($n = 50$). Response (defined as a decrease in the NIH-CPSI total score by at least 25 %) in the Eviprostat group and the pollen extract group was 88.2 and 78.1 %, respectively. There was no significant difference in the total, pain, urinary, and QOL scores of the NIH-CPSI between the two groups at 8 weeks.

This study has several limitations. Study samples were very small, it is necessary to examine the therapeutic effects of Eviprostat with a placebo control and this study was conducted in only Japanese populations.

In the present study, we conducted a prospective, randomized trial to compare the therapeutic effects of Eviprostat and Certilton, the standard treatment for CP/CPPS in Japan, and found that both agents improved CP/CPPS without any side-effects. We believe that Eviprostat is a very promising phytotherapeutic agent for the treatment of CP/CPPS in the future.

## Conclusion

Both the pollen extract and Eviprostat significantly reduced the symptoms of category III CP/CPPS without any adverse events. Eviprostat may have an identical effect on category III CP/CPPS compared the pollen extract.

### Abbreviations
CP: chronic prostatitis; CPPS: chronic pelvic pain syndrome; hps: high-power field; IPSS: International Prostate Symptom Index; MDA: malondialdehyde;

NBP: non-bacterial prostatitis; NIH: National Institutes of Health; NIH-CPSI: NIH-Chronic Prostatitis Symptom Index; PPMT: pre and post massage test; QOL: quality of life; STD: sexually transmitted disease; VB3: prostate massage urine specimen; WBC: white blood cells.

### Competing interests
The authors declare that they have no competing interests.

### Authors' contributions
CO made study conception and design. HI, TK, OS, TM, AI, SH, TY, YH and CO participated in the patient's medical treatment. HI collected data and AI performed statistical analysis. HI drafted the first version of the manuscript and TK and CO helped to draft the revised manuscript. All authors have read and approved of this submission.

### Acknowledgements
We would like to acknowledge the support and assistance provided by all the staff of the Department of Urology, Hirosaki University Graduate School of Medicine.

### References
1. Anothaisintawee T, Attia J, Nickel JC, Thammakraisorn S, Numthavaj P, McEvoy M, et al. Management of chronic prostatitis/chronic pelvic pain syndrome: a systematic review and network meta-analysis. JAMA. 2011;305(1):78–86.
2. Krieger JN, Nyberg Jr L, Nickel JC. NIH consensus definition and classification of prostatitis. JAMA. 1999;282(3):236–7.
3. Fu W, Zhou Z, Liu S, Li Q, Yao J, Li W, et al. The effect of chronic prostatitis/chronic pelvic pain syndrome (CP/CPPS) on semen parameters in human males: a systematic review and meta-analysis. PLoS One. 2014;9(4):e94991.
4. Nickel JC, Krieger JN, McNaughton-Collins M, Anderson RU, Pontari M, Shoskes DA, et al. Alfuzosin and symptoms of chronic prostatitis-chronic pelvic pain syndrome. N Engl J Med. 2008;359(25):2663–73.
5. Nickel JC. Treatment of chronic prostatitis/chronic pelvic pain syndrome. Int J Antimicrob Agents. 2008;31 Suppl 1:S112–6.

6.  Wagenlehner FM, Schneider H, Ludwig M, Schnitker J, Brahler E, Weidner W. A pollen extract (Cernilton) in patients with inflammatory chronic prostatitis-chronic pelvic pain syndrome: a multicentre, randomised, prospective, double-blind, placebo-controlled phase 3 study. Eur Urol. 2009;56(3):544–51.

7.  Thakkinstian A, Attia J, Anothaisintawee T, Nickel JC. alpha-blockers, antibiotics and anti-inflammatories have a role in the management of chronic prostatitis/chronic pelvic pain syndrome. BJU Int. 2012;110(7):1014–22.

8.  Nickel JC, Downey J, Clark J, Casey RW, Pommerville PJ, Barkin J, et al. Levofloxacin for chronic prostatitis/chronic pelvic pain syndrome in men: a randomized placebo-controlled multicenter trial. Urology. 2003;62(4):614–7.

9.  Bates SM, Hill VA, Anderson JB, Chapple CR, Spence R, Ryan C, et al. A prospective, randomized, double-blind trial to evaluate the role of a short reducing course of oral corticosteroid therapy in the treatment of chronic prostatitis/chronic pelvic pain syndrome. BJU Int. 2007;99(2):355–9.

10. Jeong CW, Lim DJ, Son H, Lee SE, Jeong H. Treatment for chronic prostatitis/chronic pelvic pain syndrome: levofloxacin, doxazosin and their combination. Urol Int. 2008;80(2):157–61.

11. Nickel JC, Narayan P, McKay J, Doyle C. Treatment of chronic prostatitis/chronic pelvic pain syndrome with tamsulosin: a randomized double blind trial. J Urol. 2004;171(4):1594–7.

12. Nickel JC, Pontari M, Moon T, Gittelman M, Malek G, Farrington J, et al. A randomized, placebo controlled, multicenter study to evaluate the safety and efficacy of rofecoxib in the treatment of chronic nonbacterial prostatitis. J Urol. 2003;169(4):1401–5.

13. Oka M, Ueda M, Oyama T, Kyotani J, Tanaka M. Effect of the phytotherapeutic agent Eviprostat on 17beta-estradiol-induced nonbacterial inflammation in the rat prostate. Prostate. 2009;69(13):1404–10.

14. Sugimoto M, Oka M, Tsunemori H, Yamashita M, Kakehi Y. Effect of a phytotherapeutic agent, Eviprostat(R), on prostatic and urinary cytokines/chemokines in a rat model of nonbacterial prostatitis. Prostate. 2011;71(4):438–44.

15. Tsunemori H, Sugimoto M, Xia Z, Taoka R, Oka M, Kakehi Y. Effect of the phytotherapeutic agent Eviprostat on inflammatory changes and cytokine production in a rat model of nonbacterial prostatitis. Urology. 2011;77(6):1507. e1515-1520.

16. Propert KJ, Alexander RB, Nickel JC, Kusek JW, Litwin MS, Landis JR, et al. Design of a multicenter randomized clinical trial for chronic prostatitis/chronic pelvic pain syndrome. Urology. 2002;59(6):870–6.

17. Monden K, Tsugawa M, Ninomiya Y, Ando E, Kumon H. A Japanese version of the National Institutes of Health Chronic Prostatitis Symptom Index (NIH-CPSI, Okayama version) and the clinical evaluation of cernitin pollen extract for chronic non-bacterial prostatitis. Nihon Hinyokika Gakkai Zasshi. 2002;93(4):539–47.

18. Homma Y, Tsukamoto T, Yasuda K, Ozono S, Yoshida M, Shinji M. Linguistic validation of Japanese version of International Prostate Symptom Score and BPH impact index. Nihon Hinyokika Gakkai Zasshi. 2002;93(6):669–80.

19. Bjerklund Johansen TE, Gruneberg RN, Guibert J, Hofstetter A, Lobel B, Naber KG, et al. The role of antibiotics in the treatment of chronic prostatitis: a consensus statement. Eur Urol. 1998;34(6):457–66.

20. Tugcu V, Tasci AI, Fazlioglu A, Gurbuz G, Ozbek E, Sahin S, et al. A placebo-controlled comparison of the efficiency of triple- and monotherapy in category III B chronic pelvic pain syndrome (CPPS). Eur Urol. 2007;51(4):1113–7. discussion 1118.

21. Nickel JC. Role of alpha1-blockers in chronic prostatitis syndromes. BJU Int. 2008;101 Suppl 3:11–6.

# 33

# Gastrointestinal cancer and bilateral hydronephrosis resulted in a high risk of ureteral stent failure

Mari Ohtaka[1†], Takashi Kawahara[1,2*†] (iD), Daiji Takamoto[1], Taku Mochizuki[1], Yusuke Hattori[1], Jun-ichi Teranishi[1], Kazuhide Makiyama[2], Yasuhide Miyoshi[1], Yasushi Yumura[1], Masahiro Yao[2] and Hiroji Uemura[1]

## Abstract

**Background:** Urologists frequently encounter malignant ureteral obstruction (MUO) caused by advanced urological or non-urological malignant disease, but the treatment policy is unclear. The present study examined the risk factors for predicting ureteral stent failure in patients with MUO after ureteral stent insertion and the change in the renal function after retrograde ureteral stent insertion in cases of bilateral hydronephrosis.

**Methods:** A total of 39 patients who required ureteral stent placement for MUO at Yokohama City University Medical Center (Yokohama, Japan) between February 2007 and May 2016 were included in this study. The age, gender, type of cancer, hydronephrosis side, pre-stenting estimated glomerular filtration rate (eGFR), and eGFR increase were assessed as predictive factors for stent failure. Among these 39 patients, 25 showed bilateral hydronephrosis. Thirteen of these patients had bilateral ureteral stents placed, and the remaining 12 had a unilateral ureteral stent placed. The renal function and overall survival (OS) were analyzed between these two groups.

**Results:** Among all 39 patients, 9 (23.1%) had stent failure. A univariate analysis revealed that causative disease (gastrointestinal cancer vs. others; $p = 0.045$) and laterality of hydronephrosis (bilateral vs. unilateral; $p = 0.05$) were associated with stent failure. A multivariate analysis revealed that only age (hazard ratio, 0.938; 95% confidence interval, 0.883–0.996; $p = 0.038$) was associated with stent failure. A Kaplan-Meier analysis and log-rank test indicated that having a unilateral ureteral stent placed was not correlated with a lower OS rate than having bilateral ureteral stents placed ($p = 0.563$). Among patients with bilateral hydronephrosis, the increase in the eGFR of those who had bilateral ureteral stents placed was not significantly different from that of those who had a unilateral ureteral stent placed ($p = 0.152$).

**Conclusions:** We revealed that age > 60 years was helpful for predicting stent failure. MUO due to gastrointestinal cancer and bilateral hydronephrosis may be predictive of stent failure. These factors may help urologists decide the optimal time to perform early percutaneous nephrostomy. These findings suggest that patients with bilateral hydronephrosis do not necessarily need to have a ureteral stent placed into both sides of the hydronephrosis.

**Keywords:** Ureteral stenting, Malignant ureteral obstruction

* Correspondence: takashi_tk2001@yahoo.co.jp
†Equal contributors
[1]Departments of Urology and Renal Transplantation, Yokohama City University Medical Center, 4-57 Urafune-cho, Minami-ku, Yokohama, Kanagawa 2320024, Japan
[2]Department of Urology, Yokohama City University Graduate School of Medicine, Yokohama, Japan

## Background

Urologists frequently encounter malignant ureteral obstruction (MUO) caused by advanced urological or non-urological malignancies. The causes of MUO are varied and include primary tumors, metastatic lymph nodes, peritoneal dissemination, and local infiltration. If untreated, progressive obstruction can result in uremia, electrolyte imbalance, urinary tract infections, and low back pain. Effective management must be attempted, but the treatment policy is unclear [1–5]. In patients with MUO, the current management options are retrograde ureteral stent (RUS) placement or percutaneous nephrostomy (PCN) under local anesthesia. RUS is usually considered as the first treatment choice because of its low rate of complications, low invasiveness, and low exchange frequency. However, the stent failure rate is high, with a mean failure rate of 12.2–34.6% [6–11]. Therefore, PCN should be used instead of RUS as the primary procedure in patients who would otherwise be at high risk of stent failure.

Previous studies have identified several factors of stent failure in patients with MUO, including the pre-stenting serum creatinine (S-Cr) level, performance states (PS), and degree of hydronephrosis [12, 13]. We can reduce the number of unnecessary procedures by carefully considering these risk factors. Sang Hoon Song et al. showed that patients with bilateral MUO, especially those ≥55 years of age or with diabetes or a poor baseline renal function, should be considered for early PCN conversion in the dominant functional kidney or in both to preserve the renal function, but few studies have explored the management of bilateral MUO [14].

The present study retrospectively reviewed our institution's experience with treating MUO using RUS and analyzed the factors predicting stent failure and the prognosis. We measured the pre- and post-baseline eGFR and analyzed the correlation between the increase in eGFR and stent failure in bilateral MUO. We also examined the risk factors predicting ureteral stent failure in MUO patients whose renal function changed after retrograde ureteral stent placement in bilateral hydronephrosis.

## Methods

### Patients

A total of 39 patients who required ureteral stent placement for MUO at Yokohama City University Medical Center (Yokohama, Japan) between February 2007 and May 2016 were retrospectively analyzed in this study. Primary indwelling ureteral stent placement was indicated for a variety of reasons, including pain control of hydronephrosis and improvement of the renal function, as well as for chemotherapy. The indication for RUS or PCN was left to the surgeon's decision. At our institute, PCN is suggested for patients with non-obstructive hydronephrosis, such as those with direct tumor invasion. In most cases, ureteral stenosis was observed between the upper and uretero-vesicle junction. At our institution, all MUO patients underwent RUS with a rigid cystoscope under local anesthesia under fluoroscopic guidance. In some male patients, we add sacral anesthesia. A 6-Fr 26-cm ureteric stent (Polaris™ Ultra; Boston Scientific, Natick, MA, USA) with a 0.035-mm SENSOR guide wire (Boston Scientific, Natick, MA, USA) was used, and the stent was changed every 3 months. At our facility, we started to use the RESONANCE metallic stent from 2016. Therefore, this study does not include any metallic stents. If RUS failed, the patients were referred for placement of a unilateral PCN tube. We defined stent failure as having to change the ureteral stent before the scheduled ureteral stent exchange time or having to perform PCN. A decreased renal function was defined as an increase in the serum creatinine level. Stent failure also included cases in which a ureteric stent could not be placed initially.

Patients' age, gender, type of cancer, hydronephrosis side, pre-stenting estimated glomerular filtration rate (eGFR), and eGFR increase were assessed as predictive factors for stent failure. The eGFR increase was defined as the difference between the pre-stenting eGFR and the best post-stenting eGFR. We also analyzed the relationship between stent failure and the overall survival (OS). In addition, from the total population, we extracted the 25 cases of bilateral hydronephrosis and compared the eGFR increase and OS in the 13 patients who received bilateral ureteral stent placement and the 12 patients who received unilateral stent placement. We usually checked the serum creatinine level and CT-KUB every 3 months. Institutional Review Board of Yokohama City University Hospital approved this study and required no written informed consent for all patients due to the retrospective observational study.

### Statistical analyses

Univariate and multivariate logistic regression analyses were performed to determine the predictors of stent failure. Odds ratios (ORs) were computed along with 95% confidence intervals (CIs). The survival duration was defined as the time between the date of RUS and death. A log-rank test was performed for comparisons between stent failure and non-failure groups. $P$ values of $< 0.05$ were considered to indicate statistical significance. The eGFR increase in patients with bilateral hydronephrosis was analyzed by the Mann-Whitney U and chi-squared tests. All statistical analyses were performed using the EZR software program (Saitama, Japan).

## Results

### Patients' characteristics

The 39 patients included 18 males and 21 females. The median age (range) was 70.0 (40–89) years, and the median observation period (range) was 141 (5–1729) days. The characteristics of the patients, including the presenting s-Cr and eGFR, eGFR increase, laterality of hydronephrosis, and causative disease, are summarized in Table 1. During the observation periods, 9 (23.1%) patients had stent failure and received placement of a unilateral PCN tube, depending on their general condition. Among the patients with colorectal cancer, three had rectal cancer, two had sigmoid cancer, and one had ascending colon cancer. The remaining cases of gastrointestinal cancer were gastric cancer. No significant differences were observed in the stent failure rate among the types of gastrointestinal cancer.

### Stent failure analyses

A univariate analysis revealed that the causative disease (gastrointestinal cancer vs. others; $p = 0.045$) and laterality of hydronephrosis (bilateral vs. unilateral; $p = 0.05$) were associated with stent failure, whereas age, gender, eGFR, and eGFR increase were not associated with the stent failure-free survival (Table 2). A multivariate analysis revealed that only age (hazard ratio [HR], 0.938;

**Table 1** Patients' clinical characteristics

| Variables | n (%) |
|---|---|
| Age (median; years) | 70.0 (40–89) |
| Gender | |
| Male | 18 (46.2%) |
| Female | 21 (53.8%) |
| Observation periods (median; days) | 141 (5–1729) |
| Serum creatinine (median; mg/dL) | 3.13 (0.81–19.21) |
| eGFR (median; ml/min/1.73 m2) | 15.6 (1.6–62.2) |
| eGFR increase rate (median; %) | 31.9 (−53.8–2606.2) |
| Laterality of Hydronephrosis | |
| Left | 5 (12.8%) |
| Right | 9 (23.1%) |
| Bilateral | 25 (64.1%) |
| Cause disease | |
| Gastrointestinal cancer | 24 (61.5%) |
| Gynecological cancer | 11 (28.2%) |
| Lung cancer | 1 (2.6%) |
| Prostate cancer | 1 (2.6%) |
| Unknown primary cancer | 2 (5.1%) |
| Stent failure | |
| Yes | 9 (23.1%) |
| No | 30 (76.9%) |

95% CI, 0.883–0.996; $p = 0.038$) was associated with stent failure (Table 2). A Kaplan-Meier analysis and log-rank test indicated that stent failure was correlated with a lower OS rate than non-stent failure ($p = 0.012$; Fig. 1).

### Bilateral hydronephrosis analyses

The eGFR increase was not significantly different between the bilateral hydronephrosis patients who underwent bilateral stenting and those that underwent unilateral stenting ($p = 0.152$; Fig. 2). In addition, a Kaplan-Meier analysis and log-rank test indicated that unilateral stenting was not correlated with a lower OS rate than bilateral stenting ($p = 0.563$; Fig. 3).

## Discussion

MUO is a frequent complication of advanced hard-to-treat malignancy and indicates a poor prognosis. However, there is no consensus on the appropriate management of MUO, as these patients' backgrounds vary widely with respect to complications, general condition, the prognosis, and quality of life issues [7, 9, 14]. MUO from malignancy may be because of compression by the primary or metastatic tumor, lymphadenopathy, or tumor direct invasion. Therefore, renal failure and associated symptoms can be improved and maintained by early optimum urinary diversion in some cases.

RUS is common in clinical practice and chosen more often than PCN when attempting to ensure the life expectancy of patients with advanced malignancies [6, 8]. However, the incidence of stent failure is high, possibly due to the high extrinsic pressure on the plastic ureteral stent or invasion of the ureter by tumors, which may lead to the stent's loss of function [15].

The present study included patients with a good general condition who had not yet received chemotherapy; this may have resulted in a relatively low stent failure rate. Furthermore, Wang et al. said that stent failure was influenced by the anesthesia used [5]. In China, the procedure is usually performed under local anesthesia in an outpatient operating room, which can lead to anxiety and pain during surgery. In Japan, most urologists perform RUS under local anesthesia in an operating room or treatment room. However, no studies have yet explored the association between stent failure and anesthesia, so the relationship remains controversial.

Some studies have reported the risk factors for stent failure. For example, Yu et al. found that middle or lower ureteral obstruction, PS ≥1, and s-Cr before ureteral stent insertion > 1.2 mg/dL were unfavorable predictors of the stent failure-free survival [16]. These factors may help urologists predict the survival time. Kamiyama et al. also showed that primary GI cancer, severe preoperative hydronephrosis, peritonitis carcinomatosa, and a poor preoperative PS were factors influencing stent

**Table 2** Univariate and multivariate analysis for stent failure

| Variables | Univariate p value | Multivariate p value | HR | 95%CI Lower | Upper |
|---|---|---|---|---|---|
| Age (≥60 years vs < 60) | 0.615 | 0.038 | 0.938 | 0.883 | 0.996 |
| Gender (Male vs Female) | 0.178 | 0.750 | 1.304 | 0.253 | 6.697 |
| eGFR (≤15.6 vs 15.6≥) | 0.5 | 0.761 | 0.798 | 0.187 | 3.407 |
| eGFR increase rate (≤31.9 vs ≥31.9) | 0.916 | 0.813 | 0.812 | 0.144 | 4.562 |
| Cause disease (GI cancer vs others) | 0.045 | 0.201 | 3.769 | 0.493 | 28.81 |
| Laterality of Hydronephrosis (Bi vs Uni) | 0.05 | 0.068 | 0.117 | 0.011 | 1.18 |

failure [17]. As these risk factors are still being discussed, there is no consensus on predicting stent failure in MUO. In the present study, the age (> 60 years), causative disease (gastrointestinal disease), and the presence of bilateral hydronephrosis were suggested to be associated with stent failure, whereas gender, pre-stenting eGFR (< 15.6 ml/min/1.73 m$^2$), and eGFR increase (< 31.9%) were not associated with stent failure. Some authors in Japan have reported that gastrointestinal disease is associated with a poorer prognosis than other types of malignancy and is reported as a risk factor of stent failure [4.5]. However, few studies have been conducted with the same parameters as those in other countries. We also examined the eGFR, not s-Cr, because of its precision in evaluating the renal function. Patients who undergo RUS for chemotherapy do not necessarily have severe renal failure, leading to a relatively low eGFR increase. This may be why eGFR was not associated with stent failure.

Song et al. suggested that patients with bilateral MUO, especially those ≥55 years of age or with diabetes or a poor baseline renal function, should be considered for early PCN conversion in the dominant functional kidney or in both to preserve the renal function [18]. However, the relative lack of studies has prevented obtaining a consensus about bilateral MUO. In the present study, we examined the eGFR increase in RUS for bilateral hydronephrosis. The increase in the eGFR and OS were not significantly different between those who had bilateral ureteral stents placed and those who had a unilateral ureteral stent placed. This suggests that bilateral stenting may not necessarily be required for bilateral MUO. PCN can be considered the first treatment approach in patients with MUO who are at risk of failure if RUS is performed. These findings suggest that patients with bilateral hydronephrosis do not necessarily need to have a ureteral stent placed into both sides of the hydronephrosis.

Several limitations associated with the present study warrant mention. First, the cases were retrospectively enrolled from only one facility, so there were few cases in our analysis. Second, the patients in whom RUS was attempted but failed because of severe obstruction were

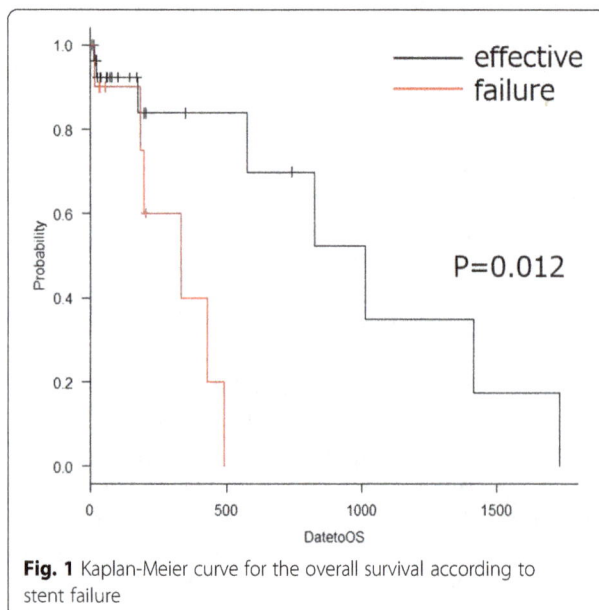

**Fig. 1** Kaplan-Meier curve for the overall survival according to stent failure

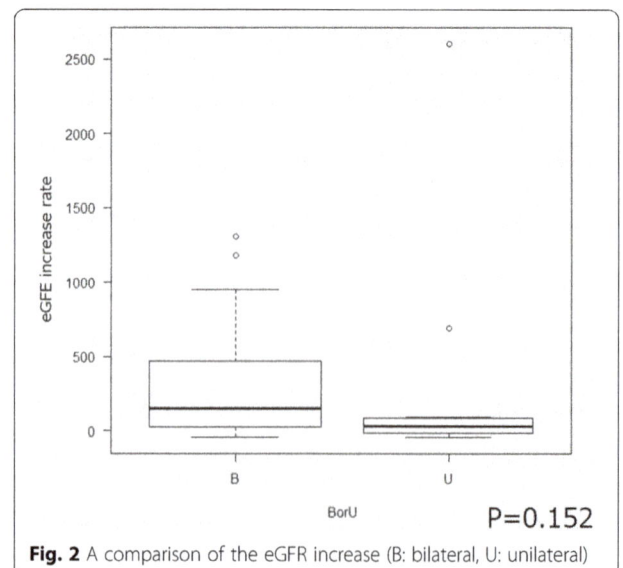

**Fig. 2** A comparison of the eGFR increase (B: bilateral, U: unilateral)

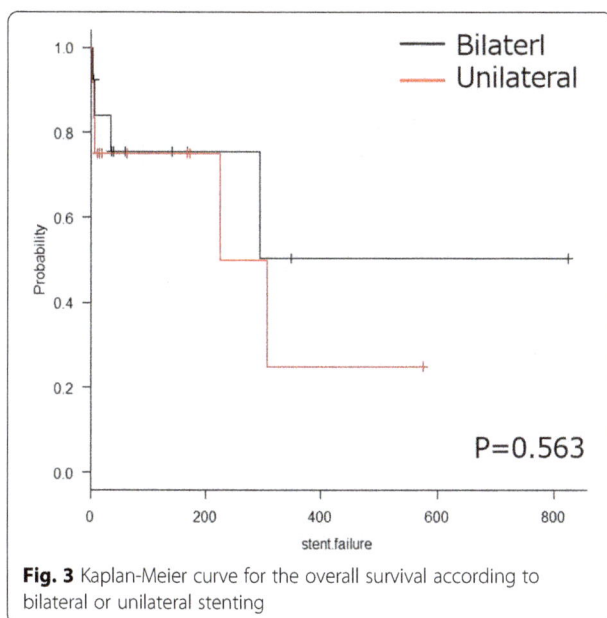

**Fig. 3** Kaplan-Meier curve for the overall survival according to bilateral or unilateral stenting

included as stent failure cases, which may have led to an increased stent failure rate. Third, we did not analyze the association between stent failure and cancer treatment, like chemotherapy or radiotherapy. Fourth, in the bilateral hydronephrosis analysis, the urologists did not share a common treatment principle concerning stenting style (bilateral or unilateral). Finally, we did not assess the split renal function. It is difficult to assess the renal function routinely in patients with MUO due to their severe performance status.

## Conclusion

This study revealed that age > 60 years, MUO due to gastrointestinal cancer, and bilateral hydronephrosis may be predictive of stent failure. These factors may help urologists decide on a treatment approach.

## Abbreviations
MUO: Malignant ureteral obstruction; PCN: Percutaneous nephrostomy; RUS: Retrograde ureteral stent

## Funding
Grants from KAKENHI grants (16 K20152) from the Ministry of Education, Culture, Sports, Science and Technology of Japan and grant for 2016–2017 Research Development Fund (Nos. WJ2810) of Yokohama City University,

## Authors' contributions
Conceived and designed the experiments: MO, TK. Analyzed data: MO, TK. Acquisition and data analysis: DT, TM, YH, JT, KM, YM, YY, MY, HU. Wrote the paper: MO, TK. All authors have read and approved of the final manuscript.

## Competing interests
The authors declare that they have no competing interests.

## References
1. Abt D, Warzinek E, Schmid HP, Haile SR, Engeler DS. Influence of patient education on morbidity caused by ureteral stents. Int J Urol. 2015;22(7):679–83.
2. Elsamra SE, Leavitt DA, Motato HA, Friedlander JI, Siev M, Keheila M, Hoenig DM, Smith AD, Okeke Z. Stenting for malignant ureteral obstruction: tandem, metal or metal-mesh stents. Int J Urol. 2015;22(7):629–36.
3. Rosenberg BH, Bianco FJ Jr, Wood DP Jr, Triest JA. Stent-change therapy in advanced malignancies with ureteral obstruction. J Endourol. 2005;19(1):63–7.
4. Yossepowitch O, Lifshitz DA, Dekel Y, Gross M, Keidar DM, Neuman M, Livne PM, Baniel J. Predicting the success of retrograde stenting for managing ureteral obstruction. J Urol. 2001;166(5):1746–9.
5. Wang JY, Zhang HL, Zhu Y, Qin XJ, Dai BO, Ye DW. Predicting the failure of retrograde ureteral stent insertion for managing malignant ureteral obstruction in outpatients. Oncol Lett. 2016;11(1):879–83.
6. Izumi K, Mizokami A, Maeda Y, Koh E, Namiki M. Current outcome of patients with ureteral stents for the management of malignant ureteral obstruction. J Urol. 2011;185(2):556–61.
7. Jeong IG, Han KS, Joung JY, Seo HK, Chung J. The outcome with ureteric stents for managing non-urological malignant ureteric obstruction. BJU Int. 2007;100(6):1288–91.
8. Wenzler DL, Kim SP, Rosevear HM, Faerber GJ, Roberts WW, Wolf JS Jr. Success of ureteral stents for intrinsic ureteral obstruction. J Endourol. 2008; 22(2):295–9.
9. Kouba E, Wallen EM, Pruthi RS. Management of ureteral obstruction due to advanced malignancy: optimizing therapeutic and palliative outcomes. J Urol. 2008;180(2):444–50.
10. Rosevear HM, Kim SP, Wenzler DL, Faerber GJ, Roberts WW, Wolf JS Jr. Retrograde ureteral stents for extrinsic ureteral obstruction: nine years' experience at University of Michigan. Urology. 2007;70(5):846–50.
11. Kanou T, Fujiyama C, Nishimura K, Tokuda Y, Uozumi J, Masaki Z. Management of extrinsic malignant ureteral obstruction with urinary diversion. Int J Urol. 2007;14(8):689–92.
12. Chung SY, Stein RJ, Landsittel D, Davies BJ, Cuellar DC, Hrebinko RL, Tarin T, Averch TD. 15-year experience with the management of extrinsic ureteral obstruction with indwelling ureteral stents. J Urol. 2004;172(2):592–5.
13. McCullough TC, May NR, Metro MJ, Ginsberg PC, Jaffe JS, Harkaway RC. Serum creatinine predicts success in retrograde ureteral stent placement in patients with pelvic malignancies. Urology. 2008;72(2):370–3.
14. Modi AP, Ritch CR, Arend D, Walsh RM, Ordonez M, Landman J, Gupta M, Knudsen BE. Multicenter experience with metallic ureteral stents for malignant and chronic benign ureteral obstruction. J Endourol. 2010;24(7):1189–93.
15. Goldsmith ZG, Wang AJ, Banez LL, Lipkin ME, Ferrandino MN, Preminger GM, Inman BA. Outcomes of metallic stents for malignant ureteral obstruction. J Urol. 2012;188(3):851–5.
16. Yu SH, Ryu JG, Jeong SH, Hwang EC, Jang WS, Hwang IS, Yu HS, Kim SO, Jung SI, Kang TW, et al. Predicting factors for stent failure-free survival in patients with a malignant ureteral obstruction managed with ureteral stents. Korean J Urol. 2013;54(5):316–21.
17. Kamiyama Y, Matsuura S, Kato M, Abe Y, Takyu S, Yoshikawa K, Arai Y. Stent failure in the management of malignant extrinsic ureteral obstruction: risk factors. Int J Urol. 2011;18(5):379–82.
18. Song SH, Pak S, Jeong IG, Kim KS, Park HK, Kim CS, Ahn H, Hong B. Outcomes of stent-change therapy for bilateral malignancy-related ureteral obstruction. Int Urol Nephrol. 2015;47(1):19–24.

# 34

# Protocol for a randomized clinical trial investigating early sacral nerve stimulation as an adjunct to standard neurogenic bladder management following acute spinal cord injury

Jeffrey D. Redshaw[1*], Sara M. Lenherr[1], Sean P. Elliott[2], John T. Stoffel[3], Jeffrey P. Rosenbluth[4], Angela P. Presson[5], Jeremy B. Myers[1] and for the Neurogenic Bladder Research Group (NBRG.org)

## Abstract

**Background:** Neurogenic bladder (NGB) dysfunction after spinal cord injury (SCI) is generally irreversible. Preliminary animal and human studies have suggested that initiation of sacral neuromodulation (SNM) immediately following SCI can prevent neurogenic detrusor overactivity and preserve bladder capacity and compliance. We designed a multicenter randomized clinical trial to evaluate the effectiveness of early SNM after acute SCI.

**Methods/Design:** The scientific protocol comprises a multi-site, randomized, non-blinded clinical trial. Sixty acute, acquired SCI patients (30 per arm) will be randomized within 12 weeks of injury. All participants will receive standard care for NGB including anticholinergic medications and usual bladder management strategies. Those randomized to intervention will undergo surgical implantation of the Medtronic PrimeAdvanced Surescan 97,702 Neurostimulator with bilateral tined leads along the S3 nerve root in a single-stage procedure. All patients will undergo fluoroscopic urodynamic testing at study enrollment, 3 months, and 1-year post randomization. The primary outcome will be changes in urodynamic maximum cystometric capacity at 1-year. After accounting for a 15% loss to follow-up, we expect 25 evaluable patients per arm (50 total), which will allow detection of a 38% treatment effect. This corresponds to an 84 mL difference in bladder capacity (80% power at a 5% significance level). Additional parameters will be assessed every 3 months with validated SCI-Quality of Life questionnaires and 3-day voiding diaries with pad-weight testing. Quantified secondary outcomes include: patient reported QoL, number of daily catheterizations, incontinence episodes, average catheterization volume, detrusor compliance, presence of urodynamic detrusor overactivity and important clinical outcomes including: hospitalizations, number of symptomatic urinary tract infections, need for further interventions, and bowel and erectile function.

**Discussion:** This research protocol is multi-centered, drawing participants from large referral centers for SCI and has the potential to increase options for bladder management after SCI and add to our knowledge about neuroplasticity in the acute SCI patient.

**Keywords:** Sacral neuromodulation, InterStim, Neurogenic bladder, Spinal cord injury, Bladder

* Correspondence: Jeff.Redshaw@hsc.utah.edu
[1]Department of Surgery, Division of Urology, University of Utah School of Medicine, 30 N. 1900 E. 3B110, Salt Lake City, UT 84132, USA
Full list of author information is available at the end of the article

## Background

Urinary bladder dysfunction and incontinence have a significant clinical, physical, and quality of life (QoL) burden in patients with spinal cord injury (SCI). Contemporary studies report bladder problems are the second leading reason SCI patients seek medical care. Almost 80% of SCI patients report some degree of bladder dysfunction within 1 year of injury and 42% are hospitalized for urinary problems every year [1–4]. Renal failure and urinary sepsis historically were the major causes of death in SCI patients after recovery from the initial injury [5]. Advances in urologic care, specifically the introduction of clean intermittent catheterization (CIC) in the 1970's revolutionized the care of SCI patients [6, 7]. However, there is a significant inconvenience, potential dependence on others, and often continued leakage that leads to patient non-compliance and discontinuation of CIC [4, 8, 9]. The currently established goals of neurogenic bladder (NGB) management include; prevention of renal insufficiency or failure by keeping bladder pressures low, preservation of urinary continence, and optimization of QoL. Current available treatments including pharmacologic therapy, injection of botulinum toxin, and surgical bladder augmentation or urinary diversion all address NGB physiology at the bladder level rather than the neurologic injury leading to NGB.

Largely, NGB cannot be reversed and prevention of the development of some of the worst aspects of NGB such as poor compliance, high intravesical filling pressures, and spasticity by trying to address the neurologic cause of these sequelae is a unique research approach. Over the past 20 years sacral neuromodulation (SNM) has become an established treatment for refractory urinary urge incontinence, urinary frequency/urgency syndrome, non-obstructive idiopathic urinary retention and chronic fecal incontinence [10–13]. The surgical procedure is minimally invasive and has few risks. Recent animal and human pilot data suggest that SNM implemented in the acute setting after SCI may preserve bladder compliance, bladder volume, and reduce urinary tract infections [14–16].

Based on this encouraging preliminary data, we designed a prospective, randomized, multicenter clinical trial to assess the efficacy and safety of SNM for treating neurogenic bladder dysfunction in patients with spinal cord injuries. The study hypothesizes that sacral neuromodulation, initiated during the acute phase following spinal cord injury, can decrease bladder spasticity preserving bladder compliance, bladder volume, and low bladder filling pressures. This will result in improvements in both objective quantifiable clinical outcomes, as well as subjective patient reported quality of life compared with standard neurogenic bladder management.

## Methods and design

### Study design

Patients will be randomized to standard neurogenic bladder management or standard management plus sacral neuromodulation (via S3 nerve root stimulation) in a parallel non-blinded fashion with the intent to demonstrate the superiority of sacral neuromodulation plus standard management over standard management alone. Patients randomized to the intervention arm, will undergo implantation of the PrimeAdvanced Surescan 97702 Neurostimulator (Medtronic, Minneapolis, MN) with bilateral tined leads within 12 weeks of spinal cord injury.

### Study locations

The study will take place at the Universities of Michigan, Minnesota, and Utah. All three of these sites are large volume academic hospitals that see a high volume of patients with SCI and are associated with acute rehabilitation centers that treat SCI immediately after hospitalization from injury.

### Study population and recruitment

Patients will initially be identified with the assistance of our colleagues in either Physical Medicine & Rehabilitation or Neurosurgery according to the inclusion and exclusion criteria in Table 1. All consecutive patients will be eligible for screening and approached for enrollment.

### Investigations

Sixty patients will be enrolled and randomized (30 per arm). A timeline and an overview of the procedures and diagnostic studies that will occur during the course of the study are shown in Fig. 1. The PrimeAdvanced Surescan 97702 Neurostimulator (Medtronic, Minneapolis, MN, USA) with bilateral tined leads will be implanted in patients randomized to the intervention arm using a standard surgical technique. Because the study hypothesis dictates early stimulation of the sacral nerve roots with a primary outcome evaluated 1 year post implant, the quadripolar tined leads and pulse generator will be placed in the same procedure. Food and drug administration (FDA) approved programming parameters for the InterStim II system will be utilized in this study.

All patients will receive usual standard of care bladder management for neurogenic bladder. Specifically, standard treatment entails the following: [1] clean intermittent catheterization (CIC) at regular timed intervals, [2] treatment with anticholinergic medicine or botulinum toxin as indicated to increase bladder compliance, decrease urinary leakage, and lower bladder pressures to prevent renal damage, [3] routine follow up in the urology and physical medicine and rehabilitation clinic [17].

At enrollment, all participants will complete the following: [1] standardized 3-day voiding diary to annotate

**Table 1** Study inclusion and exclusion criteria

Inclusion criteria

  Age > 18 years

  Ability to implant device less than 12 weeks post-SCI

  Presence of acute SCI at or above T12

  ASIA scale A or B

  Expectation to perform CIC personally or have caretaker perform CIC

  Medically stable to discharge to a rehab setting

Exclusion criteria

  Inability to perform CIC or have caregiver perform it

  Pre-existing SCI

  Pre-existing progressive neurological disorder

  Autonomic dysreflexia

  Prior sacral back surgery

  Posterior pelvic fracture with distortion of the sacroiliac joint

  Prior urethral sphincter or bladder dysfunction

  Chronic urinary tract infections prior to SCI

  Pregnancy at the time of enrollment

  Presence of coagulation disorder or need for anticoagulation that they cannot be stopped temporarily for procedure

  Any significant co-morbidity or illness that would preclude their participation or increase the risk to them having a surgical procedure

  Active untreated infection

  Traumatic injury to the genitourinary system

  Prior pelvic radiation, bladder cancer or other surgical procedure to the bladder that would effect baseline bladder physiology

the catheterization time, amount and time of fluid intake, and incontinence events, [2] 24 h pad weight test, [3] 3-day bowel diary to quantify baseline bowel habits, [4] inventory of current medications, [5] the Neurogenic Bladder Symptom Score (NBSS), [6] Spinal Cord Injury Quality of Life questionnaire (SCI-QoL) Bladder Management Difficulties, [7] SCI-QoL Bladder Complications, [7] the Neurogenic Bowel Dysfunction Score, [8] a non-validated questionnaire about autonomic dysreflexia impact, [9] Sexual Health Inventory for Men (SHIM), and [18] baseline urodynamic testing. Repeat measurements, other than urodynamic testing, will be obtained during clinic visits at 3, 6, 9, and 12 months after enrollment. For patients randomized to the intervention arm, urodynamic testing will be completed less than 2 weeks before implantation of the device. Urodynamic testing will be repeated at 3 months and then again at 12 months.

At each time point, a retrospective review since the prior time point will be performed in order to capture major events such as urinary tract infection (UTI), hospitalizations, additional surgery, as well as additional subjective data. Those additional subjective data will include: (1) current usage of anti-cholinergic medications and/or botulinum toxin treatment (2) bowel program including

use of medication and mechanical aids (i.e. digital stimulation, enemas, etc.), (3) use of medications for sexual function, (4) symptomatic UTIs requiring antibiotic treatment, (4) complications attributable to the device, (5) need for revision of device or leads. A renal ultrasound will be obtained at the end of 12 months to evaluate for the development of hydronephrosis. This will be compared with baseline CT or US imaging obtained during their initial trauma evaluation. Serum creatinine as an estimate of renal function will be collected annually. Variables to be collected during the course of the study and timeline for collecting them is shown in Table 2.

**Safety**

The study safety monitoring committee will consist of a study investigator, a non-investigator urologist familiar with SNM, and an independent safety monitor (ISM) (a non-investigator familiar with randomized trial design). The safety committee will meet semi-annually and the ISM will have the authority to halt the study. Videos of the 1st procedures and two other randomly assigned procedures of the 10 expected from each center will be produced and viewed by the safety monitoring committee to assure consistency in placement of the SNM device. The following criteria will be used to evaluate the surgical technique used for the procedures.

*Video evaluation criteria for device implantation:*

- Maintenance of sterile procedure and use of a double prep with an iodine skin protective cover.
- Placement of electrodes appropriately using fluoroscopy in the S3 foramen.
- Adequate testing for motor response indicating close proximity of the nerve and appropriate placement in the S3 foramen.
- Correctly attaching electrodes to the IPG device and tunneling of electrodes.
- Appropriate closure of all incisions in a manner consistent with preventing erosions of the electrodes or generator.

Reportable safety concerns will be any of the following: (1) device infection requiring antibiotics or removal (significant rates triggering a full review and report will be greater than 5% infection rate), (2) revision of device and reason for revision accounting for surgical, device, or patient factors (significant rates triggering a full review of the device use will be greater than a 30% revision rate over the course of study), (3) autonomic dysreflexia rates in patients within both arms of the study as assessed by the autonomic dysreflexia specific questionnaires and any autonomic dysreflexia, which causes patients to turn off the device for more than a few minutes, not use the device as intended, or are the reason for explantation, (4) the need for removal of the

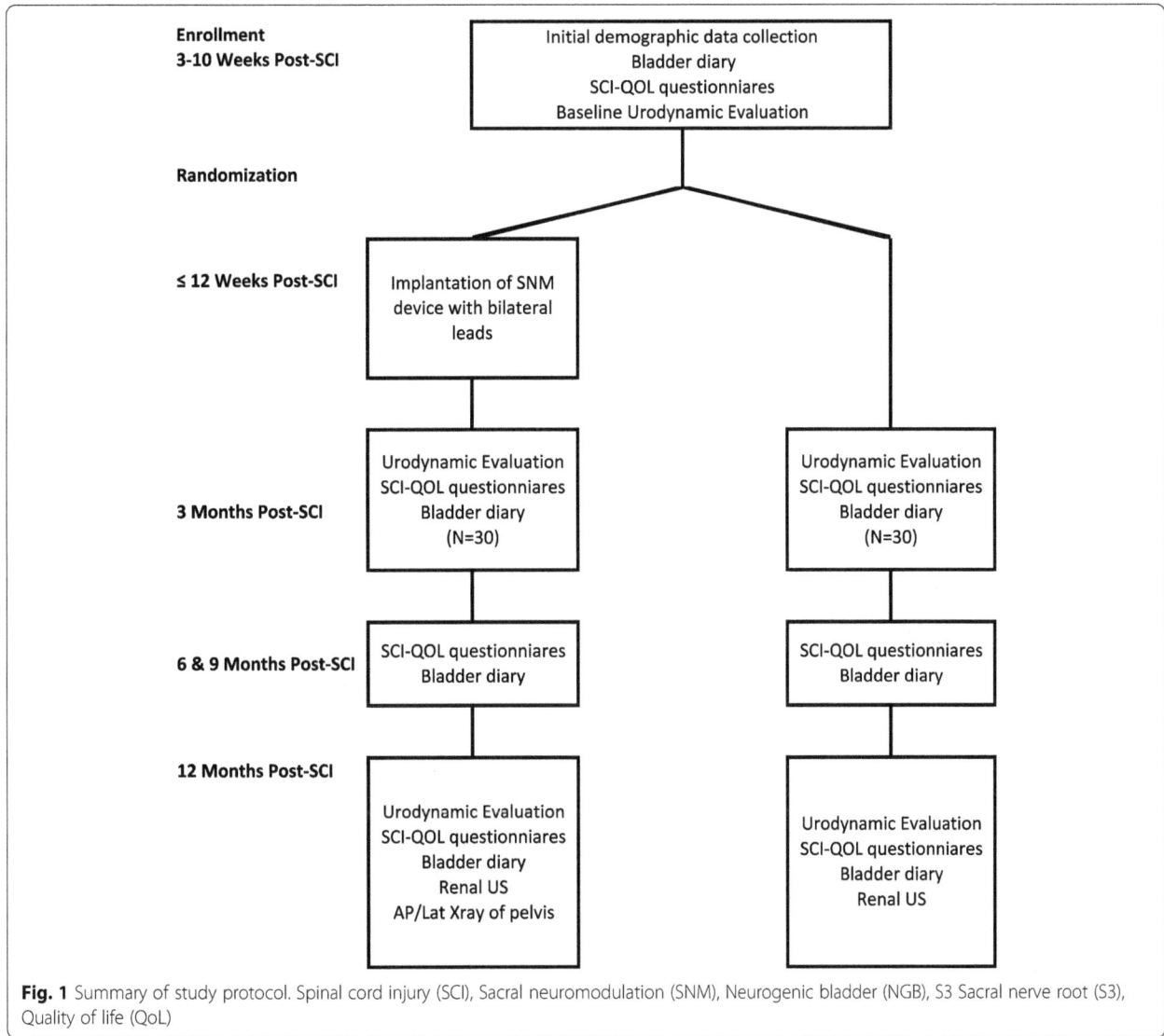

**Fig. 1** Summary of study protocol. Spinal cord injury (SCI), Sacral neuromodulation (SNM), Neurogenic bladder (NGB), S3 Sacral nerve root (S3), Quality of life (QoL)

device for erosion or pressure ulcers, (5) the need to remove the device due to the need for MRI imaging, (6) surgical complications within 6 weeks as classified by the Clavien-Dindo classification. Any events in category 1–6 will be reviewed by the study investigators as a whole during a semi-annual report from the safety committee. Event rates 1–6 will be disclosed to participants in the study during the consent process after they have been reviewed by the safety committee and investigators.

Safety committee will include reports to the FDA, institutional IRB's, and to the funding agency (the Department of Defense) at 6 month intervals or as specified by the rules of each organization. A written report of all adverse events will be created every 3 months and a log maintained with study documents.

An interim analysis will be conducted at 50% enrollment ($N = 26$ after loss to follow-up, 13 patients per arm) accrual, and the decision to stop early will be governed by a significance level of 0.003. The ISM decision to stop early will be guided both by interim results and clinical judgment, especially in the context of emerging, relevant literature.

## Study device

The PrimeAdvanced Surescan 97702 Neurostimulator is an implantable device marketed by Medtronic (Minneapolis, MN, USA) for use in the United States. It is FDA approved for spinal cord stimulation rather than sacral nerve root stimulation, which is the intention of this study, however, it is conceptually and functionally, similar to the InterStim II Model 3058 neurostimulator, which is FDA approved for sacral neurostimulation in the United States. Importantly, unlike the InterStim II, the PrimeAdvanced has the ability to accommodate and simultaneously stimulate bilateral leads. All the preliminary studies in acute spinal cord injury have utilized bilateral sacral

**Table 2** Primary and secondary outcome variables. UDS (urodynamic study), NBSS (Neurogenic Bladder Symptom Score), SCI-QoL (spinal cord injury quality of life measurement system bladder management difficulties and bladder complications), SHIM (sexual health inventory for men)

| | Collection method | Time points (month) | Variable type | Analyzed At |
|---|---|---|---|---|
| Urodynamic parameters – aim 1 | | | | |
| Primary | | | | |
| Maximum cystometric capacity | UDS | 0,12 m | Continuous | 12 m |
| Secondary | | | | |
| Maximum cystometric at 3 months | UDS | 0,3 m | Continuous | 3 m |
| Bladder compliance | UDS | 0,3,12 m | Continuous | 3 m, 12 m |
| Presence of detrusor overactivity | UDS | 0,3,12 m | Binary | 3 m, 12 m |
| Volume & pressure at first detrusor contraction | UDS | 0,3,12 m | Continuous | 3 m, 12 m |
| Quality of Life – Aim 2 | | | | |
| Primary | | | | |
| Difference in mean NBSS, SCI-QoL questionnaires | Questionnaire | 3,6,9,12 m | Continuous | 3,6,9,12 m |
| Secondary | | | | |
| Daily number of catheterizations, | Bladder diary | 3,6,9,12 m | Continuous | 3,6,9,12 m |
| Average catheterization volume, | Bladder diary | 3,6,9,12 m | Continuous | 3,6,9,12 m |
| Urinary incontinence episodes per day | Bladder diary | 3,6,9,12 m | Continuous | 3,6,9,12 m |
| 24 h pad weight test | 24 h pad | 3,6,9,12 m | Continuous | 3,6,9,12 m |
| Clinical – Aim 3 | | | | |
| Primary | | | | |
| # of UTIs requiring antibiotics | Chart review | 12 m | Continuous | 12 m |
| Secondary | | | | |
| Development of hydronephrosis | Renal ultrasound | 12 m | Categorical | 12 m |
| Need for anticholinergic medication | Chart review | 12 m | Binary | 12 m |
| Botulinum toxin injection | Chart review | event | Binary | 12 m |
| Need for device revision | Chart review | event | Binary | 12 m |
| Device explanation | Chart review | event | Binary | 12 m |
| Use of medications / mechanical bowel stimulation | Chart review | event | Continuous | 12 m |
| SHIM | Chart review | event | Continuous | 12 m |
| Erectile dysfunction medications | Chart review | event | Continuous | 12 m |

stimulation, which we believe offers a certain amount of redundancy defending against failure due to lead migration or malfunction and possibly increased efficacy.

Implantation is usually accomplished via a two-step process involving a placement of the permanent quadripolar electrode alongside the S3 nerve root under local or general anesthesia. This permanent lead is controlled by a temporary external programming device for 7–14 days. If greater than 50% improvement in clinical symptoms over that test period, the internal pulse generator (IPG) is implanted subcutaneously under during a second surgical procedure. Because the study hypothesis dictates early stimulation of the sacral nerve roots with a primary outcome evaluated 1 year post implant, the quadripolar electrical lead and IPG will be placed in the same procedure. This will avoid delay in stimulation of the sacral nerves

during the critical window for preventing adverse neuroplastic changes. Patients will be mostly insensate due to their SCI or being under general anesthesia for the procedure. Therefore, to confirm intraoperative placement we will rely upon expected motor responses associated with S3 stimulation (anal bellows and toe flexion). If correct motor responses cannot be elicited intraoperatively than the patients will not undergo implantation and will be included in the randomized arm but in an 'intention-to-treat' manner.

FDA approved programming parameters for the InterStim II system will be utilized in this study as follows. The device will provide continuous stimulation (i.e. always on) without discrete treatment periods. The PrimeAdvanced Surescan IPG is capable of generating a maximum voltage of 10.5 V, 2 V higher than the InterStim II system, however, it will be programed to function within the normal InterStim II system parameters (maximum 8.5 V). Additionally, it will be programed to use the same stimulation pulsewidth (210 msec) and frequency (14 Hz) as the InterStim II system. The area under the stimulation curve will be the same or less than intended by the InterStim II parameters.

Each patient will be evaluated intraoperatively as is standard clinical practice to select stimulation parameters that result in typical, consistent physiological responses (e.g. anal bellows and first toe flexion). The default 14 Hz frequency will be maintained. The electrode with the lowest amplitude stimulation as a proxy for the most closely placed electrode to the S3 nerve. This electrode will be trialed first. The stimulation amplitude will be set at 0.7 V per protocol as was utilized in the one prior bilateral SNM study in acute SCI. Note: If the subject has S3 sensation (incomplete SCI), the amplitude will be set 0.1 V lower than the level of sensation. In such sensate patients, each lead will be programmed individually and then both leads will be activated simultaneously to determine whether further amplitude reduction is needed. These parameters will be set during the initial programming session and will remain constant for the duration of the study. All study centers will utilize the same protocol.

## Statistical analyses and outcomes

Sample size calculations for this study were based on the preliminary research by Sievert et al., and a feasibility of enrolling 30 patients per arm within the study period [16]. After accounting for a 15% loss to follow-up we expect 25 evaluable patients per arm. Using thresholds for study power of 80% (5% significance level) we would detect a 38% treatment effect (84 mL difference in bladder capacity).

### Aim 1: To determine the effect of sacral neuromodulation on urodynamic parameters in the setting of acute spinal cord injury

The efficacy of SNM on the following urodynamic parameters will be evaluated at 3 months and 1 year post-injury: (1) maximum cystometric capacity, (2) bladder compliance, (3) presence of detrusor overactivity, and (4) volume and pressure for first detrusor contraction. Maximum cystometric capacity at 1 year is the *primary outcome*, and it will be compared between SNM and control arms using restricted maximum likelihood estimation under a linear mixed model controlling for institution [19]. Both an intention to treat and per-protocol analysis will be performed to account for any patients who were randomized to the intervention arm, but were unable to undergo placement of the device due to poor motor response intraoperatively.

### Aim 2: To assess the impact of sacral neuromodulation on patient-reported quality of life after acute spinal cord injury

Patient-reported QoL will be assessed using the Neurogenic Bladder Symptom Score (NBSS) and the two bladder specific item banks from the spinal cord injury quality of life measurement system (SCI-QoL) Bladder Management Difficulties and Bladder Complications. We will use a similar linear mixed model framework as described in Aim 1 to compare the mean questionnaire scores at each follow-up assessment between the intervention (SNM) and control arms. *The primary outcome* will be the difference in mean questionnaire scores. *Secondary outcomes* will include daily number of catheterizations, average catheterization volume, and episodes of incontinence per day will be compared between groups. The primary efficacy will be evaluated at 1 year between the randomized groups. Secondary contrasts will evaluate intermediate treatment effects at earlier time points, and on average across all time points.

### Aim 3: To examine the impact of sacral neuromodulation on quantifiable clinical outcomes

Patients will be followed longitudinally during the study period and assessed for the following: (1) number of symptomatic UTIs per year, (2) need for anti-cholinergic medications and/or botulinum toxin treatment, (3) complications attributable to the device, (4) need for revision of device or leads due to lead migration or failure, (5) development of hydronephrosis, (6) the need for medications and or mechanical aids (i.e. digital stimulation, enemas, etc.) for bowel program (7) SHIM scores, and (8) use of medications for erectile function. Our primary outcome will be the rate of symptomatic UTIs requiring antibiotic treatment over the 12-month study period. UTIs and many of our secondary complications can be experienced multiple times throughout the year. As a result, we will use a frailty model to handle complications that are potentially recurring events [20]. This method allows for heterogeneity among the evaluable subjects in terms of their differences in complication risk, as it is likely that some subjects will be more prone to UTIs (and other complications) than others. Events such as the use of anticholinergic medicines for control of detrusor overactivity are simply yes/no indicators during the annual period, and are thus more meaningfully modeled in the typical Cox regression framework for analyzing single rather than recurrent events. Again, all analyses will control for institution.

## Ethics and dissemination

An investigational device exemption (G160136/A002) was obtained from the FDA. A centralized IRB (based at the University of Utah) will approve a data and safety monitoring plan to the risks and complexity of this trial. Approval from the USAMRC ORP Human Research Protection Office has also been granted. This trial will be performed in accordance with the guidelines for Good Clinical Practice in Clinical Trials. Handling of all personal data will strictly comply with the Health Insurance Portability and Accountability Act. The trial has been registered at clinicaltrials.gov (https://clinicaltrials.gov/ct2/show/NCT03083366).

## Discussion

Sacral neuromodulation has a very well established track record in the treatment of patients with non-neurogenic urinary and fecal dysfunction. In the US, the InterStim Therapy System (Medtronic, Minneapolis, MN, USA) has been FDA approved for use in idiopathic overactive bladder since 1997, urinary frequency/urgency syndrome and non-obstructive idiopathic urinary retention since 1999, and for chronic fecal incontinence since 2011 [21–24]. Efficacy is well established for all three uses. In idiopathic overactive bladder, SNM achieves sustained therapeutic success in 85% of patients with a greater than 60% reduction in leaks per day. From a quality of life standpoint, 80% of subjects report significant improvement in their urinary symptoms [23]. Similar improvements with SNM are noted when treating chronic fecal incontinence, with 86% of patients achieving therapeutic success [25].

Once changes in the neurological control of the bladder have occurred following SCI they are in most cases irreversible. As a result, treatments must be directed at the local muscle level in order to control the high bladder pressures, incontinence and other symptoms. Consequently, the majority of research into the effects of spinal cord injury on the urinary bladder has focused on patients with well-established chronic neurogenic bladder physiology. Interventions during the acute phase of SCI aimed at preventing the development of, or reducing the symptoms of NGB, has not been extensively studied.

SNM implemented during the acute phase of SCI has good theoretical and experimental support in both animal and human clinical studies. In an animal model of complete spinal cord injury, Shi et al. demonstrated that SNM, could reduce peak bladder pressures and uninhibited detrusor contractions during bladder filling [14]. In vitro on a tissue level, in isometric relaxation experiments complete spinal cord transection caused a decrease in β-adrenergic relaxation responses which was shown to be muted by SNM in an animal model [15].

In humans, a pilot feasibility study has also demonstrated efficacy of SNM in the acute phase of SCI. Sixteen patients with traumatic complete SCI were enrolled during the acute bladder-areflexia phase [16]. Ten of these patients were implanted with bilateral sacral neuromodulators in a non-randomized fashion less than 3 months after their initial spinal cord injury. Six patients who met inclusion criteria, but did not wish to undergo treatment were used as controls. At 1 year follow-up, urodynamic studies showed an increased capacity (582 mL vs 294 mL), improved compliance and end filling pressures. The patients who underwent SNM had fewer UTIs (0.5/yr. vs. 3.8/yr) and hospital admissions. Other benefits of SNM included elimination of incontinence, in fact, none of the patients in the SNM group experienced incontinence, compared to 100% of the control group. Additional evidence for improvement in bladder pressures was the decreased need for anti-cholinergic medications (20% in the SNM group vs. 100% in controls).

This research protocol is multi-centered, drawing participants from large academic referral centers for SCI and has the potential to increase options for bladder management after SCI and add to our knowledge about neuroplasticity in the acute SCI patient.

## Abbreviations

CIC: Clean intermittent catheterization; FDA: Food and drug administration; IPG: Internal pulse generator; ISM: Independent safety monitor; NBSS: Neurogenic bladder symptom score; NGB: Neurogenic bladder; QoL: Quality of life; SCI: Spinal cord injury; SHIM: Sexual health inventory for men; SNM: Sacral neuromodulation; UTI: Urinary tract infection

## Acknowledgements

This project was supported by Department of Defense Grant Spinal Cord Injury Research Program grant (SC150071).

## Funding

Department of Defense Grant Spinal Cord Injury Research Program grant (SC150071) provided funding for this project. The Department of Defense had no input on the design of the study, collection of date, analysis, interpretation of data, or in writing the manuscript.

## Authors' contributions

All authors participated in creating the study design. JDR, SML, and JBM drafted the manuscript. SPE, JTS, JPR, APP provided a critical revision of the manuscript. JDR, SML, and JBM obtained the funding of this study. All the authors read, approved the final manuscript, and agreed to be accountable for all aspects of the work.

## Competing interests

The authors declare that they have no competing interests.

## Author details

[1]Department of Surgery, Division of Urology, University of Utah School of Medicine, 30 N. 1900 E. 3B110, Salt Lake City, UT 84132, USA. [2]Department of Urology, University of Minnesota, Minneapolis, MN, USA. [3]Department of Urology, University of Michigan, Ann Arbor, MI, USA. [4]University of Utah School of Medicine, Physical Medicine and Rehabilitation, Salt Lake City, UT, USA. [5]Division of Epidemiology, University of Utah, Salt Lake City, UT, USA.

## References

1. Sekhon LH, Fehlings MG. Epidemiology, demographics, and pathophysiology of acute spinal cord injury. Spine. 2001;26:S2–12.
2. Ku JH. The management of neurogenic bladder and quality of life in spinal cord injury. BJU Int. 2006;98:739–45.

3.  Ginsberg D. The epidemiology and Pathophysiologyof neurogenic bladder. Am J Manag Care. 2013;19:191–6.
4.  Manack A, Motsko SP, Haag-Molkenteller C, et al. Epidemiology and healthcare utilization of neurogenic bladder patients in a us claims database. Neurourol Urodyn. 2010;30:395–401.
5.  Strauss DJ, DeVivo MJ, Paculdo DR, et al. Trends in life expectancy after spinal cord injury. Arch Phys Med Rehabil. 2006;87:1079–85.
6.  Bloom DA, McGuire EJ, Lapides J. A brief history of urethral catheterization. JURO. 1994;151:317–25.
7.  Larsen LD, Chamberlin DA, Khonsari F, et al. Retrospective analysis of urologic complications in male patients with spinal cord injury managed with and without indwelling urinary catheters. URL. 1997;50:418–22.
8.  Cameron AP, Clemens JQ, Latini JM, et al. Combination drug therapy improves compliance of the neurogenic bladder. JURO. 2009;182:1062–7.
9.  Wyndaele JJ. Complications of intermittent catheterization: their prevention and treatment. Spinal Cord. 2002;40:536–41.
10. Tanagho EA, Schmidt RA. Electrical stimulation in the clinical management of the neurogenic bladder. JURO. 1988;140:1331–9.
11. Wöllner J, Krebs J, Pannek J. Sacral neuromodulation in patients with neurogenic lower urinary tract dysfunction. Spinal Cord. 2016;54:137–40.
12. Joussain C, Denys P. Electrical management of neurogenic lower urinary tract disorders. Annals Phys Rehab Med. 2015;58:245–50.
13. Banakhar M, Hassouna M. Sacral neuromodulation for genitourinary problems. Prog Neurol Surg. 2015;29:192–9.
14. Shi P, Zhao X, Wang J, et al. Effects of acute sacral neuromodulation on bladder reflex in complete spinal cord injury rats. Neuromodul Technol Neural Interface. 2012;16:583–9.
15. Kumsar Ş, Keskin U, Akay A, et al. Effects of sacral neuromodulation on isolated urinary bladder function in a rat model of spinal cord injury. Neuromodul Technol Neural Interface. 2014;18:67–75.
16. Sievert K-D, Amend B, Gakis G, et al. Early sacral neuromodulation prevents urinary incontinence after complete spinal cord injury. Ann Neurol. 2010;67: 74–84.
17. Cameron AP, Rodriguez GM, Schomer KG. Systematic review of urological followup after spinal cord injury. J Urol. 2012;187:391–7.
18. Redshaw JD, Elliott SP, Rosenstein DI, et al. Procedures needed to maintain functionality of adult continent Catheterizable channels: a comparison of continent cutaneous Ileal Cecocystoplasty with tunneled Catheterizable channels. JURO. 2014;192:821–6.
19. Harville DA. Maximum likelihood approaches to variance component estimation and to related problems. J Am Stat Assoc. 1977;72:320–38.
20. Vaupel JW, Manton KG, Stallard E. The impact of heterogeneity in individual frailty on the dynamics of mortality. Demography. 1979;16(3):439–54.
21. Wexner SD, Coller JA, Devroede G, et al. Sacral nerve stimulation for fecal incontinence: results of a 120-patient prospective multicenter study. Ann Surg. 2010;251:441–9.
22. Cameron AP, Anger JT, Madison R, et al. National Trends in the usage and success of sacral nerve test stimulation. JURO. 2011;185:970–5.
23. Noblett K, Siegel S, Mangel J, et al. Results of a prospective, multicenter study evaluating quality of life, safety, and efficacy of sacral neuromodulation at twelve months in subjects with symptoms of overactive bladder. Neurourol Urodyn. 2016;35(2):246–21.
24. Peters KM, Kandagatla P, Killinger KA, et al. Clinical outcomes of sacral neuromodulation in patients with neurologic conditions. Urology. 2013;81: 738–43.
25. Mellgren A, Wexner SD, Coller JA, et al. Long-term efficacy and safety of sacral nerve stimulation for fecal incontinence. Dis Colon Rectum. 2011;54: 1065–75.

# Permissions

All chapters in this book were first published in UROLOGY, by BioMed Central; hereby published with permission under the Creative Commons Attribution License or equivalent. Every chapter published in this book has been scrutinized by our experts. Their significance has been extensively debated. The topics covered herein carry significant findings which will fuel the growth of the discipline. They may even be implemented as practical applications or may be referred to as a beginning point for another development.

The contributors of this book come from diverse backgrounds, making this book a truly international effort. This book will bring forth new frontiers with its revolutionizing research information and detailed analysis of the nascent developments around the world.

We would like to thank all the contributing authors for lending their expertise to make the book truly unique. They have played a crucial role in the development of this book. Without their invaluable contributions this book wouldn't have been possible. They have made vital efforts to compile up to date information on the varied aspects of this subject to make this book a valuable addition to the collection of many professionals and students.

This book was conceptualized with the vision of imparting up-to-date information and advanced data in this field. To ensure the same, a matchless editorial board was set up. Every individual on the board went through rigorous rounds of assessment to prove their worth. After which they invested a large part of their time researching and compiling the most relevant data for our readers.

The editorial board has been involved in producing this book since its inception. They have spent rigorous hours researching and exploring the diverse topics which have resulted in the successful publishing of this book. They have passed on their knowledge of decades through this book. To expedite this challenging task, the publisher supported the team at every step. A small team of assistant editors was also appointed to further simplify the editing procedure and attain best results for the readers.

Apart from the editorial board, the designing team has also invested a significant amount of their time in understanding the subject and creating the most relevant covers. They scrutinized every image to scout for the most suitable representation of the subject and create an appropriate cover for the book.

The publishing team has been an ardent support to the editorial, designing and production team. Their endless efforts to recruit the best for this project, has resulted in the accomplishment of this book. They are a veteran in the field of academics and their pool of knowledge is as vast as their experience in printing. Their expertise and guidance has proved useful at every step. Their uncompromising quality standards have made this book an exceptional effort. Their encouragement from time to time has been an inspiration for everyone.

The publisher and the editorial board hope that this book will prove to be a valuable piece of knowledge for researchers, students, practitioners and scholars across the globe.

# List of Contributors

Carsten Frohme, Friederike Ludt, Peter J Olbert, Rainer Hofmann and Axel Hegele
Department of Urology and Pediatric Urology, University hospital Marburg, Philipps University, Marburg, Germany

Zoltan Varga
Department of Urology, District hospital Sigmaringen, Sigmaringen, Germany

Mauro Gacci, Omar Saleh, Claudia Giannessi, Vincenzo Li Marzi, Andrea Minervini, Marco Carini and Sergio Serni
Department of Urology, University of Florence, Careggi Hospital, Largo Brambilla 3, Urologic Clinic San Luca, Florence 50100, Italy

Beatrice Detti, Lorenzo Livi, Eleonora Monteleone Pasquetti and Tatiana Masoni
Department of Radiation Therapy, University of Florence, Careggi Hospital, Largo Brambilla 3, Florence, Italy

Enrico Finazzi Agro
Department of Urology, Tor Vergata University, Via di Tor Vergata, Rome, Italy

Stavros Gravas
Department of Urology, University Hospital of Larissa, Larissa, Greece

Matthias Oelke
Department of Urology, Hannover Medical School, Hannover, Germany

Lorenz Leitner, Matthias Walter, Patrick Freund, Ulrich Mehnert and Thomas M Kessler
Neuro-Urology, Spinal Cord Injury Centre & Research, University of Zürich, Balgrist University Hospital, Forchstrasse 340, 8008 Zürich, Switzerland

Lars Michels and Spyros Kollias
Institute of Neuro-Radiology, University of Zürich, University Hospital Zürich, Zürich, Switzerland

Gianluca Baio and Maria De Iorio
Department of Statistics, University College London, London, UK

Scott S Wildman
Medway School of Pharmacy, The Universities of Kent and Greenwich at Medway, Chatham, Kent, UK

Kiren Gill, Harry Horsley, Anthony S Kupelian, Sanchutha Sathiananamoorthy, Rajvinder Khasriya, Jennifer L Rohn and James Malone-Lee
Division of Medicine, University College London, Archway Campus, London, UK
Research Department of Clinical Medicine, Division of Medicine, University College London, Wolfson House, 2 – 10 Stephenson Way, NW1 2HE London, UK

Dong-Seok Han, Hoon Jang, Chang-Shik Youn and Seung-Mo Yuk
The Catholic University of Korea, Daejeon Saint Mary's Hospital, 64, Daeheung-ro, Jung-gu, Daejeon 301-723, Republic of Korea

Riccardo Giovannone, Stefano Tricarico, Francesco Del Giudice, Vincenzo Gentile and Ettore De Berardinis
Department of Urology, Sapienza Rome University, Rome, Italy

Matteo Ferro, Deliu Victor Matei and Ottavio De Cobelli
Department of Urology, European Oncology Institute, Milan, Italy

Gian Maria Busetto
Department of Urology, Sapienza Rome University, Rome, Italy
Policlinico Umberto I, Sapienza Rome University, viale del Policlinico, 155, 00161 Rome, Italy

Gen Ishii, Kanako Kasai, Kenichi Hata, Hiroshi Omono and Masayasu Suzuki
Atsugi City Hospital, 1-16-36 Mizuhiki, zip 243-8588 Atsugi City, Kanagawa, Japan

Takehito Naruoka, Takahiro Kimura and Shin Egawa
Jikei University School of Medicine, 3-25-8 Nishishinbashi minato-ku, zip 105-8461 Tokyo, Japan

Michael A. Moriarty, Matthew A. Uhlman, Megan T. Bing, Michael A. O'Donnell, James A. Brown, Chad R. Tracy, Sundeep Deorah, Kenneth G. Nepple and Amit Gupta
Department of Urology, University of Iowa, 200 Hawkins Drive, 3RCP, Iowa City, IA 52242, USA

Anna Masajtis-Zagajewska, Ilona Kurnatowska, Malgorzata Wajdlich and Michal Nowicki
Department of Nephrology, Hypertension and Kidney Transplantation, University Hospital and Education Centre of the Medical University of Lodz, Pomorska 251, 92-213 Lodz, Poland

Mauro Gacci, Arcangelo Sebastianelli, Matteo Salvi, Marco Carini and Sergio Serni
Department of Urology, University of Florence, Careggi Hospital, Viale S. Luca – 50134, Florence, Italy

Giacomo Novara
Department of Surgical, Oncological and Gastroenterological sciences, Urology clinic, University of Padua, Padua, Italy

Cosimo De Nunzio and Andrea Tubaro
Department of Urology, Sant'Andrea Hospital, University 'La Sapienza', Rome, Italy

Riccardo Schiavina and Eugenio Brunocilla
Department of Urology, University of Bologna, Bologna, Italy

Matthias Oelke
Department of Urology, Hannover Medical School, Hannover, Germany

Stavros Gravas
Department of Urology, University Hospital of Larissa, Larissa, Greece

Masahiro Yashi, Tomoya Mizuno, Hideo Yuki, Akinori Masuda, Tsunehito Kambara, Hironori Betsunoh, Hideyuki Abe, Yoshitatsu Fukabori and Takao Kamai
Department of Urology, Dokkyo Medical University, 880 Kitakobayashi, Mibu, Shimotsuga, Tochigi 321-0293, Japan

Osamu Muraishi
Department of Urology, St. Luke's International Hospital, Tokyo, Japan

Koyu Suzuki
Department of Pathology, St. Luke's International Hospital, Tokyo, Japan

Yoshimasa Nakazato
Department of Pathology, Dokkyo Medical University, Tochigi, Japan

Dongliang Hu, Tongzu Liu and Xinghuan Wang
Department of Urology, Zhongnan Hospital of Wuhan University, Wuhan, China

Bo Yang and Qiang Dong
Department of Urology, West China Hospital, Sichuan University, Chengdu 610041, China

Yuan Yang, Wenling Tu and Ying Shen
Department of Medical Genetics, West China Hospital, Sichuan University, Chengdu 610041, China

Luca Topazio, Valentina Maurelli, Gabriele Gaziev and Valerio Iacovelli
School of Specialization in Urology, Tor Vergata University, Rome, Italy

Roberto Miano
Department of Experimental Medicine and Surgery, Tor Vergata University, Rome, Italy

Mauro Gacci
Department of Urology, University of Florence, Florence, Italy

Enrico Finazzi-Agrò
Department of Experimental Medicine and Surgery, Tor Vergata University, Rome, Italy
Unit for Functional Urology, Department of Urology, Policlinico Tor Vergata, Rome, Italy

Giovanni Saredi, Andrea Pacchetti and Alberto Mario Marconi
Department of Urology, Ospedale di Circolo e Fondazione Macchi, Varese, Italy

Giacomo Maria Pirola
Department of Urology, University of Modena e Reggio Emilia, viale Borri, 57, 21100 Varese, Modena, Italy

Jon Alexander Lovisolo
Department of Urology, Ospedale di Circolo di Busto Arsizio, Saronno, Italy

**Giacomo Borroni**
Department of Surgery, Ospedale di Circolo e Fondazione Macchi, Varese, Italy

**Federico Sembenini**
Department of Statistics, Bicocca University, Milan, Italy

**Atsushi Fujiwara, Junko Nakahira, Toshiyuki Sawai and Toshiaki Minami**
Department of Anesthesiology, Osaka Medical College, 2-7 Daigaku-machi, Takatsuki, Osaka 569-8686, Japan

**Teruo Inamoto**
Department of Urology, Osaka Medical College, 2-7 Daigaku-machi, Takatsuki, Osaka 569-8686, Japan

**Gautier Müllhaupt, Daniel S. Engeler, Hans-Peter Schmid and Dominik Abt**
Department of Urology, Cantonal Hospital St. Gallen, Rorschacherstrasse 95, 9007 St. Gallen, Switzerland

**Darshan P. Patel, Sara M. Lenherr and Jeremy B. Myers**
Division of Urology, Department of Surgery, University of Utah Health Care, 30 North 1900 East, Room #3B420, Salt Lake City, UT 84132, USA

**John T. Stoffel**
Department of Urology, University of Michigan, Ann Arbor, Michigan, USA

**Sean P. Elliott**
Department of Urology, University of Minnesota, Minneapolis, Minnesota, USA

**Blayne Welk**
Divsion of Urology, University of Western Ontario, London, Ontario, Canada

**Angela P. Presson**
Divsion of Epidemiology, Department of Internal Medicine, University of Utah Health Care, Salt Lake City, Utah, USA

**Amitabh Jha and Jeffrey Rosenbluth**
Department of Physical Medicine and Rehabilitation, University of Utah Health Care, Salt Lake City, Utah, USA

**Mingming Yu, Geng Ma, Zheng Ge, Rugang Lu, Yongji Deng and Yunfei Guo**
Department of Urology, Nanjing Children's Hospital Affiliated to Nanjing Medical University, Nanjing, Jiangsu 210029, China

**Dong Sup Lee, Hyun-Sop Choe, Hee Youn Kim and Seung-Ju Lee**
Department of Urology, St. Vincent's Hospital, The Catholic University of Korea, College of Medicine, 93-6 Ji-dong Paldal-gu, Suwon 442-723, South Korea

**Sun Wook Kim**
Department of Urology, Yeouido St. Mary's Hospital, The Catholic University of Korea, College of Medicine, Seoul, South Korea

**Sang Rak Bae**
Department of Urology, Uijeongbu St. Mary's Hospital, The Catholic University of Korea, College of Medicine, Uijeongbu, South Korea

**Byung Il Yoon**
Department of Urology, International St. Mary's Hospital, Catholic Kwandong University, Incheon, South Korea

**Kai Li, Xuedong Wei, Miao Li, Xuefeng Zhang, Chenhao Zhou, Jianquan Hou and Hexing Yuan**
Department of Urology, The First Affiliated Hospital of Soochow University, NO.188 Shizi Road, Suzhou 215006, Jiangsu, China

**Guangbo Zhang**
The Institute of Clinical Immunology, The First Affiliated Hospital of Soochow University, NO. 708 Renmin Road, Suzhou 215006, China

**Hideo Fukuhara, Keiji Inoue and Taro Shuin**
Department of Urology, Kochi Medical School, Kohasu, Oko, Nankoku, Kochi 783-8505, Japan

**Atsushi Kurabayashi and Mutsuo Furihata**
Department of Pathology, Kochi Medical School, Kohasu, Oko, Nankoku, Kochi 783-8505, Japan

**Kyu-Sung Lee**
Department of Urology, Samsung Medical Center, Sungkyunkwan University School of Medicine, Seoul, Korea

**Tag Keun Yoo**
Department of Urology, Nowon Eulji Medical Center, Eulji University School of Medicine, 68, Hangeulbiseok-ro, Nowon-gu, Seoul, Korea

**Limin Liao**
Department of Urology, China Rehabilitation Research Center, Capital Medical University, Beijing, China

**Jianye Wang**
Department of Urology, Beijing Hospital, Beijing, China

**Yao-Chi Chuang**
Department of Urology, Kaohsiung Chang Gung Memorial Hospital, Chang Gung University College of Medicine, Kaohsiung, Taiwan

**Shih-Ping Liu**
Department of Urology, National Taiwan University Hospital and College of Medicine, Taipei, Taiwan

**Budiwan Sumarsono**
Astellas Pharma Singapore Pte. Ltd., Singapore, Singapore

**Romeo Chu**
Astellas Pharma Singapore Pte. Ltd., Singapore, Singapore
Pemimpin Drive, #19-03 Seasons View, Singapore, Singapore

**Qinyu Liu, Banghua Liao, Ruochen Zhang, Tao Jin, Liang Zhou, Deyi Luo, Jiaming Liu, Hong Li and Kunjie Wang**
Department of Urology, Institute of Urology (Laboratory of Reconstructive Urology), West China Hospital, Sichuan University, Chengdu 610041, Sichuan, People's Republic of China

**Kazutoshi Fujita, Motohide Uemura and Nonomura Norio**
Department of Urology, Osaka University Graduate School of Medicine, 2-2 Yamada-oka, Suita, Osaka 565-0871, Japan

**Kei Taneishi and Yasushi Okuno**
Department of Clinical System Onco-Informatics, Graduate School of Medicine, Kyoto University, Kyoto, Japan

**Teruo Inamoto and Haruhito Azuma**
Department of Urology, Osaka Medical College, Takatsuki, Osaka, Japan

**Yu Ishizuya**
Department of Urology, Osaka Medical Center for Cancer and Cardiovascular Diseases, Osaka, Japan

**Shingo Takada**
Department of Urology, Osaka General Medical Center, Osaka, Japan

**Masao Tsujihata**
Department of Urology, Osaka Police Hospital, Osaka, Japan

**Go Tanigawa**
Department of Urology, Sumitomo Hospital, Osaka, Japan

**Noriko Minato**
Department of Urology, Osaka Rosai Hospital, Sakai, Osaka, Japan

**Shigeaki Nakazawa**
Department of Urology, Nishinomiya Prefectural Hospital, Nishinomiya, Japan

**Tsuyoshi Takada**
Department of Urology, Minoh Municipal Hospital, Minoh, Japan

**Toshichika Iwanishi**
Department of Urology, Higashi Osaka General Medical Center, Higashi-, Osaka, Japan

**Andrew P. Smith**
Centre for Occupational and Health Psychology, School of Psychology, Cardiff University, 63 Park Place, Cardiff CF10 3AS, UK

**Shuji Isotani, Akira Horiuchi, Masayuki Koja, Takahiro Noguchi, Shouichiro Sugiura, Shino Tokiwa, Keisuke Saito, Masaki Kimura, Hisamitsu Ide, Satoru Muto and Raizo Yamaguchi**
Department of Urology, Teikyo University, Kaga 2-11-1, Itabashi-ku, Tokyo, Japan

**Hirofumi Shimoyama, Yasuhiro Noma, Kousuke Kitamura, Toshiyuki China, Shin-ichi Hisasue and Shigeo Horie**
Department of Urology, Juntendo University, Graduate School of Medicine, Tokyo, Japan

**Tony Lough, Qingyang Luo, Alastair Anderson, Jimmy Suttie and David Darling**
Pacific Edge Limited, 87 St David Street, Dunedin 9016, New Zealand

**Carthika Luxmanan**
Pacific Edge Limited, 87 St David Street, Dunedin 9016, New Zealand
University of Otago, Dunedin, New Zealand

**Paul O'Sullivan**
Pacific Edge Limited, 87 St David Street, Dunedin 9016, New Zealand
Merck, Sharpe & Dohme, Auckland, New Zealand

**Zhipeng Chen and Al-dhabi Mokhtar**
China Medical University, No. 77 Puhe Road, Shenyang North New Area 110122, Shenyang, Liaoning Province, People's Republic of China

**Chuize Kong and Zhe Zhang**
Department of Urology, The First Affiliated Hospital of China Medical University, No. 155 Nanjing North Street, Heping District 110001, Shenyang, Liaoning Province, People's Republic of China

**Shuqi Du**
China Medical University, No. 77 Puhe Road, Shenyang North New Area 110122, Shenyang, Liaoning Province, People's Republic of China
Department of Urology, The First Affiliated Hospital of China Medical University, No. 155 Nanjing North Street, Heping District 110001, Shenyang, Liaoning Province, People's Republic of China

**Anna H. de Vries and Ad J. M. Hendrikx**
Department of Urology, Catharina Hospital, Eindhoven, The Netherlands

**Scheltus J. van Luijk**
Academy of Post-graduate Education, Maastricht University Medical Centre, Maastricht, The Netherlands

**Albert J. J. A. Scherpbier**
Faculty of Health, Medicine and Life Sciences, Maastricht University Medical Centre, Maastricht, The Netherlands

**Evert L. Koldewijn**
Department of Urology, Catharina Hospital, Eindhoven, The Netherlands
Faculty of Health, Medicine and Life Sciences, Maastricht University Medical Centre, Maastricht, The Netherlands

**Cordula Wagner**
Department of Public and Occupational Health, EMGO Institute for Health and Care Research, Amsterdam, The Netherlands

Netherlands Institute for Health Services Research (NIVEL), Utrecht, The Netherlands

**Barbara M. A. Schout**
Netherlands Institute for Health Services Research (NIVEL), Utrecht, The Netherlands
Department of Urology, St. Antonius Hospital, Nieuwegein, The Netherlands

**Wilbert Sybesma, Marc P. Schneider, Andrea Sartori, Ulrich Mehnert and Thomas M. Kessler**
Neuro-Urology, Spinal Cord Injury Center & Research, University of Zürich, Balgrist University Hospital, Zürich, Switzerland

**Lorenz Leitner**
Neuro-Urology, Spinal Cord Injury Center & Research, University of Zürich, Balgrist University Hospital, Zürich, Switzerland
Department of Urology, University Hospital Basel, Basel, Switzerland

**Nina Chanishvili and Marina Goderdzishvili**
The Eliava Institute of Bacteriophage, Microbiology, and Virology, Tbilisi, Georgia

**Archil Chkhotua and Aleksandre Ujmajuridze**
Tsulukidze National Center of Urology, Tbilisi, Georgia

**Lucas M. Bachmann**
Medignition Inc., Research Consultants, Zürich, Switzerland

**Hiromichi Iwamura, Takuya Koie, Osamu Soma, Teppei Matsumoto, Atsushi Imai, Shingo Hatakeyama, Takahiro Yoneyama, Yasuhiro Hashimoto and Chikara Ohyama**
Department of Urology, Hirosaki University Graduate School of Medicine, 5 Zaifucho, Hirosaki, Aomori 036-8562, Japan

**Mari Ohtaka, Daiji Takamoto, Taku Mochizuki, Yusuke Hattori, Jun-ichi Teranishi, Yasuhide Miyoshi, Yasushi Yumura and Hiroji Uemura**
Departments of Urology and Renal Transplantation, Yokohama City University Medical Center, 4-57 Urafune-cho, Minami-ku, Yokohama, Kanagawa 2320024, Japan

**Kazuhide Makiyama and Masahiro Yao**
Department of Urology, Yokohama City University Graduate School of Medicine, Yokohama, Japan

**Takashi Kawahara**
Departments of Urology and Renal Transplantation, Yokohama City University Medical Center, 4-57 Urafune-cho, Minami-ku, Yokohama, Kanagawa 2320024, Japan
Department of Urology, Yokohama City University Graduate School of Medicine, Yokohama, Japan

**Jeffrey D. Redshaw, Sara M. Lenherr and Jeremy B. Myers**
Department of Surgery, Division of Urology, University of Utah School of Medicine, 30 N. 1900 E. 3B110, Salt Lake City, UT 84132, USA

**Sean P. Elliott**
Department of Urology, University of Minnesota, Minneapolis, MN, USA

**John T. Stoffel**
Department of Urology, University of Michigan, Ann Arbor, MI, USA

**Jeffrey P. Rosenbluth**
University of Utah School of Medicine, Physical Medicine and Rehabilitation, Salt Lake City, UT, USA

**Angela P. Presson**
Division of Epidemiology, University of Utah, Salt Lake City, UT, USA

# Index

www.ingramcontent.com/pod-product-compliance
Lightning Source LLC
Chambersburg PA
CBHW061259190326
41458CB00011B/3711